RADCLIFF & OGDEN'S

CALCULATION
OF DRUG DOSAGES

An Interactive Workbook

SIXTH EDITION

RADCLIFF & OGDEN'S

CALCULATION
OF DRUG DOSAGES
An Interactive Workbook

SIXTH EDITION

Sheila J. Ogden, RN, MSN

Clinical Manager
Clarian Health—Indiana University
Indianapolis, Indiana

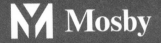 Mosby

St. Louis Baltimore Boston Carlsbad Chicago Minneapolis New York Philadelphia Portland
London Milan Sydney Tokyo Toronto

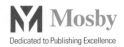
Dedicated to Publishing Excellence

A Times Mirror
Company

Editor-in-Chief: Sally Schrefer
Editor: Jeanne Allison
Associate Developmental Editor: Jeff Downing
Project Manager: John Rogers
Senior Production Editor: Helen Hudlin
Designer: Kathi Gosche, Cover; Pati Pye, Interior
Manufacturing Supervisor: Karen Boehme

SIXTH EDITION

Composition by Graphic World Inc.
Printing/binding by Von Hoffmann Press

Mosby, Inc.
11830 Westline Industrial Drive
St. Louis, Missouri 63146

Library of Congress Cataloging-in-Publication Data

Ogden, Sheila J.
    Radcliff & Ogden's calculation of drug dosages :   an interactive
workbook. — 6th ed. / Sheila J. Ogden.
        p.   cm.
    Includes index.
    ISBN 0-323-00698-1
    1. Pharmaceutical arithmetic—Programmed instruction.
I. Radcliff, Ruth K. Calculation of drug dosages.
II. Title.   III. Title: Radcliff and Ogden's calculation of drug
dosages.   IV. Title: Calculation of drug dosages.
    [DNLM: 1. Pharmaceutical Preparations—administration & dosage
problems.   2. Mathematics problems.   QV 18.2 034r 1999]
RS57.R33   1999
615′.14—dc21
DNLM/DLC
for Library of Congress   98-54874
                                                                                      CIP

99   00   01   02   03   /   9 8 7 6 5 4 3 2 1

To
my children—John, Amy, and Justin—
for your patience and understanding
and

To
David—my husband, best friend, and love—
for his ever constant support, without which the project
could not have been completed.
S.J.O.

Reviewers

Teri Boese, MSN, RN
Learning Resource Services Coordinator
College of Nursing
University of Iowa
Iowa City, Iowa

Jean Park Brown, MS, RN, C
Clinical Nurse Specialist
Shriners Hospitals for Children
Greenville, South Carolina

Laura Clayton, RN, MSN
Assistant Professor of Nursing Education
Shepherd College
Shepherdstown, West Virginia

Joan LaRue, RN, BSN, MN
Instructor/Supervisor
Mary Grimes School of Nursing
Neosho County Community College
Chanute, Kansas

Barbara May, MSN, MEd, RN
Associate Professor
Department of Nursing
Fitchburg State College
Fitchburg, Massachusetts

Donna S. Thomas, RN, MSN
Director of Nursing Education
St. Louis College of Health Careers
St. Louis, Missouri

Patricia P. Wickham, RN, MSN
Instructor
Practical Nursing Program
Center for Arts and Technology
Brandywine Campus
Coatesville, Pennsylvania

Preface

This workbook was designed for students in professional and vocational schools of nursing and for nurses returning to practice after being away from the clinical setting. It can be used in the classroom or for individual study. The workbook contains an extensive review of basic mathematics to assist students who have not mastered the subject in previous educational experiences. It can also be used for those who have not attended school for a number of years and feel deficient in mathematics. It may be that a person has not needed mathematics. Today we are very dependent on modern technology; a calculator is used in most activities involving numbers.

To become skilled in mathematics, extensive practice is necessary. Each chapter begins with a pretest for evaluating present skills. Learning objectives are listed so the student will know the goals that must be achieved, the subject matter is introduced, and examples for solving the various types of problems are provided. Work sheets give the student an opportunity to practice solving realistic problems. Two tests evaluate the student's learning. The student skilled in mathematics can easily adapt to applying the skills to solving problems of drug dosages.

The sixth edition of this workbook retains many important features of the fifth edition such as the mathematics pretest and posttest in Part I.

Part II continues to begin with use of the metric system that is predominant in the medical field. The apothecaries' system is still used and must also be learned. These chapters remain separate because each system must be learned separately before it can be manipulated in conversions.

Part III emphasizes interpretation of the physician's orders and how to read drug labels. The actual number of drug label reprints has been increased in all of the chapters dealing with the calculation of drug dosages. Dosages measured in units and intravenous flow rates have been expanded. The chapter on pediatric dosages includes calculations related to body surface area. Two new chapters have been added. Chapter 15 covers a new method of performing calculation of drug dosages. Chapter 16 introduces the use of the automated drug dispensing system. With the aging of the general population as a concern, the chapter on special considerations for the elderly has been enhanced. Further the home care considerations chapter has been expanded and chapters have been added on dimensional analysis and automated medication dispensing systems. All problems relating to drug dosages continue to represent actual physicians' orders in various health care settings in Indianapolis, Indiana.

In conclusion, a comprehensive posttest has been provided for the student. The questions asked help the student assess total learning of the process of calculation of drug dosages. A Glossary has been included to define important terms.

I want to thank the following pharmaceutical companies that have allowed us to use their medication labels in the book to provide a more realistic representation of medication administration.

Adria Laboratories (Erbamont Inc.)
Beecham (SmithKline Beecham Pharmaceuticals)
Boots Pharmaceuticals, Inc.
Bristol (Bristol-Myers Squibb Company)
Burroughs Wellcome Company
Dista (Eli Lilly and Company)
DuPont Pharmaceuticals
Elkins-Sinn, Inc.

Geigy (Ciba-Geigy Corporation)
Hoeschst-Roussel Pharmaceuticals Inc.
Knoll Pharmaceuticals
Lederle Laboratories (American Cyanamid Company)
Eli Lilly and Company
LyphoMed
McNeil Pharmaceutical
Meed Johnson Pharmaceuticals (Bristol-Myers Squibb Company)
Merck & Co., Inc.
Norwich Eaton (Procter & Gamble Pharmaceuticals, Inc.)
Parke-Davis (Warner-Lambert Company)
Pfizer Inc.
A.H. Robins Company, Inc.
Roche Products, Inc.
Roerig (Pfizer Inc.)
Roxane Laboratories
Sandoz Pharmaceuticals
Schering Corporation
Scot-Tussin
SmithKline & French (SmithKline Beecham Inc.)
Squibb (Bristol-Myers Squibb Company)
The Upjohn Company
Warner Chilcott (Warner-Lambert Company)
Wyeth-Ayerst Laboratories (American Home Products Corporation)

I appreciate the physicians, nurses, pharmacists, and representatives of various health care agencies who took time to discuss topics with me. I am grateful to my students, from whom I have learned so much. They have helped me understand the problems students have with basic mathematics as well as with the calculation of drug dosages. I hope this book will provide its readers with a feeling of confidence when working with a variety of mathematical problems.

Sheila J. Ogden

Introduction

The purpose of this book is to provide the student in a school of nursing with a systematic review of mathematics and a simplified method of calculating drug dosages.

To attain the maximum benefit from this workbook, begin at the beginning and work through the book in the order presented. Extensive practice is essential for mastery of mathematics.

Each chapter in Parts I and II begins with a pretest to evaluate previous learning. If the grade on the pretest is acceptable (an acceptable score is noted at the top of the test), you may continue to the pretest in the next chapter. If the score on the pretest indicates a need for further study, read the introduction to the chapter, study the method of solving the problems, and complete the work sheet. If you have difficulty with a problem, refer to the examples in the introduction.

On completion of the work sheet, refer to the Answer Key to verify that the answers are correct. Rework all the incorrect problems to find the error. It may be necessary to refer again to the examples in each chapter. Take posttest 1, and grade the test. If the grade is acceptable, as indicated at the top of the test, continue to the next chapter. If the grade is less than acceptable, rework all incorrect problems to find the error. Review as necessary before completing posttest 2. Again verify that your answers are correct. At this point, if you have followed the system of study, the grade on the second posttest should be more than acceptable. Follow the same system of study in each of the following chapters.

When all the chapters in the workbook are completed with acceptable scores (between 90% and 100%), you should be proficient in solving problems relating to drug dosage; more importantly, you will have completed the first step toward becoming a safe practitioner of medication administration.

On completion of the materials provided in this workbook, you will have mastered the following mathematical concepts for the accurate performance of computations:

1. Solve problems using fractions, decimals, percents, ratios, and proportions
2. Solve problems involving the apothecaries', metric, and household systems of measurements
3. Solve problems measured in units and milliequivalents
4. Solve problems related to oral and parenteral dosages
5. Solve problems involving intravenous flow rates
6. Solve problems confirming the correct dosage of pediatric medications
7. Solve problems by use of the dimensional analysis method

You are now ready to begin Chapter 1.

Detailed Contents

PART II UNITS AND MEASUREMENTS FOR THE CALCULATION OF DRUG DOSAGES

CHAPTER 6 METRIC AND HOUSEHOLD MEASUREMENTS, 137

CHAPTER 7 APOTHECARIES' AND HOUSEHOLD MEASUREMENTS, 153

CHAPTER 8 EQUIVALENTS BETWEEN APOTHECARIES' AND METRIC MEASUREMENTS, 167

PART III   CALCULATION OF DRUG DOSAGES

Part *I* Review of Mathematics

Chapters

PRETEST

Name _____

Date _____

ACCEPTABLE SCORE __**68**__

YOUR SCORE _____

Directions: Add and reduce fractions to lowest terms.

1. $\frac{3}{8} + \frac{1}{3} =$ _____

2. $2\frac{3}{7} + 1\frac{2}{3} =$ _____

3. $\frac{4}{5} + \frac{5}{9} =$ _____

4. $1\frac{3}{5} + \frac{7}{8}\big/\frac{1}{3} =$ _____

Directions: Add the following decimal fractions.

5. $1.03 + 2.2 + 1.134 =$ _____

6. $30.962 + 0.57 + 2.3 =$ _____

7. $6.88 + 4.5 + 1.678 =$ _____

8. $1.479 + 28.68 + 4.5 =$ _____

Directions: Subtract and reduce fractions to lowest terms.

9. $2\frac{1}{4} - \frac{7}{9}/\frac{2}{3} =$ _____

10. $\frac{14}{15} - \frac{1}{6} =$ _____

11. $5\frac{1}{4} - 4\frac{5}{8} =$ _____

12. $2\frac{1}{3} - \frac{1}{2} =$ _____

Directions: Subtract the following decimal fractions.

13. $2.04 - 0.987 =$ _____

14. $43.597 - 42.843 =$ _____

15. $8.53 - 7.945 =$ _____

16. $2.006 - 0.589 =$ _____

Directions: Multiply and reduce fractions to lowest terms.

17. $3 \times \frac{4}{7} =$ _____

18. $\frac{2}{3} \times \frac{5}{6} =$ _____

19. $2\frac{1}{2} \times 3\frac{3}{5} =$ _____

20. $4\frac{7}{10} \times 1\frac{3}{4} =$ _____

Directions: Multiply the following decimal fractions.

21. $3.47 \times 7.9 = $ _____

22. $0.315 \times 5.8 = $ _____

23. $4.884 \times 6.51 = $ _____

24. $235 \times 6.72 = $ _____

Directions: Divide and reduce fractions to lowest terms.

25. $\frac{3}{5} \div \frac{5}{6} = $ _____

26. $\frac{1}{8} \div \frac{3}{10} = $ _____

27. $\frac{1}{150} \div \frac{1}{20} = $ _____

28. $2\frac{3}{4} \div 6\frac{2}{3} = $ _____

Directions: Divide the following decimal fractions.

29. $241.73 \div 9.3 = $ _____

30. $0.9412 \div 4.16 = $ _____

31. $128.24 \div 6 = $ _____

32. $22.67 \div 3.5 = $ _____

Directions: Circle the decimal fraction that has the *least* value.

33. 0.3, 0.03, 0.003

34. 0.9, 0.45, 0.66

35. 0.72, 0.721, 0.0072

36. 0.058, 0.1001, 0.07

Directions: Circle the decimal fraction that has the *greatest* value.

37. 0.1, 0.15, 0.155

38. 0.4, 0.8, 0.21

39. 0.249, 0.1587, 0.00633

40. 2.913, 2.99, 2.9

Directions: Change the following fractions to decimals.

41. $^5\!/_8$ = _____

42. $^3\!/_4$ = _____

43. $^{11}\!/_{20}$ = _____

44. $^{17}\!/_{25}$ = _____

Directions: Change the following decimals to fractions reduced to lowest terms.

45. 0.875 = _____

46. 0.375 = _____

47. 0.05 = _____

48. 0.125 = _____

Directions: Calculate the following problems.

49. Express 0.432 as a percent.

50. Express 65% as a proper fraction and reduce to the lowest terms.

51. Express 0.3% as a ratio.

52. Express ⅛ as a percent.

53. What percent of 2.5 is 0.5?

54. What percent of ¾ is ⅜?

55. What percent of 160 is 12?

56. What is ¼% of 60?

57. What is 4½% of 940?

58. What is 65% of 450?

Directions: Change the following fractions and decimals to ratios reduced to lowest terms.

59. $^9/_{42}$ = _____

60. $1\frac{1}{2}/2\frac{2}{3}$ = _____

61. 0.8225 = _____

62. $^{125}/_{275}$ = _____

63. 0.34 = _____

Directions: Find the value of x.

64. $7 : ^7/_{100} :: x : 4$

65. $x : 40 :: 7 : 56$

66. $2.5 : 6 :: 10 : x$

67. $x : \frac{1}{4}\% :: 9.6 : \frac{1}{300}$

68. $\frac{1}{150} : \frac{1}{100} :: x : 30$

69. $25 : x :: 5 : 400$

70. $0.10 : 0.20 :: x : 200$

71. $\frac{1}{200} : \frac{1}{40} :: 100 : x$

72. $x : 85 :: 6 : 10$

73. $\frac{1}{20}/\frac{1}{5} : 5 :: x : 50$

74. $100 : 5 :: x : 3.4$

75. $72 : \frac{1}{9} :: x : 56$

Answers on p. 411.

PRETEST

Name _____

Date _____

ACCEPTABLE SCORE __**36**__

YOUR SCORE _____

Directions: Perform the indicated calculations and reduce fractions to lowest terms.

1. $\frac{1}{8} + \frac{2}{3} =$ _____

2. $\frac{5}{7} + \frac{4}{9} =$ _____

3. $6\frac{3}{5} + 2\frac{3}{4} =$ _____

4. $2\frac{1}{2} + 8\frac{1}{6} =$ _____

5. $3\frac{13}{20} + 1\frac{3}{10} + 4\frac{4}{5} =$ _____

6. $2\frac{5}{16} + 3\frac{1}{4} =$ _____

7. $5\frac{6}{11} + 3\frac{1}{2} =$ _____

8. $3\frac{2}{3} + 4\frac{2}{9} =$ _____

9. $2\frac{5}{8} + 1\frac{5}{24} =$ _____

10. $1\frac{3}{4} + 2\frac{3}{8} + 1\frac{5}{6} =$ _____

11. $\frac{9}{10} - \frac{3}{5} =$ _____

12. $2\frac{1}{4} - 1\frac{3}{8} =$ _____

13. $2\frac{2}{3} - 1\frac{4}{5} = $ _____

14. $6\frac{1}{8} - 3\frac{1}{2} = $ _____

15. $9\frac{1}{2} - 3\frac{5}{13} = $ _____

16. $4\frac{5}{6} - 2\frac{1}{8} = $ _____

17. $3\frac{3}{4} - 1\frac{11}{12} = $ _____

18. $7\frac{1}{2} - 5\frac{7}{10} = $ _____

19. $5\frac{1}{4} - 3\frac{15}{16} = $ _____

20. $6\frac{1}{2} - 4\frac{2}{3} = $ _____

21. $\frac{4}{5} \times \frac{1}{12} = $ _____

22. $\frac{3}{8} \times \frac{7}{10} = $ _____

23. $1\frac{1}{3} \times 3\frac{3}{4} = $ _____

24. $3\frac{2}{7} \times 2\frac{2}{9} = $ _____

25. $\frac{5}{8} \times 1\frac{5}{7} = $ _____

26. $\frac{1}{1000} \times \frac{1}{10} = $ _____

27. $2\frac{4}{9} \times 1\frac{3}{4} = $ _____

28. $3\frac{7}{15} \times 1\frac{3}{5} =$ _____

29. $4\frac{1}{6} \times 2\frac{9}{10} =$ _____

30. $1\frac{1}{8} \times 2\frac{4}{7} =$ _____

31. $\frac{1}{4} \div \frac{4}{5} =$ _____

32. $1\frac{5}{9} \div 2\frac{4}{7} =$ _____

33. $2\frac{1}{6} \div 1\frac{5}{8} =$ _____

34. $\frac{1}{3} \div \frac{1}{100} =$ _____

35. $1\frac{3}{4} \div 2 =$ _____

36. $\frac{4}{5} / \frac{3}{5} =$ _____

37. $\frac{1}{16} / \frac{3}{4} =$ _____

38. $\frac{1}{3} / \frac{3}{5} =$ _____

39. $2\frac{5}{6} / 1\frac{2}{3} =$ _____

40. $4\frac{1}{2} / 2\frac{1}{4} =$ _____

Answers on p. 411.

Chapter *1* | *Fractions*

Learning Objectives

On completion of the materials provided in this chapter, you will be able to perform computations accurately by mastering the following mathematical concepts:

1. Changing an improper fraction to a mixed number
2. Changing a mixed number to an improper fraction
3. Changing a fraction to an equivalent fraction with the lowest common denominator
4. Changing a mixed number to an equivalent fraction with the lowest common denominator
5. Adding fractions having the same denominator, unlike denominators, or involving whole numbers and unlike denominators
6. Subtracting fractions having the same denominator, unlike denominators, or involving whole numbers and unlike denominators
7. Multiplying fractions and mixed numbers
8. Dividing fractions and mixed numbers
9. Reducing a complex fraction
10. Reducing a complex fraction involving mixed numbers

A **fraction** indicates the number of equal parts of a whole. An example is ¾, which means three of four equal parts.

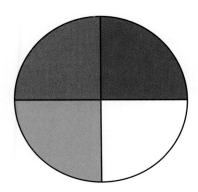

The **denominator** indicates the number of parts into which a whole has been divided. The denominator is the number *below* the fraction line. The **numerator** designates the number of parts that you have of a divided whole. It is the number *above* the fraction line. The line also indicates division to be performed and can be read as "divided by." The example ¾, or three fourths, can therefore be read as "three divided by four." In other words the numerator is "divided by" the denominator. The numerator is the **dividend,** and the denominator is the **divisor.**

A fraction can often be expressed in smaller numbers without any change in its real value. This is what is meant by the direction "Reduce to lowest terms." The reduction is accomplished by dividing both numerator and denominator by the same number.

Example: ⁶⁄₈   **Example:** ³⁄₉   **Example:** ⁴⁄₁₀

$6 \div 2 = 3$ $3 \div 3 = 1$ $4 \div 2 = 2$

$8 \div 2 = 4$ $9 \div 3 = 3$ $10 \div 2 = 5$

$$\frac{6}{8} = \frac{3}{4}$$ $$\frac{3}{9} = \frac{1}{3}$$ $$\frac{4}{10} = \frac{2}{5}$$

There are several different types of fractions. A **proper fraction** is one in which the numerator is smaller than the denominator. A proper fraction is sometimes called a *common* or *simple fraction.*

Examples: ⅔,   ⅛,   ⁵⁄₁₂

An **improper fraction** is a fraction whose numerator is larger than or equal to the denominator.

Examples: ⁸⁄₇,   ⁶⁄₆,   ⁴⁄₂

A **complex fraction** is one that contains a fraction in its numerator, its denominator, or both.

Examples: 2⅓/3,   2/1½,   ¾/⅜

Sometimes a fraction is seen in conjunction with a whole number. This combination is called a **mixed number.**

Examples: 2⅜,   4⅓,   6½

Changing an Improper Fraction to a Mixed Number

1. Divide the numerator by the denominator.
2. Place any remainder over the denominator and write this proper fraction beside the whole number found in step 1.

Example: ⁵⁄₃   **Example:** ⁷⁄₂

$$\begin{array}{r} 1 \\ 3)\overline{5} \\ \underline{3} \\ 2 \end{array} \text{ remainder } 2 = 1\frac{2}{3}$$ $$\begin{array}{r} 3 \\ 2)\overline{7} \\ \underline{6} \\ 1 \end{array} \text{ remainder } 1 = 3\frac{1}{2}$$

When an improper fraction is reduced, it will *always* result in a mixed number or in a whole number.

Changing a Mixed Number to an Improper Fraction

1. Multiply the denominator of the fraction by the whole number.
2. Add the product to the numerator of the fraction.
3. Place the sum over the denominator.

Example: $3\frac{1}{4}$

$4 \times 3 = 12$

$12 + 1 = 13$

$3\frac{1}{4} = \frac{13}{4}$

Example: $1\frac{3}{8}$

$8 \times 1 = 8$

$8 + 3 = 11$

$1\frac{3}{8} = \frac{11}{8}$

Example: $2\frac{7}{10}$

$10 \times 2 = 20$

$20 + 7 = 27$

$2\frac{7}{10} = \frac{27}{10}$

If fractions are to be added or subtracted, it is necessary for their *denominators to be the same.*

LOWEST COMMON DENOMINATOR

Computations are facilitated when the lowest common denominator is used. The term **lowest common denominator** is defined as the smallest whole number that can be divided evenly by all denominators within the problem.

When trying to determine the lowest common denominator, first observe whether one of the denominators in the problem is evenly divisible by each of the other denominators. If so, this will be the lowest common denominator for the problem.

Example: $\frac{2}{3}$ and $\frac{5}{12}$
You find that 12 is evenly divisible by 3; therefore 12 is the lowest common denominator.

Example: $\frac{1}{2}$ and $\frac{3}{8}$
You find that 8 is evenly divisible by 2; therefore 8 is the lowest common denominator.

Example: $\frac{2}{7}$ and $\frac{5}{14}$ and $\frac{1}{28}$
You find that 28 is evenly divisible by 7 and 14; therefore 28 is the lowest common denominator.

Changing a Fraction to an Equivalent Fraction with the Lowest Common Denominator

1. Divide the lowest common denominator by the denominator of the fraction to be changed.
2. Multiply the quotient by the numerator of the fraction to be changed.
3. Place the product over the lowest common denominator.

Example: $\frac{2}{3} = \frac{?}{12}$

$12 \div 3 = 4$

$4 \times 2 = 8$

$\frac{2}{3} = \frac{8}{12}$

Example: $\frac{1}{2} = \frac{?}{8}$

$8 \div 2 = 4$

$4 \times 1 = 4$

$\frac{1}{2} = \frac{4}{8}$

Example: $\frac{2}{7} = \frac{?}{14}$

$14 \div 7 = 2$

$2 \times 2 = 4$

$\frac{2}{7} = \frac{4}{14}$

Changing a Mixed Number to an Equivalent Fraction with the Lowest Common Denominator

1. Change the mixed number to an improper fraction.
2. Divide the lowest common denominator by the denominator of the fraction.
3. Multiply the quotient by the numerator of the improper fraction.
4. Place the product over the lowest common denominator.

Example: 1¾ and 5/12   **Example:** 3⅔ and 4/9

$1\dfrac{3}{4} = \dfrac{?}{12}$ $3\dfrac{2}{3} = \dfrac{?}{9}$

$4 \times 1 = 4$ $3 \times 3 = 9$

$4 + 3 = 7$ $9 + 2 = 11$

$\dfrac{7}{4} = \dfrac{?}{12}$ $\dfrac{11}{3} = \dfrac{?}{9}$

$12 \div 4 = 3$ $9 \div 3 = 3$

$3 \times 7 = 21$ $3 \times 11 = 33$

$1\dfrac{3}{4} = \dfrac{21}{12}$ $3\dfrac{2}{3} = \dfrac{33}{9}$

If one of the denominators in the problem is not the lowest common denominator for all, you must look further. One suggestion is to multiply two of the denominators together and if possible use that number as the lowest common denominator.

Example: 3½ and ⅔
Multiply the two denominators: $2 \times 3 = 6$

$3\dfrac{1}{2} = \dfrac{?}{6}$ $\dfrac{2}{3} = \dfrac{?}{6}$

$2 \times 3 = 6$ $6 \div 3 = 2$

$6 + 1 = 7$ $2 \times 2 = 4$

$\dfrac{7}{2} = \dfrac{?}{6}$ $\dfrac{2}{3} = \dfrac{4}{6}$

$6 \div 2 = 3$

$3 \times 7 = 21$

$3\dfrac{1}{2} = \dfrac{21}{6}$

Another method is to multiply one of the denominators by 2, 3, or 4. Determine whether the resulting number can be used as a common denominator.

Example: ¾ and ⅛ and 5/12
Multiply the denominator 8 by 3: $8 \times 3 = 24$

$\dfrac{3}{4} = \dfrac{?}{24}$ $\dfrac{1}{8} = \dfrac{?}{24}$ $\dfrac{5}{12} = \dfrac{?}{24}$

$24 \div 4 = 6$ $24 \div 8 = 3$ $24 \div 12 = 2$

$6 \times 3 = 18$ $3 \times 1 = 3$ $2 \times 5 = 10$

$\dfrac{3}{4} = \dfrac{18}{24}$ $\dfrac{1}{8} = \dfrac{3}{24}$ $\dfrac{5}{12} = \dfrac{10}{24}$

ADDITION OF FRACTIONS

Addition of Fractions Having the Same Denominator

1. Add the numerators.
2. Place the sum over the common denominator.
3. Reduce to lowest terms.

Example: $1/7 + 2/7 =$ _____

$$\frac{1}{7} + \frac{2}{7} =$$

$$\frac{1+2}{7} =$$

$$\frac{3}{7}$$

Example: $1/8 + 3/8 =$ _____

$$\frac{1}{8} + \frac{3}{8} =$$

$$\frac{1+3}{8} =$$

$$\frac{4}{8} = \frac{1}{2}$$

Addition of Fractions with Unlike Denominators

1. Change the fractions to equivalent fractions with the lowest common denominator.
2. Add the numerators.
3. Place the sum over the lowest common denominator.
4. Reduce to lowest terms.

Example: $2/3 + 1/5 =$ _____

$$\frac{2}{3} + \frac{1}{5} =$$

To find the lowest common denominator, multiply the two denominators together.

$$3 \times 5 = 15$$

Change each fraction to an equivalent fraction with 15 as the denominator.

$$\frac{2}{3} = \frac{?}{15}$$

$$15 \div 3 = 5$$

$$5 \times 2 = 10$$

$$\frac{2}{3} = \frac{10}{15}$$

$$\frac{1}{5} = \frac{?}{15}$$

$$15 \div 5 = 3$$

$$3 \times 1 = 3$$

$$\frac{1}{5} = \frac{3}{15}$$

$$\frac{10}{15} + \frac{3}{15} =$$

$$\frac{10+3}{15} = \frac{13}{15}$$

Example: ⅙ + ¼ + ⅓ = _____

To find a common denominator, try multiplying two of the denominators together and check to see if that number is divisible by the other denominator.

$$4 \times 3 = 12$$

Is 12 divisible by the other denominator, 6? The answer is YES.

$$\frac{1}{6} = \frac{?}{12} \qquad\qquad \frac{1}{4} = \frac{?}{12} \qquad\qquad \frac{1}{3} = \frac{?}{12}$$

$$12 \div 6 = 2 \qquad\qquad 12 \div 4 = 3 \qquad\qquad 12 \div 3 = 4$$

$$2 \times 1 = 2 \qquad\qquad 3 \times 1 = 3 \qquad\qquad 4 \times 1 = 4$$

$$\frac{1}{6} = \frac{2}{12} \qquad\qquad \frac{1}{4} = \frac{3}{12} \qquad\qquad \frac{1}{3} = \frac{4}{12}$$

$$\frac{2}{12} + \frac{3}{12} + \frac{4}{12} =$$

$$\frac{2 + 3 + 4}{12} = \frac{9}{12}$$

$$\frac{9}{12} = \frac{3}{4} \text{ (reduced to lowest terms)}$$

Addition of Fractions Involving Whole Numbers and Unlike Denominators

1. Change the fractions to equivalent fractions with the lowest common denominator.
2. Add the numerators.
3. Place the sum over the lowest common denominator.
4. Reduce to lowest terms.
5. Write the reduced fraction next to the sum of the whole numbers.

Example: 1⅓ + 2⅜ = _____

To find the lowest common denominator, multiply the two denominators together.

$$3 \times 8 = 24$$

Change the fractions ⅓ and ⅜ to equivalent fractions with 24 as their denominators.

$$\frac{1}{3} = \frac{?}{24} \qquad\qquad\qquad \frac{3}{8} = \frac{?}{24}$$

$$24 \div 3 = 8 \qquad\qquad\qquad 24 \div 8 = 3$$

$$8 \times 1 = 8 \qquad\qquad\qquad 3 \times 3 = 9$$

$$\frac{1}{3} = \frac{8}{24} \qquad\qquad\qquad \frac{3}{8} = \frac{9}{24}$$

$$1\frac{8}{24} + 2\frac{9}{24} =$$

$$\begin{array}{r} 1\dfrac{8}{24} \\[2mm] + 2\dfrac{9}{24} \\[1mm] \hline 3\dfrac{17}{24} \end{array}$$

Example: $5\frac{1}{2} + 3\frac{3}{10} = $ _____

Because 10 is evenly divisible by 2, 10 is the lowest common denominator. Therefore ½ needs to be changed to an equivalent fraction with 10 as the denominator.

$$\frac{1}{2} = \frac{?}{10}$$

$$10 \div 2 = 5$$

$$5 \times 1 = 5$$

$$\frac{1}{2} = \frac{5}{10}$$

$$5\frac{5}{10} + 3\frac{3}{10} =$$

$$5\frac{5}{10}$$

$$+ 3\frac{3}{10}$$

$$8\frac{8}{10} = 8\frac{4}{5} \text{ (reduced to lowest terms)}$$

SUBTRACTION OF FRACTIONS

Subtraction of Fractions Having the Same Denominators

1. Subtract the numerator of the **subtrahend** from the numerator of the **minuend**.
2. Place the difference over the common denominator.
3. Reduce to lowest terms.

Example: $\frac{6}{8} - \frac{4}{8} = $ _____

$$\frac{6}{8} - \frac{4}{8} =$$

$$\frac{6-4}{8} =$$

$$\frac{2}{8} = \frac{1}{4} \text{ (reduced to lowest terms)}$$

Example: $\frac{7}{12} - \frac{1}{12} = $ _____

$$\frac{7}{12} - \frac{1}{12} =$$

$$\frac{7-1}{12} =$$

$$\frac{6}{12} = \frac{1}{2} \text{ (reduced to lowest terms)}$$

Subtraction of Fractions with Unlike Denominators

1. Change the fractions to equivalent fractions with the lowest common denominator.
2. Subtract the numerator of the subtrahend from that of the minuend.
3. Place the difference over the lowest common denominator.
4. Reduce to lowest terms.

Example: $\frac{2}{3} - \frac{1}{6} = $ _____

The lowest common denominator is 6, because 6 is evenly divisible by 3. Therefore the fraction $\frac{2}{3}$ needs to be changed to an equivalent fraction with 6 as the denominator.

Step 1: $\frac{2}{3} = \frac{?}{6}$

$6 \div 3 = 2$

$2 \times 2 = 4$

$\frac{2}{3} = \frac{4}{6}$

Step 2: $\frac{4}{6} - \frac{1}{6} =$

$\frac{4 - 1}{6} =$

$\frac{3}{6} = \frac{1}{2}$ (reduced to lowest terms)

Example: $\frac{7}{10} - \frac{3}{5} = $ _____

The lowest common denominator is 10, because 10 is evenly divisible by 5. Therefore the fraction $\frac{3}{5}$ needs to be changed to an equivalent fraction with 10 as the denominator.

Step 1: $\frac{3}{5} = \frac{?}{10}$

$10 \div 5 = 2$

$2 \times 3 = 6$

$\frac{3}{5} = \frac{6}{10}$

Step 2: $\frac{7}{10} - \frac{6}{10} =$

$\frac{7 - 6}{10} = \frac{1}{10}$

Subtraction of Fractions Involving Whole Numbers and Unlike Denominators

1. Change the fractions to equivalent fractions with the lowest common denominator.
2. Subtract the numerator of the subtrahend from the minuend, borrowing one from the whole number if necessary.
3. Place the difference over the lowest common denominator.
4. Reduce to lowest terms.
5. Write the reduced fraction next to the difference of the whole numbers.

Example: $3\frac{2}{3} - 1\frac{1}{4} = $ _____

The lowest common denominator is 12 (determined by multiplying 3×4). Each fraction needs to be changed to an equivalent fraction with 12 as the common denominator.

$\frac{2}{3} = \frac{?}{12}$

$12 \div 3 = 4$

$4 \times 2 = 8$

$\frac{2}{3} = \frac{8}{12}$

$\frac{1}{4} = \frac{?}{12}$

$12 \div 4 = 3$

$3 \times 1 = 3$

$\frac{1}{4} = \frac{3}{12}$

$$3\frac{8}{12} - 1\frac{3}{12} =$$

$$3\frac{8}{12}$$

$$-1\frac{3}{12}$$

$$\overline{2\frac{5}{12}}$$

Example: $8\frac{1}{2} - 3\frac{4}{7} =$ _____

The lowest common denominator is 14 (determined by multiplying 2×7). Each fraction needs to be changed to an equivalent fraction with 14 as the common denominator.

$$\frac{1}{2} = \frac{?}{14} \qquad\qquad \frac{4}{7} = \frac{?}{14}$$

$$14 \div 2 = 7 \qquad\qquad 14 \div 7 = 2$$

$$7 \times 1 = 7 \qquad\qquad 2 \times 4 = 8$$

$$\frac{1}{2} = \frac{7}{14} \qquad\qquad \frac{4}{7} = \frac{8}{14}$$

$$8\frac{7}{14} - 3\frac{8}{14} =$$

To perform the subtraction, it is necessary to borrow one from the whole number. "One" for this problem can be expressed as $\frac{14}{14}$. Therefore $8\frac{7}{14} = 7\frac{21}{14}$. Now the mathematics may be completed.

$$
\begin{array}{ccc}
8\dfrac{7}{14} & & 7\dfrac{21}{14} \\[2ex]
-\,3\dfrac{8}{14} & = & -\,3\dfrac{8}{14} \\[2ex]
\hline
& & 4\dfrac{13}{14}
\end{array}
$$

MULTIPLICATION OF FRACTIONS

1. Multiply the numerators.
2. Multiply the denominators.
3. Place the product of the numerators over the product of the denominators.
4. Reduce to lowest terms.

Example: $\frac{2}{3} \times \frac{3}{5} =$ _____

$$\frac{2}{3} \times \frac{3}{5} =$$

$$\frac{2 \times 3}{3 \times 5} = \frac{6}{15}$$

$$\frac{6}{15} = \frac{2}{5} \text{ (reduced to lowest terms)}$$

Example: $\frac{4}{9} \times \frac{4}{5} =$ _____

$$\frac{4}{9} \times \frac{4}{5} =$$

$$\frac{4 \times 4}{9 \times 5} = \frac{16}{45} \text{ (reduced to lowest terms)}$$

The process of multiplying fractions may be shortened by **canceling**. In other words, numbers common to the numerators and denominators may be divided or canceled out.

Example: $\frac{2}{3} \times \frac{3}{5} =$ _____

$$\overset{1}{\underset{1}{\frac{2}{3}}} \times \frac{\cancel{3}}{5} = \frac{2 \times 1}{1 \times 5} = \frac{2}{5}$$

Example: $\frac{7}{20} \times \frac{2}{5} \times \frac{3}{14} =$ _____

$$\overset{1}{\underset{10}{\frac{\cancel{7}}{20}}} \times \overset{1}{\underset{}{\frac{\cancel{2}}{5}}} \times \underset{2}{\frac{3}{14}} =$$

$$\frac{1 \times 1 \times 3}{10 \times 5 \times 2} = \frac{3}{100}$$

Example: $\frac{2}{6} \times \frac{3}{4} =$ _____

$$\overset{1}{\underset{2}{\cancel{\frac{2}{6}}}} \times \overset{1}{\underset{2}{\cancel{\frac{3}{4}}}} = \frac{1 \times 1}{2 \times 2} = \frac{1}{4}$$

Multiplication of Mixed Numbers

1. Change each mixed number to an improper fraction.
2. Multiply the numerators.
3. Multiply the denominators.
4. Place the product of the numerators over the product of the denominators.
5. Reduce to lowest terms.

Example: $1\frac{1}{2} \times 2\frac{1}{4} =$ _____

$$\frac{3}{2} \times \frac{9}{4} =$$

$$\frac{3 \times 9}{2 \times 4} = \frac{27}{8} = 3\frac{3}{8} \text{ (reduced to lowest terms)}$$

Example: $2 \times 3\frac{5}{6} =$ _____

$$\frac{2}{1} \times \frac{23}{6} =$$

$$\underset{1}{\cancel{\frac{2}{1}}} \times \underset{3}{\cancel{\frac{23}{6}}} =$$

$$\frac{1 \times 23}{1 \times 3} = \frac{23}{3} = 7\frac{2}{3} \text{ (reduced to lowest terms)}$$

DIVISION OF FRACTIONS

1. Invert (or turn upside down) the divisor.
2. Multiply the two fractions.
3. Reduce to lowest terms.

Example: $\frac{2}{3} \div \frac{6}{8} =$ _____

$$\frac{2}{3} \div \frac{6}{8} =$$

$$\frac{2}{3} \times \frac{8}{6} =$$

$$\underset{3}{\cancel{\frac{2}{3}}} \times \overset{1}{\cancel{\frac{8}{6}}} = \frac{1 \times 8}{3 \times 3} = \frac{8}{9}$$

Example: $\frac{3}{4} \div \frac{8}{9} =$ _____

$$\frac{3}{4} \div \frac{8}{9} =$$

$$\frac{3}{4} \times \frac{9}{8} =$$

$$\frac{3 \times 9}{4 \times 8} = \frac{27}{32}$$

Division of Mixed Numbers

1. Change each mixed number to an improper fraction.
2. Invert (or turn upside down) the divisor.
3. Multiply the two fractions.
4. Reduce to lowest terms.

Example: $1\frac{3}{4} \div 2\frac{1}{8} =$ _____

$$\frac{7}{4} \div \frac{17}{8} =$$

$$\frac{7}{\overset{}{\underset{1}{4}}} \times \frac{\overset{2}{8}}{17} = \frac{7 \times 2}{1 \times 17} = \frac{14}{17}$$

Example: $\frac{1}{7} \div 7 =$ _____

$$\frac{1}{7} \div \frac{7^*}{1} =$$

$$\frac{1}{7} \times \frac{1}{7} = \frac{1 \times 1}{7 \times 7} = \frac{1}{49}$$

*Remember the denominator of a whole number is always 1.

$$6 = \frac{6}{1}$$

$$12 = \frac{12}{1}$$

REDUCTION OF A COMPLEX FRACTION

1. Rewrite the complex fraction as a division problem.
2. Invert (or turn upside down) the divisor.
3. Multiply the two fractions.
4. Reduce to lowest terms.

Example: $\frac{3}{8} \big/ \frac{1}{4} =$ _____

$$\frac{3}{8} \div \frac{1}{4} =$$

$$\frac{3}{8} \times \frac{4}{1} =$$

$$\frac{3}{\underset{2}{8}} \times \frac{\overset{1}{4}}{1} = \frac{3 \times 1}{2 \times 1} = \frac{3}{2} = 1\frac{1}{2} \text{ (reduced to lowest terms)}$$

Example: $\frac{1}{2} \big/ \frac{2}{7} =$ _____

$$\frac{1}{2} \div \frac{2}{7} =$$

$$\frac{1}{2} \times \frac{7}{2} =$$

$$\frac{1 \times 7}{2 \times 2} = \frac{7}{4} = 1\frac{3}{4} \text{ (reduced to lowest terms)}$$

Reduction of a Complex Fraction with Mixed Numbers

1. Change the mixed numbers to improper fractions.
2. Rewrite the complex fraction as a division problem.
3. Invert (or turn upside down) the divisor.
4. Multiply the two fractions.
5. Reduce to lowest terms.

Example: $2\frac{1}{2} \big/ 1\frac{1}{3} =$ _____

$$2\frac{1}{2} \div 1\frac{1}{3} =$$

$$\frac{5}{2} \div \frac{4}{3} =$$

$$\frac{5}{2} \times \frac{3}{4} =$$

$$\frac{5 \times 3}{2 \times 4} = \frac{15}{8} = 1\frac{7}{8} \text{ (reduced to lowest terms)}$$

Example: $3\frac{3}{4} \big/ 2\frac{1}{6} =$ _____

$$3\frac{3}{4} \div 2\frac{1}{6} =$$

$$\frac{15}{4} \div \frac{13}{6} =$$

$$\frac{15}{4} \times \frac{6}{13} =$$

$$\frac{15 \times \overset{3}{6}}{\underset{2}{4} \times 13} = \frac{45}{26} = 1\frac{19}{26} \text{ (reduced to lowest terms)}$$

Study the introductory material for fractions. The processes for the calculation of fraction problems are listed in steps. Memorize the steps for each type of calculation before beginning the work sheet. Complete the following work sheet, which provides extensive practice in the manipulation of fractions. Check your answers. If you have difficulties, go back and review the steps for that type of calculation. When you feel ready to evaluate your learning, take the first posttest. Check your answers. An acceptable score (number of answers correct) as indicated on the posttest signifies that you are ready for the next chapter. An unacceptable score signifies a need for further study before taking the second posttest.

WORK SHEET

Directions: Change the following improper fractions to mixed numbers.

1. $4/3 =$ _____

2. $6/2 =$ _____

3. $9/4 =$ _____

4. $16/5 =$ _____

5. $17/10 =$ _____

6. $3/2 =$ _____

7. $10/7 =$ _____

8. $13/4 =$ _____

9. $10/3 =$ _____

10. $19/9 =$ _____

11. $15/10 =$ _____

12. $9/8 =$ _____

13. $10/6 =$ _____

14. $26/12 =$ _____

15. $19/3 =$ _____

16. $22/7 =$ _____

17. $35/13 =$ _____

18. $21/6 =$ _____

19. $14/3 =$ _____

20. $11/8 =$ _____

21. $7/2 =$ _____   **22.** $112/100 =$ _____   **23.** $37/15 =$ _____   **24.** $9/6 =$ _____

Directions: Change the following mixed numbers to improper fractions.

1. $1\frac{1}{2} =$ _____   **2.** $3\frac{3}{4} =$ _____   **3.** $2\frac{2}{3} =$ _____   **4.** $4\frac{1}{8} =$ _____

5. $7\frac{2}{9} =$ _____   **6.** $5\frac{3}{10} =$ _____   **7.** $2\frac{5}{6} =$ _____   **8.** $1\frac{3}{5} =$ _____

9. $3\frac{4}{7} =$ _____   **10.** $7\frac{1}{3} =$ _____   **11.** $4\frac{7}{8} =$ _____   **12.** $5\frac{1}{2} =$ _____

13. $9\frac{2}{3} =$ _____   **14.** $6\frac{4}{11} =$ _____   **15.** $3\frac{7}{100} =$ _____   **16.** $4\frac{3}{7} =$ _____

17. $1\frac{1}{3} =$ _____   **18.** $2\frac{7}{10} =$ _____   **19.** $6\frac{5}{8} =$ _____   **20.** $2\frac{3}{13} =$ _____

21. $1\frac{3}{25} =$ _____   **22.** $4\frac{1}{4} =$ _____   **23.** $5\frac{3}{8} =$ _____   **24.** $2\frac{4}{9} =$ _____

Directions: Add and reduce fractions to lowest terms.

1. $\frac{2}{3} + \frac{5}{6} =$ _____   **2.** $\frac{2}{5} + \frac{3}{7} =$ _____   **3.** $3\frac{1}{8} + \frac{2}{3} =$ _____

4. $1\frac{1}{3} + \frac{5}{9} =$ _____   **5.** $2\frac{1}{2} + \frac{3}{4} =$ _____   **6.** $\frac{4}{7} + \frac{3}{11} =$ _____

7. $2\frac{1}{4} + 3\frac{2}{5} =$ _____   **8.** $1\frac{6}{13} + 1\frac{2}{3} =$ _____   **9.** $1\frac{1}{16} + 2\frac{3}{8} =$ _____

10. $3\frac{3}{5} + 2\frac{7}{10} + 4\frac{1}{2} =$ _____   **11.** $2\frac{5}{12} + \frac{5}{6} + 3\frac{1}{4} =$ _____   **12.** $4\frac{2}{3} + 2\frac{4}{15} =$ _____

13. $1\frac{1}{2} + 3\frac{3}{4} + 2\frac{3}{8} =$ _____   **14.** $4\frac{3}{11} + 2\frac{1}{2} =$ _____   **15.** $2\frac{2}{3} + 3\frac{7}{9} =$ _____

16. $1\frac{3}{10} + 4\frac{2}{5} + \frac{2}{3} = $ _____   **17.** $2\frac{1}{4} + \frac{5}{8} + 1\frac{5}{6} = $ _____   **18.** $3\frac{3}{5} + 2\frac{7}{8} = $ _____

19. $1\frac{2}{3} + 2\frac{1}{6} + 2\frac{4}{5} = $ _____   **20.** $\frac{5}{6} + \frac{3}{4} = $ _____   **21.** $1\frac{2}{5} + 2\frac{3}{4} = $ _____

22. $3\frac{1}{2} + 2\frac{5}{6} + 2\frac{2}{3} = $ _____   **23.** $2\frac{4}{9} + 3\frac{5}{7} = $ _____   **24.** $5\frac{5}{6} + 2\frac{2}{5} = $ _____

Directions: Subtract and reduce fractions to lowest terms.

1. $\frac{2}{3} - \frac{3}{7} = $ _____   **2.** $\frac{7}{8} - \frac{5}{16} = $ _____   **3.** $\frac{9}{16} - \frac{5}{12} = $ _____

4. $1\frac{1}{3} - \frac{5}{6} = $ _____   **5.** $\frac{7}{10} - \frac{1}{2} = $ _____   **6.** $\frac{15}{24} - \frac{7}{16} = $ _____

7. $2\frac{17}{20} - 1\frac{3}{4} = $ _____   **8.** $3\frac{1}{2} - 2\frac{1}{3} = $ _____   **9.** $4\frac{3}{8} - 1\frac{3}{5} = $ _____

10. $2\frac{7}{8} - 1\frac{5}{6} =$ _____

11. $\frac{15}{16} - \frac{1}{4} =$ _____

12. $4\frac{1}{6} - 2\frac{5}{8} =$ _____

13. $5\frac{1}{4} - 3\frac{5}{16} =$ _____

14. $5\frac{3}{8} - 4\frac{3}{4} =$ _____

15. $3\frac{1}{4} - 1\frac{11}{12} =$ _____

16. $6\frac{1}{2} - 3\frac{7}{8} =$ _____

17. $3\frac{3}{8} - 2\frac{7}{12} =$ _____

18. $5\frac{3}{16} - 3\frac{2}{3} =$ _____

19. $4\frac{1}{6} - 2\frac{3}{4} =$ _____

20. $2\frac{3}{8} - 1\frac{1}{12} =$ _____

21. $3\frac{5}{6} - 2\frac{3}{4} =$ _____

22. $5\frac{2}{3} - 3\frac{7}{8} =$ _____

23. $4\frac{1}{2} - 2\frac{9}{10} =$ _____

24. $2\frac{5}{16} - 1\frac{3}{8} =$ _____

Directions: Multiply and reduce fractions to lowest terms.

1. $\frac{1}{3} \times \frac{4}{5} =$ _____

2. $\frac{5}{12} \times \frac{4}{9} =$ _____

3. $\frac{7}{8} \times \frac{2}{3} =$ _____

4. $\frac{4}{5} \times \frac{5}{7} = $ _____

5. $6 \times \frac{2}{3} = $ _____

6. $\frac{3}{8} \times 4 = $ _____

7. $2\frac{1}{3} \times 3\frac{3}{4} = $ _____

8. $1\frac{4}{5} \times 3\frac{3}{7} = $ _____

9. $4\frac{3}{8} \times 2\frac{5}{7} = $ _____

10. $2\frac{3}{5} \times 2\frac{3}{10} = $ _____

11. $1\frac{5}{6} \times 2\frac{4}{5} = $ _____

12. $2\frac{5}{12} \times 5\frac{1}{4} = $ _____

13. $1\frac{3}{5} \times 2\frac{2}{3} = $ _____

14. $\frac{3}{4} \times 2\frac{3}{8} = $ _____

15. $2\frac{1}{2} \times 2\frac{1}{4} = $ _____

16. $\frac{3}{8} \times \frac{4}{5} \times \frac{2}{3} = $ _____

17. $1\frac{5}{8} \times 2\frac{3}{4} = $ _____

18. $\frac{1}{10} \times \frac{3}{100} = $ _____

19. $1\frac{9}{10} \times 2\frac{3}{19} = $ _____

20. $1\frac{3}{4} \times 2\frac{3}{7} = $ _____

21. $1\frac{5}{8} \times 1\frac{5}{7} = $ _____

22. $3\frac{1}{2} \times 1\frac{5}{6} =$ _____

23. $1\frac{2}{3} \times 2\frac{1}{5} =$ _____

24. $2\frac{4}{9} \times 1\frac{3}{11} =$ _____

Directions: Divide and reduce fractions to lowest terms.

1. $1\frac{2}{3} \div 3\frac{1}{2} =$ _____

2. $2\frac{2}{5} \div 1\frac{1}{3} =$ _____

3. $5\frac{1}{2} \div 2\frac{1}{2} =$ _____

4. $2\frac{1}{8} \div \frac{3}{4} =$ _____

5. $3\frac{1}{2} \div 2\frac{1}{4} =$ _____

6. $3\frac{6}{7} \div 1\frac{3}{5} =$ _____

7. $4\frac{3}{8} \div 1\frac{3}{4} =$ _____

8. $3\frac{1}{2} \div 1\frac{6}{7} =$ _____

9. $7\frac{1}{3} \div 2\frac{3}{5} =$ _____

10. $\frac{9}{10} \div \frac{2}{3} =$ _____

11. $3 \div 1\frac{5}{6} =$ _____

12. $4\frac{1}{2} \div 2\frac{2}{5} =$ _____

13. $2\frac{7}{8} \div 1\frac{2}{3} =$ _____

14. $6\frac{2}{3} \div 1\frac{7}{10} =$ _____

15. $5\frac{1}{8} \div 4\frac{2}{5} =$ _____

16. $^7/_8 / ^1/_4 =$ _____

17. $6^1/_2 / 2^5/_6 =$ _____

18. $8^1/_2 / 1^5/_7 =$ _____

19. $4^3/_8 / 2^3/_4 =$ _____

20. $5^1/_2 / 2^2/_3 =$ _____

21. $3^1/_3 / 1^7/_{12} =$ _____

22. $3^7/_{10} / 2^4/_5 =$ _____

23. $2^2/_3 / 1^7/_9 =$ _____

24. $4^1/_2 / 2^3/_{10} =$ _____

Answers on p. 412.

POSTTEST 1

Name _____

Date _____

ACCEPTABLE SCORE ___**36**___

YOUR SCORE _____

Directions: Perform the indicated calculations and reduce fractions to lowest terms.

1. $\frac{2}{3} + \frac{4}{9} =$ _____

2. $\frac{3}{8} + \frac{1}{3} =$ _____

3. $2\frac{3}{4} + 2\frac{1}{3} =$ _____

4. $1\frac{7}{10} + 2\frac{3}{5} =$ _____

5. $2\frac{2}{3} + \frac{3}{7} =$ _____

6. $3\frac{4}{21} + 1\frac{2}{7} =$ _____

7. $\frac{3}{4} + \frac{3}{100} =$ _____

8. $\frac{5}{8} + 3\frac{1}{6} =$ _____

9. $4\frac{2}{5} + 3\frac{3}{4} =$ _____

10. $4\frac{1}{6} + \frac{2}{3} + 2\frac{3}{4} =$ _____

11. $\frac{8}{9} - \frac{3}{4} =$ _____

12. $1\frac{3}{10} - \frac{2}{5} =$ _____

13. $2\frac{1}{2} - 1\frac{2}{3} =$ _____

14. $\frac{5}{7} - \frac{1}{2} =$ _____

15. $5\frac{1}{9} - 3\frac{2}{3} =$ _____

16. $3\frac{1}{2} - 1\frac{9}{16} =$ _____

17. $2\frac{5}{7} - 1\frac{2}{9} =$ _____

18. $3\frac{3}{5} - 2\frac{3}{20} =$ _____

19. $9\frac{1}{5} - 3\frac{1}{2} =$ _____

20. $2\frac{1}{4} - \frac{7}{9}/\frac{2}{3} =$ _____

21. $\frac{3}{4} \times \frac{6}{7} =$ _____

22. $3 \times \frac{4}{5} =$ _____

23. $\frac{4}{5} \times \frac{1}{2} =$ _____

24. $\frac{2}{9} \times 9 =$ _____

25. $2\frac{3}{4} \times 1\frac{1}{6} =$ _____

26. $1\frac{1}{4} \times 2\frac{2}{3} =$ _____

27. $10\frac{1}{2} \times 1\frac{2}{5} =$ _____

28. $5\frac{6}{7} \times \frac{3}{5} =$ _____

29. $\frac{1}{4} \times 3\frac{1}{2} =$ _____

30. $7\frac{1}{2} \times 5\frac{2}{3} =$ _____

31. $\frac{2}{3} \div \frac{5}{8} =$ _____

32. $\frac{1}{5} \div \frac{1}{50} =$ _____

33. $\frac{1}{3} \div \frac{1}{2} =$ _____

34. $5/6 \div 2/3 =$ _____

35. $3/10 \div 2 =$ _____

36. $6/7 / 1\frac{1}{3} =$ _____

37. $1/5 / 1/3 =$ _____

38. $1\frac{1}{5} / 8/9 =$ _____

39. $3/4 / 1/6 =$ _____

40. $3\frac{1}{8} / 2\frac{3}{4} =$ _____

Answers on p. 413.

POSTTEST 2

Name _____

Date _____

ACCEPTABLE SCORE ___**36**___

YOUR SCORE _____

Directions: Perform the indicated calculations and reduce fractions to lowest terms.

1. $\frac{1}{4} + \frac{5}{6} =$ _____

2. $2\frac{3}{5} + 1\frac{1}{2} =$ _____

3. $\frac{2}{3} + 2\frac{3}{7} =$ _____

4. $4\frac{2}{3} + 2\frac{6}{15} =$ _____

5. $1\frac{7}{8} + 3\frac{2}{5} =$ _____

6. $1\frac{3}{4} + \frac{5}{8} + 2\frac{5}{12} =$ _____

7. $10\frac{1}{2} + 1\frac{3}{10} =$ _____

8. $4\frac{4}{9} + 2\frac{1}{4} =$ _____

9. $1\frac{5}{14} + 2\frac{3}{21} =$ _____

10. $2\frac{1}{8} + 1\frac{7}{20} =$ _____

11. $\frac{4}{9} - \frac{1}{3} =$ _____

12. $2\frac{3}{4} - \frac{7}{8} =$ _____

13. $3\frac{1}{2} - 1\frac{2}{3} =$ _____

14. $1\frac{5}{7} - \frac{4}{5} =$ _____

15. $3\frac{5}{8} - 1\frac{5}{16} =$ _____

16. $5\frac{1}{8} - 4\frac{1}{2} = $ _____

17. $7\frac{1}{3} - 5\frac{5}{6} = $ _____

18. $7\frac{7}{10} - 3\frac{4}{5} = $ _____

19. $3\frac{4}{15} - 2\frac{2}{3} = $ _____

20. $8\frac{1}{2} - 3\frac{4}{7} = $ _____

21. $\frac{2}{7} \times \frac{2}{3} = $ _____

22. $3\frac{4}{9} \times 1\frac{4}{5} = $ _____

23. $2 \times \frac{2}{3} = $ _____

24. $3\frac{1}{2} \times 2\frac{3}{11} = $ _____

25. $\frac{5}{6} \times 2\frac{1}{3} = $ _____

26. $\frac{1}{100} \times \frac{1}{10} = $ _____

27. $1\frac{4}{5} \times 3\frac{7}{11} = $ _____

28. $6\frac{3}{4} \times 5\frac{1}{3} = $ _____

29. $2\frac{5}{8} \times 1\frac{1}{3} = $ _____

30. $3\frac{1}{2} \times 3\frac{3}{14} = $ _____

31. $\frac{3}{4} \div \frac{8}{9} = $ _____

32. $1\frac{1}{2} \div 1\frac{6}{7} = $ _____

33. $2\frac{1}{3} \div \frac{3}{8} = $ _____

34. $\frac{1}{7} \div 7 =$ _____

35. $\frac{5}{6}/1\frac{1}{3} =$ _____

36. $1\frac{1}{2}/2\frac{2}{7} =$ _____

37. $1\frac{3}{8}/\frac{4}{5} =$ _____

38. $2\frac{1}{4}/1\frac{1}{3} =$ _____

39. $3\frac{3}{4}/2\frac{1}{6} =$ _____

40. $\frac{3}{8}/\frac{3}{9} =$ _____

Answers on p. 413.

PRETEST

Name _____

Date _____

ACCEPTABLE SCORE ___**63**___

YOUR SCORE _____

Directions: Write the following numbers in words.

1. 0.04 _____

2. 1.6 _____

3. 16.06734 _____

_____

4. 1.015 _____

5. 0.009 _____

Directions: Circle the decimal with the *least value*.

6. 0.2, 0.25, 0.025, 0.02

7. 0.4, 0.48, 0.04, 0.004

8. 1.6, 1.64, 1.682, 1.69

9. 2.8, 2.82, 2.082, 2.822

10. 0.3, 0.33, 0.003, 0.033

Directions: Perform the indicated calculations.

11. 184.36 + 2.031 + 1236.987 + 6.043 = _____

12. 2.43 + 140.59 + 839.78 + 0.999 = _____

13. 6.8 + 2.986 + 14.7 + 0.89 = _____

14. 141.71 + 84.98 + 9.98 + 87.63 = _____

15. 2.5 + 17.292 + 12.63 + 3.6874 = _____

16. 1006.48 + 0.008 + 6.2 + 0.179 = _____

17. $47.21 + 48.496 +$
$0.2976 + 54.67 =$ _____

18. $67.276 + 918.9495 +$
$12.76 + 4.628 =$ _____

19. $5.971 + 63.1 +$
$8.264 + 7.23 =$ _____

20. $188.646 + 334.72 +$
$1.3666 + 27.4 =$ _____

21. $2.176 - 1.098 =$ _____

22. $912.13 - 48.68 =$ _____

23. $2.006 - 0.998 =$ _____

24. $836.2 - 76.8 =$ _____

25. $100.3 - 98.6 =$ _____

26. $20.48 - 8.79 =$ _____

27. $0.375 - 0.296 =$ _____

28. $12.6 - 1.654 =$ _____

29. $2.4 - 1.92 =$ _____

30. $34.9 - 26.84 =$ _____

31. $0.63 \times 0.09 =$ _____

32. $41.545 \times 0.16 =$ _____

33. $0.76 \times 0.08 =$ _____

34. $8.053 \times 0.024 =$ _____

35. $5.25 \times 0.37 =$ _____

36. $4.18 \times 0.78 =$ _____

37. $44.08 \times 0.67 =$ _____

38. $56.7 \times 3.29 =$ _____

39. $8.45 \times 0.08 =$ _____

40. $52.9 \times 6.74 =$ _____

41. $0.89 \div 4.32 =$ _____

42. $1.436 \div 0.08 =$ _____

43. $216.48 \div 55 =$ _____

44. $248 \div 0.008 =$ _____

45. $0.689 \div 62.8 =$ _____

46. $3.59 \div 0.4 =$ _____

47. $12.54 \div 0.02 =$ _____

48. $13.26 \div 18.9 =$ _____

49. $1.304 \div 0.032 =$ _____

50. $23 \div 1236 =$ _____

Directions: Change the following decimal fractions to proper fractions.

51. 0.2 = _____   **52.** 0.45 = _____   **53.** 0.008 = _____   **54.** 0.25 = _____

55. 0.322 = _____   **56.** 0.27 = _____   **57.** 0.3 = _____   **58.** 0.004 = _____

59. 0.34 = _____   **60.** 0.95 = _____

Directions: Change the following proper fractions to decimal fractions.

61. $^3/_5$ = _____   **62.** $^2/_3$ = _____   **63.** $^3/_{500}$ = _____   **64.** $^7/_{20}$ = _____

65. $^1/_{12}$ = _____   **66.** $^5/_8$ = _____   **67.** $^1/_{32}$ = _____   **68.** $^3/_8$ = _____

69. $^1/_{120}$ = _____   **70.** $^4/_{25}$ = _____

Answers on p. 413.

Chapter 2 | *Decimals*

Learning Objectives

On completion of the materials provided in this chapter, you will be able to perform computations accurately by mastering the following mathematical concepts:

1 | Reading and writing decimal numbers
2 | Determining the value of decimal fractions
3 | Adding, subtracting, multiplying, and dividing decimals
4 | Rounding decimal fractions to an indicated place value
5 | Multiplying and dividing decimals by 10 or a power of 10
6 | Multiplying and dividing decimals by 0.1 or a multiple of 0.1
7 | Converting a decimal fraction to a proper fraction
8 | Converting a proper fraction to a decimal fraction

Decimals are used in the metric system of measurement. The nurse uses the metric system in the calculation of drug dosages. Therefore it is essential for the nurse to be able to manipulate decimals easily and accurately.

Each **decimal fraction** consists of a numerator that is expressed in numerals, a decimal point placed so that it designates the value of the denominator, and the denominator, which is understood to be 10 or some power of 10. In writing a decimal fraction, always place a zero to the left of the decimal point so that the decimal point can readily be seen. Some examples are as follows:

Fraction	Decimal fraction
$\dfrac{7}{10}$	0.7
$\dfrac{13}{100}$	0.13
$\dfrac{227}{1000}$	0.227

Decimal numbers include an integer, a decimal point, and a decimal fraction. The value of the combined integer and decimal fraction is determined by the placement of the decimal point. Whole numbers are written to the *left* of the decimal point and decimal fractions to the *right*. The diagram included on the next page illustrates the place occupied by the numeral that has the value indicated.

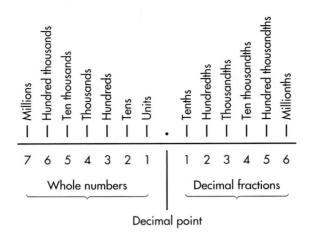

Reading Decimal Numbers

The reading of a decimal number is determined by the place value of the integers and decimal fractions.
1. Read the whole number.
2. Read the decimal point as "and."
3. Read the decimal fraction.

Examples: 0.4   four tenths
              0.86   eighty-six hundredths
              3.659   three and six hundred fifty-nine thousandths
           182.0012   one hundred eighty-two and twelve ten-thousandths
            9.47735   nine and forty-seven thousand seven hundred thirty-five one hundred-thousandths

Determining the Values of Decimal Fractions

1. Place the numbers in a vertical column with the decimal points in a vertical line.
2. Add zeros on the right in the decimal fractions to make columns even.
3. The largest number in a column to the right of the decimal point has the *greatest* value.
4. If two numbers in a column are of equal value, examine the next column to the right and so on.
5. The smallest number in the column to the right of the decimal point has the *least* value. If two numbers in the first column are of equal value, examine the second column to the right and so on.

Example: Of the following fractions (0.623, 0.841, 0.0096, 0.432), which has the greatest value? the least value?

0.6320

0.8410

0.0096

0.4320

0.841 has the greatest value; 0.0096 has the least value.

Note: In mixed numbers the values of both the integer and the fraction are considered.

Example: Which decimal number (0.4, 0.25, 1.2, 1.002) has the greatest value? the least value?

0.400

0.250

1.200

1.002

1.2 has the greatest value; 0.25 has the least value.

ADDITION AND SUBTRACTION OF DECIMALS

1. Write the numerals in a vertical column with the decimal points in a straight line.
2. Add zeros as needed to complete the columns.
3. Add or subtract each column as indicated by the symbol.
4. Place the decimal point in the sum or difference directly below the decimal points in the column.
5. Place a zero to the left of the decimal point in a decimal fraction.

Example: Add: 14.8 + 6.29 + 3.028   **Example:**   Subtract: 5.163 − 4.98

$$\begin{array}{r} 14.800 \\ 6.290 \\ +\ 3.028 \\ \hline 24.118 \end{array}$$

$$\begin{array}{r} 5.163 \\ -\ 4.980 \\ \hline 0.183 \end{array}$$

MULTIPLICATION OF DECIMALS

1. Place the smaller group of numbers under the larger group of numbers.
2. Multiply.
3. Add the number of places to the right of the decimal point in the multiplicand and the multiplier (i.e., the numbers being multiplied). The sum determines the placement of the decimal point within the product.
4. Count from right to left the value of the sum and place the decimal point.

Example: 0.19 × 0.24

$$\begin{array}{r} 0.19 \quad \text{two place values} \\ \times\ 0.24 \quad \text{two place values} \\ \hline 076 \\ 038 \\ 000 \\ \hline 0.0456 \quad \text{four place values} \end{array}$$

Example: 0.459 × 0.52

$$\begin{array}{r} 0.459 \quad \text{three place values} \\ \times\ 0.52 \quad \text{two place values} \\ \hline 0918 \\ 2295 \\ 0000 \\ \hline 0.23868 \quad \text{five place values} \end{array}$$

Example: 8.265 × 4.36

$$\begin{array}{r} 8.265 \quad \text{three place values} \\ \times\ 4.36 \quad \text{two place values} \\ \hline 49590 \\ 24795 \\ 33060 \\ \hline 36.03540 \quad \text{five place values} \end{array}$$

Example: 160.41 × 3.527

$$\begin{array}{r} 160.41 \quad \text{two place values} \\ \times\ 3.527 \quad \text{three place values} \\ \hline 112287 \\ 32082 \\ 80205 \\ 48123 \\ \hline 565.76607 \quad \text{five place values} \end{array}$$

Multiplying a Decimal by 10 or a Power of 10 (100, 1000, 10,000, 100,000)

1. Move the decimal point to the right the same number of places as there are zeros in the multiplier.
2. Zeros may be added as indicated.

Example: $0.132 \times 10 = 1.32$ **Example:** $0.053 \times 100 = 5.3$

Example: $2.64 \times 1000 = 2640$ **Example:** $49.6 \times 10,000 = 496,000$

Multiplying a Whole Number or Decimal by 0.1 or a Multiple of 0.1 (0.01, 0.001, 0.0001, or 0.00001)

1. Move the decimal point to the left the same number of spaces as there are numbers to the right of the decimal point in the multiplier.
2. Zeros may be added as indicated.

Example: $354.86 \times 0.0001 = 0.035486$ **Example:** $0.729 \times 0.1 = 0.0729$

Example: $12.73 \times 0.01 = 0.1273$ **Example:** $5.752 \times 0.001 = 0.005752$

ROUNDING A DECIMAL FRACTION

1. Find the number to the right of the place value desired.
2. If the number is 5, 6, 7, 8, or 9, add one to the number in the place value desired and drop the rest of the numbers.
3. If the number is 0, 1, 2, 3, or 4, remove all numbers to the right of the desired place value.

Example: Round the following decimal fractions to the nearest tenth.

    A. 0.268

        0.2)68   6 is the number to the right of the tenth place. Therefore 1 should be added to the number 2 and the 68 dropped.

        0.3   correct answer

    B. 4.374

        4.3)74   7 is the number to the right of the tenth place. Therefore 1 should be added to the number 3 and the 74 dropped.

        4.4   correct answer

    C. 5.723

        5.7)23   2 is the number to the right of the tenth place. Therefore all numbers to the right of the tenth place should be removed.

        5.7   correct answer

Example: Round the following decimal fractions to the nearest hundredth.

    A. 0.876

        0.87)6   6 is the number to the right of the hundredths place. Therefore 1 should be added to the number 7 and the 6 dropped.

        0.88   correct answer

    B. 2.3249

        2.32)49   4 is the number to the right of the hundredths place. Therefore all numbers to the right of the hundredths place should be removed.

        2.32   correct answer

Example: Round the following decimal fractions to the nearest thousandth.

    A. 3.1325

        3.132)5   5 is the number to the right of the thousandths place. Therefore 1 should be added to the number 2 and the 5 dropped.

        3.133   correct answer

    B. 0.4674

        0.467)4   4 is the number to the right of the thousandths place. Therefore all numbers to the right of the thousandths place should be removed.

        0.467   correct answer

Rounding numbers helps to estimate values, compare values, have more realistic and workable numbers, and spot errors. Decimal fractions may be rounded to any designated place value.

DIVISION OF DECIMALS

1. Place a caret to the right of the last number in the divisor, signifying the movement of the decimal point that will make the divisor a whole number.
2. Count the number of spaces that the decimal point is moved in the divisor.
3. Count to the right an equal number of spaces in the dividend and place a caret to signify the movement of the decimal.
4. Place a decimal point on the quotient line directly above the caret.
5. Divide, extending the decimal fraction three places to the right of the decimal point.
6. Zeros may be added as indicated to extend the decimal fraction dividend.
7. Round the quotient to the nearest hundredth.

Example: 8.326 ÷ 1.062

$$
\begin{array}{r}
7.839 \text{ or } 7.84 \\
1.062 \wedge \overline{)8.326 \wedge 000} \\
\underline{7\ 434} \\
892\ 0 \\
\underline{849\ 6} \\
42\ 40 \\
\underline{31\ 86} \\
10\ 540 \\
\underline{9\ 558}
\end{array}
$$

Example: 386 ÷ 719

$$
\begin{array}{r}
0.536 \text{ or } 0.54 \\
719\overline{)386.000} \\
\underline{359\ 5} \\
26\ 50 \\
\underline{21\ 57} \\
4\ 930 \\
\underline{4\ 314}
\end{array}
$$

Note: The decimal fraction is emphasized by the placement of a zero to the left of the decimal point.

Dividing a Decimal by 10 or a Multiple of 10 (100, 1000, 10,000, 100,000)

1. Move the decimal point to the left the same number of places as there are zeros in the divisor.
2. Zeros may be added as indicated.

Example: 6.41 ÷ 10 = 0.641   **Example:**   358.0 ÷ 100 = 3.58

Dividing a Whole Number or a Decimal Fraction by 0.1 or a Multiple of 0.1 (0.01, 0.001, 0.0001, 0.00001)

1. Move the decimal point to the right as many places as there are numbers in the divisor.
2. Zeros may be added as indicated.

Example: $5.897 \div 0.01 = 589.7$ **Example:** $46.31 \div 0.001 = 46{,}310$

CONVERSION

Converting a Decimal Fraction to a Proper Fraction

1. Remove the decimal point and the zero preceding it.
2. The numerals are the numerator.
3. The placement of the decimal point has indicated what the denominator will be.
4. Reduce to lowest terms.

Example: 0.3   **Example:** 0.86   **Example:** 0.375

$$\frac{3}{10}$$ $$\frac{86}{100} = \frac{43}{50}$$ $$\frac{375}{1000} = \frac{3}{8}$$

Converting a Proper Fraction to a Decimal Fraction

1. Divide the numerator by the denominator.
2. Extend the decimal the desired number of places (often three).
3. Place a zero to the left of the decimal point in a decimal fraction.

Example: $\frac{4}{5}$ **Example:** $\frac{7}{8}$

```
      0.8                                0.875
   5)4.0                               8)7.000
     4 0                                 6 4
                                         60
   4/5 = 0.8                             56
                                         40
                                         40

                                      7/8 = 0.875
```

Study the introductory material for decimals. The processes for the calculation of decimal problems are listed in steps. Memorize the steps for each calculation before beginning the work sheet. Complete the following work sheet, which provides for extensive practice in the manipulation of decimals. Check your answers. If you have difficulties, go back and review the steps for that type of calculation. When you feel ready to evaluate your learning, take the first posttest. Check your answers. An acceptable score as indicated on the posttest signifies that you are ready for the next chapter. An unacceptable score signifies a need for further study before taking the second posttest.

WORK SHEET

Directions: Write the following numbers in words.

1. 0.2 _____

2. 9.68 _____

3. 186.935 _____
_____

4. 0.00008 _____

5. 0.86931 _____
_____

6. 698,437.15 _____
_____

7. 0.0003 _____

8. 12,375.7 _____
_____

9. 6.004 _____

10. 1,968.342 _____
_____

11. 0.02 _____

12. 35.4726 _____
_____

Directions: Circle the decimal numbers with the *greatest value.*

13. 0.2, 0.15, 0.1, 0.25   **14.** 0.4, 0.45, 0.04, 0.042   **15.** 0.9, 0.09, 0.95, 0.98

16. 0.5, 0.065, 0.58, 0.68   **17.** 1.8, 1.08, 1.18, 1.468   **18.** 7.4, 7.42, 7.423, 7.44

Directions: Circle the decimal numbers with the *least value.*

19. 0.6, 0.66, 0.666, 0.6666   **20.** 0.3, 0.03, 0.003, 0.0003   **21.** 1.2, 1.22, 1.022, 1.0022

22. 0.8, 0.08, 0.868, 0.859   **23.** 0.75, 0.07, 0.007, 0.0075   **24.** 3.015, 3.1, 3.006, 3.02

Directions: Add the following decimal problems.

1. 1.080 + 31.2 +
0.065 + 9.41 = _____

2. 2.2 + 355.6 +
8.125 + 6.75 = _____

3. 24.684 + 5.3697 +
8.025 + 2.9 = _____

4. 58.7 + 2.5397 +
4.63 + 822.73 = _____

5. 18.95 + 1.903 +
8.82 + 9.4 = _____

6. 5.291 + 17.54 +
1.32 + 3.7 = _____

7. 7.043 + 0.67 +
13.006 + 1.2 = _____

8. 3.096 + 5.892 +
1.9 + 6.02 = _____

9. 1.069 + 2.5 +
1.43 + 49.034 = _____

10. 56.93 + 765.7 +
64.882 + 7.33 = _____

11. 0.3 + 0.874 +
2.763 + 63.2 = _____

12. 9.2 + 2.88 +
4.31 + 21.004 = _____

13. 5.693 + 1.5 +
1.44 + 14.2 = _____

14. 4.6 + 3.291 +
102.8269 + 0.874 = _____

15. 13.5 + 1.023 +
8.83 + 3.267 = _____

16. 1.95 + 14.271 +
5.37 + 1.8 = _____

17. 8.25 + 6.326 +
6.2 + 20.6521 = _____

18. 3.6 + 8.25 +
2.05 + 24 = _____

19. $25.82 + 432.7 +$
      $64.993 + 2.66 = $ _____

20. $0.6 + 0.985 +$
      $1.432 + 52.1 = $ _____

21. $63.65 + 11.73 +$
      $4.005 + 136.895 = $ _____

22. $1.29 + 17.5 +$
      $32.44 + 0.325 = $ _____

23. $3.75 + 0.718 +$
      $136.95 + 0.8 = $ _____

24. $3.64 + 10.49 +$
      $8.65 + 195.27 = $ _____

Directions: Subtract the following decimal problems.

1. $1321.52 - 63.65 = $ _____

2. $4.745 - 2.896 = $ _____

3. $1.8 - 1.09 = $ _____

4. $42.571 - 9.825 = $ _____

5. $250.7 - 75.896 = $ _____

6. $24.186 - 16.768 = $ _____

7. $1.943 - 0.864 = $ _____

8. $6.33 - 2.186 = $ _____

9. $0.486 - 0.025 = $ _____

10. $1 - 0.012 = $ _____

11. $3.4 - 0.068 = $ _____

12. $8.96 - 2.067 = $ _____

13. $114.3 - 63.625 = $ _____   **14.** $63 - 0.978 = $ _____   **15.** $300 - 12.629 = $ _____

16. $0.386 - 0.199 = $ _____   **17.** $44.892 - 34.943 = $ _____   **18.** $5.003 - 2.064 = $ _____

19. $1.84 - 0.96 = $ _____   **20.** $0.013 - 0.004 = $ _____   **21.** $1036.88 - 117.31 = $ _____

22. $708.6 - 48.86 = $ _____   **23.** $2.436 - 1.989 = $ _____   **24.** $47.56 - 29.89 = $ _____

Directions: Multiply the following decimal problems.

1. $14.376 \times 8.025 = $ _____   **2.** $1.3 \times 12.5 = $ _____   **3.** $29.6 \times 5.4 = $ _____

4. $16.4 \times 0.4 = $ _____   **5.** $127 \times 4.8 = $ _____   **6.** $1.69 \times 30.8 = $ _____

7. $105 \times 0.25 =$ _____

8. $120 \times 5.8 =$ _____

9. $9.08 \times 6.18 =$ _____

10. $52.4 \times 0.8 =$ _____

11. $7.31 \times 1.6 =$ _____

12. $28.9 \times 0.04 =$ _____

13. $3.61 \times 9.33 =$ _____

14. $10.2 \times 3.5 =$ _____

15. $420 \times 0.08 =$ _____

16. $2.3 \times 45.21 =$ _____

17. $325 \times 40.87 =$ _____

18. $7.46 \times 54.83 =$ _____

19. $0.64 \times 0.8 =$ _____

20. $5.72 \times 7.6 =$ _____

21. $6953.64 \times 92.5 =$ _____

22. $1.19 \times 0.127 =$ _____

23. $187.5 \times 38.12 =$ _____

24. $7.85 \times 3.006 =$ _____

Directions: Multiply the following numbers by 10 by moving the decimal point.

1. 0.09 _____   **2.** 0.2 _____   **3.** 0.18 _____
4. 0.3 _____   **5.** 0.625 _____   **6.** 2.33 _____

Directions: Multiply the following numbers by 100 by moving the decimal point.

1. 0.023 _____   **2.** 1.5 _____   **3.** 0.004 _____
4. 0.125 _____   **5.** 8.65 _____   **6.** 76.4 _____

Directions: Multiply the following numbers by 1000 by moving the decimal point.

1. 0.2 _____   **2.** 0.005 _____   **3.** 0.187 _____
4. 9.65 _____   **5.** 0.46 _____   **6.** 0.489 _____

Directions: Multiply the following numbers by 0.1 by moving the decimal point.

1. 30.0 _____   **2.** 0.69 _____   **3.** 1.7 _____
4. 0.95 _____   **5.** 0.138 _____   **6.** 5.67 _____

Directions: Multiply the following numbers by 0.01 by moving the decimal point.

1. 0.26 _____   **2.** 90.8 _____   **3.** 5.5 _____
4. 11.2 _____   **5.** 0.875 _____   **6.** 63.3 _____

Directions: Multiply the following numbers by 0.001 by moving the decimal point.

1. 56.0 _____   **2.** 12.55 _____   **3.** 126.5 _____
4. 33.3 _____   **5.** 9.684 _____   **6.** 241 _____

Directions: Round the following decimal fractions to the nearest tenth.

1. 0.33 _____   **2.** 0.913 _____   **3.** 2.359 _____
4. 0.66 _____   **5.** 58.36 _____   **6.** 8.092 _____

Directions: Round the following decimal fractions to the nearest hundredth.

1. 2.555 _____   **2.** 4.275 _____   **3.** 0.284 _____
4. 3.923 _____   **5.** 6.534 _____   **6.** 2.988 _____

Directions: Round the following decimal fractions to the nearest thousandth.

1. 27.86314 _____   **2.** 5.9246 _____   **3.** 2.1574 _____
4. 0.8493 _____   **5.** 321.0869 _____   **6.** 455.7682 _____

Directions: Divide. Round the quotient to the nearest hundredth.

1. $7.02 \div 6 =$ _____   **2.** $124.2 \div 0.03 =$ _____   **3.** $5.46 \div 0.7 =$ _____

4. $0.145 \div 5 =$ _____

5. $24 \div 0.06 =$ _____

6. $67.2 \div 8 =$ _____

7. $5.44 \div 3.2 =$ _____

8. $0.986 \div 7.36 =$ _____

9. $3.7 \div 0.02 =$ _____

10. $24 \div 1500 =$ _____

11. $4.6 \div 35.362 =$ _____

12. $4.13 \div 0.05 =$ _____

13. $2.22 \div 0.003 =$ _____

14. $0.412 \div 8 =$ _____

15. $0.21 \div 0.42 =$ _____

16. $9.08 \div 2.006 =$ _____

17. $4.5 \div 3.1 =$ _____

18. $6.1732 \div 0.355 =$ _____

19. $63 \div 132.3 =$ _____

20. $0.56 \div 0.7 =$ _____

21. $21.25 \div 8.43 =$ _____

22. 9.2 ÷ 3.5 = _____   **23.** 75.2 ÷ 1.6 = _____   **24.** 8.075 ÷ 0.462 = _____

Directions: Divide the following numbers by 10 by moving the decimal point.

1. 6.0 _____   **2.** 0.2 _____   **3.** 9.8 _____
4. 0.05 _____   **5.** 0.375 _____   **6.** 0.99 _____

Directions: Divide the following numbers by 100 by moving the decimal point.

1. 0.7 _____   **2.** 8.11 _____   **3.** 700.0 _____
4. 0.19 _____   **5.** 12.0 _____   **6.** 30.2 _____

Directions: Divide the following numbers by 1000 by moving the decimal point.

1. 1.8 _____   **2.** 360.0 _____   **3.** 0.25 _____
4. 54.6 _____   **5.** 7.5 _____   **6.** 7140 _____

Directions: Divide the following numbers by 0.1 by moving the decimal point.

1. 2.8 _____   **2.** 0.1 _____   **3.** 0.65 _____
4. 0.987 _____   **5.** 15.0 _____   **6.** 8.25 _____

Directions: Divide the following numbers by 0.01 by moving the decimal point.

1. 36.0 _____   **2.** 0.16 _____   **3.** 0.48 _____
4. 9.59 _____   **5.** 0.8 _____   **6.** 0.097 _____

Directions: Divide the following numbers by 0.001 by moving the decimal point.

1. 6.2 _____   **2.** 839.0 _____   **3.** 5.0 _____
4. 0.86 _____   **5.** 13.8 _____   **6.** 0.0156 _____

Directions: Change the following decimal fractions to proper fractions.

1. 0.06 _____   **2.** 0.095 _____   **3.** 0.8 _____   **4.** 0.68 _____

5. 0.125 _____   **6.** 0.74 _____   **7.** 0.0025 _____   **8.** 0.85 _____

9. 0.5 _____

10. 0.625 _____

11. 0.25 _____

12. 0.9 _____

13. 0.004 _____

14. 0.12 _____

15. 0.055 _____

16. 0.875 _____

17. 0.64 _____

18. 0.75 _____

19. 0.16 _____

20. 0.22 _____

21. 0.005 _____

22. 0.01 _____

23. 0.044 _____

24. 0.2 _____

Directions: Change the following proper fractions to decimal fractions.

1. ⅛ _____

2. ¹¹⁄₂₀ _____

3. ⅔ _____

4. ⅜ _____

5. ¹⁶⁄₂₅ _____

6. ¼ _____

7. ¹⁸⁄₇₅ _____

8. ⅗ _____

9. $8/200$ _____   **10.** $1/3$ _____   **11.** $6/7$ _____   **12.** $1/12$ _____

13. $1/2$ _____   **14.** $9/10$ _____   **15.** $4/5$ _____   **16.** $3/20$ _____

17. $7/8$ _____   **18.** $13/52$ _____   **19.** $3/4$ _____   **20.** $17/50$ _____

21. $1/200$ _____   **22.** $11/125$ _____   **23.** $5/6$ _____   **24.** $19/20$ _____

Answers on pp. 414-415.

POSTTEST 1

Name _____

Date _____

ACCEPTABLE SCORE __**63**__

YOUR SCORE _____

Directions: Write the following numbers in words.

1. 42.68593 _____

_____

2. 634.18 _____

_____

3. 0.9 _____

4. 0.003 _____

5. 64.231 _____

_____

Directions: Circle the decimal fractions with the *greatest value*.

6. 0.15, 0.25, 0.045, 0.0048

7. 0.1, 0.01, 0.15, 0.015

8. 0.666, 0.068, 0.006, 0.66

9. 0.4, 0.08, 0.6, 0.03

10. 0.525, 5.5, 0.5252, 0.52

Directions: Perform the indicated calculations.

11. $1.342 + 0.987 + 8.062 + 44.269 =$ _____

12. $2.6 + 4.83 + 0.8 + 0.005 =$ _____

13. $63.9 + 850.6 + 3.8 + 7.743 =$ _____

14. $0.004 + 1.2 + 16.5 + 5.2 =$ _____

15. $0.6 + 0.45 + 2.9 + 4.94 =$ _____

16. $1280.49 + 630.51 + 49.98 + 93.76 =$ _____

17. $11.33 + 9.2 +$
   $88.75 + 29.16 =$ _____

18. $3.004 + 0.848 +$
   $0.9 + 1.6 =$ _____

19. $2.875 + 0.75 +$
   $0.094 + 2.385 =$ _____

20. $1981.62 + 4.876 +$
   $146.35 + 19.78 =$ _____

21. $93.712 - 4.73 =$ _____

22. $26.521 - 19.384 =$ _____

23. $1 - 0.661 =$ _____

24. $8 - 2.68 =$ _____

25. $2.46 - 1.0068 =$ _____

26. $844.6 - 521.52 =$ _____

27. $1.6 - 0.972 =$ _____

28. $36.892 - 15.942 =$ _____

29. $43.69 - 0.0823 =$ _____

30. $0.9 - 0.689 =$ _____

31. $72.8 \times 9.649 =$ _____

32. $1.58 \times 0.088 =$ _____

33. $6.25 \times 0.875 =$ _____

34. $125.929 \times 18.789 =$ _____

35. $360 \times 0.45 =$ _____

36. $0.949 \times 0.896 =$ _____

37. $26.2 \times 1.69 =$ _____

38. $1.5 \times 0.39 =$ _____

39. $9846.29 \times 93.888 =$ _____

40. $2.6 \times 8.42 =$ _____

41. $268.8 \div 16 =$ _____

42. $2984 \div 0.64 =$ _____

43. $8.89 \div 0.006 =$ _____

44. $7.52 \div 0.004 =$ _____

45. $462 \div 0.009 =$ _____

46. $12.54 \div 0.02 =$ _____

47. $56.4 \div 40 =$ _____

48. $165.9 \div 3.006 =$ _____

49. $0.7 \div 0.35 =$ _____

50. $45 \div 0.09 =$ _____

Directions: Change the following decimal fractions to proper fractions.

51. 0.09 _____   **52.** 0.625 _____   **53.** 0.16 _____   **54.** 0.5 _____

55. 0.0025 _____   **56.** 0.55 _____   **57.** 0.375 _____   **58.** 0.4 _____

59. 0.006 _____   **60.** 0.75 _____

Directions: Change the following proper fractions to decimal fractions.

61. $5/7$ _____   **62.** $11/50$ _____   **63.** $17/20$ _____   **64.** $1/100$ _____

65. $4/5$ _____   **66.** $5/16$ _____   **67.** $1/3$ _____   **68.** $1/250$ _____

69. $1/8$ _____   **70.** $3/32$ _____

Answers on p. 416.

POSTTEST 2

Name _____

Date _____

ACCEPTABLE SCORE __**63**__

YOUR SCORE _____

Directions: Write the following numbers in words.

1. 0.5 _____
_____

2. 8.2658 _____
_____

3. 4.0002 _____

4. 123.69 _____
_____

5. 2.405 _____
_____

Directions: Circle the decimal with the *greatest value.*

6. 0.3, 0.6, 0.8, 0.1   **7.** 0.25, 0.5, 0.75, 0.9

8. 0.04, 0.45, 0.8, 0.86   **9.** 0.006, 0.065, 0.65, 0.659

10. 1.202, 1.22, 1.2, 1.222

Directions: Perform the indicated calculations.

11. 1.2791 + 327.8 +
123.07 + 4.67 = _____

12. 101.98 + 4.6 +
9.005 + 14.9987 = _____

13. 6.95 + 0.8 +
0.625 + 7.68 = _____

14. 19.29 + 3.5 +
5.869 + 4.55 = _____

15. 3.75 + 186.857 +
83.3 + 6.988 = _____

16. 198.5 + 14.271 +
29.28 + 43.54 = _____

17. $823.68 + 459.75 + 723.8 + 4.076 =$ _____

18. $1.5 + 6.3 + 10.46 + 29.465 =$ _____

19. $19.29 + 16.5 + 462.833 + 9.006 =$ _____

20. $322 + 0.95 + 6.45 + 9.6 =$ _____

21. $632.838 - 19.869 =$ _____

22. $32.8 - 4.9 =$ _____

23. $1.572 - 0.985 =$ _____

24. $16.486 - 8.697 =$ _____

25. $6.4 - 3.634 =$ _____

26. $2.6 - 0.087 =$ _____

27. $91.18 - 9.39 =$ _____

28. $11.6 - 7.76 =$ _____

29. $4.819 - 3.734 =$ _____

30. $291.84 - 67.86 =$ _____

31. $14.26 \times 2.004 =$ _____

32. $57.6 \times 2.9 =$ _____

33. $149.36 \times 700 =$ _____

34. $45.5 \times 5.45 =$ _____

35. $13.39 \times 2.062 =$ _____ **36.** $56.43 \times 0.018 =$ _____ **37.** $62.41 \times 4.428 =$ _____

38. $12.8 \times 6.5 =$ _____ **39.** $800 \times 3.2 =$ _____ **40.** $27.5 \times 5.89 =$ _____

41. $32.8 \div 0.04 =$ _____ **42.** $5.9 \div 5.3 =$ _____ **43.** $0.295 \div 0.059 =$ _____

44. $537.6 \div 1120 =$ _____ **45.** $4.89 \div 1.2 =$ _____ **46.** $124 \div 0.008 =$ _____

47. $5 \div 2.5 =$ _____ **48.** $9.6 \div 0.8 =$ _____ **49.** $0.7 \div 2.3 =$ _____

50. $5.928 \div 2.4 =$ _____

Directions: Change the following decimal fractions to proper fractions.

51. 0.04 _____   **52.** 0.005 _____   **53.** 0.35 _____   **54.** 0.125 _____

55. 0.9 _____   **56.** 0.85 _____   **57.** 0.003 _____   **58.** 0.8 _____

59. 0.22 _____   **60.** 0.6 _____

Directions: Change the following proper fractions to decimal fractions.

61. $^{11}/_{20}$ _____   **62.** $^1/_6$ _____   **63.** $^1/_{400}$ _____   **64.** $^7/_8$ _____

65. $^2/_5$ _____   **66.** $^3/_4$ _____   **67.** $^1/_{150}$ _____   **68.** $^1/_2$ _____

69. $^1/_{125}$ _____   **70.** $^3/_{16}$ _____

Answers on pp. 416-417.

PRETEST

Name _____

Date _____

ACCEPTABLE SCORE __36__

YOUR SCORE _____

Directions: Change the following fractions to percents.

1. 1/60 _____

2. 5/7 _____

3. 1/8 _____

4. 3/10 _____

5. 4/3 _____

Directions: Change the following decimals to percents.

6. 0.006 _____

7. 0.35 _____

8. 0.427 _____

9. 3.821 _____

10. 0.7 _____

Directions: Change the following percents to proper fractions.

11. 0.5% _____

12. 75% _____

13. 9½% _____

14. 24.8% _____

15. ⅜% _____

Directions: Change the following percents to decimals.

16. 1⅙% _____

17. 7.5% _____

18. 13³⁄₁₀% _____

19. ⅚% _____

20. 63% _____

Directions: What percent of

21. 1.60 is 6 _____

22. ¾ is ⅛ _____

23. 100 is 65 _____

24. 500 is 1 _____

25. 4.5 is 1.5 _____

26. 37.8 is 4.6 _____

27. $1\frac{4}{9}$ is $\frac{5}{8}$ _____

28. 1000 is 100 _____

29. $3\frac{1}{2}$ is $\frac{1}{4}$ _____

30. 9.7 is $\frac{1}{6}$ _____

Directions: What is

31. 3% of 60 _____

32. $\frac{1}{4}$% of 60 _____

33. 4.5% of 57 _____

34. $2\frac{1}{8}$% of 32 _____

35. 4% of 77 _____

36. 9.3% of 46 _____

37. $\frac{3}{7}$% of 14 _____

38. 22% of 88 _____

39. 7.6% of 156 _____

40. 5% of 300 _____

Answers on p. 417.

Chapter 3 | *Percents*

Learning Objectives

On completion of the materials provided in this chapter, you will be able to perform computations accurately by mastering the following mathematical concepts:

1 | Changing a fraction or decimal to a percent
2 | Changing a percent to a fraction or decimal
3 | Changing a percent containing a fraction to a decimal
4 | Finding what percent one number is of another
5 | Finding the given percent of a number

A **percent** is a third way of showing a fractional relationship. Fractions, decimals, and percents can all be converted from one form to the others. Conversions of fractions and decimals are discussed in Chapter 2. A percent indicates a value equal to the number of hundredths. Therefore, when a percent is written as a fraction, the denominator is *always* 100. The number beside the % sign becomes the numerator.

Changing a Fraction to a Percent

1. Multiply by 100.
2. Add the percent sign (%).

Example: ²/₅

$$\frac{2}{\overset{1}{\cancel{5}}} \times \frac{\overset{20}{100}}{1} =$$

$$\frac{2 \times 20}{1 \times 1} = 40$$

40%

Example: ³/₁₀

$$\frac{3}{\underset{1}{\cancel{10}}} \times \frac{\overset{10}{100}}{1} =$$

$$\frac{3 \times 10}{1 \times 1} = 30$$

30%

Example: 1¼

$$\frac{5}{\overset{\scriptstyle 25}{\cancel{4}}_{\,1}} \times \frac{100}{1} =$$

$$\frac{5 \times 25}{1 \times 1} = 125$$

125%

Example: ⅓

$$\frac{1}{3} \times \frac{100}{1} =$$

$$\frac{1 \times 100}{3 \times 1} = \frac{100}{3} = 33\frac{1}{3}$$

33⅓%

Changing a Decimal to a Percent

1. Multiply by 100 (by moving the decimal point two places to the right).
2. Add the percent sign (%).

Example: 0.421

0.421 × 100 = 42.1

42.1%

Example: 0.2

0.2 × 100 = 20

20%

Example: 0.98

0.98 × 100 = 98

98%

Example: 1.1212

1.1212 × 100 = 112.12

112.12%

Changing a Percent to a Fraction

1. Drop the % sign.
2. Write the remaining number as the fraction's numerator.
3. Write 100 as the denominator. (The denominator will *always* be 100.)
4. Reduce to lowest terms.

Example: 45%

$$\frac{45}{100} = \frac{9}{20} \text{ (reduced to lowest terms)}$$

Example: 3½%

$$\frac{3\frac{1}{2}}{100} = \frac{7/2}{100}$$

$$\frac{7}{2} \div \frac{100}{1} =$$

$$\frac{7}{2} \times \frac{1}{100} = \frac{7}{200}$$

Example: 0.3%

$$\frac{0.3}{100} =$$

$$\frac{\frac{3}{10}}{100}$$

$$\frac{3}{10} \div \frac{100}{1} =$$

$$\frac{3}{10} \times \frac{1}{100} = \frac{3}{1000}$$

Changing a Percent to a Decimal

1. Drop the % sign.
2. Divide the remaining number by 100 (by moving the decimal point two places to the left).
3. Express the quotient as a decimal. Place a zero before the decimal if there are no whole numbers.

Example: 32%

0.32

Example: 125%

1.25

Changing a Percent Containing a Fraction to a Decimal

1. Drop the % sign.
2. Change the mixed number to an improper fraction.
3. Divide by 100. Remember, the denominator of all whole numbers is one.
4. Reduce to lowest terms.
5. Divide the numerator by the denominator, expressing the quotient as a decimal.

Example: $12\frac{1}{2}\%$

$$\frac{25}{2} \div \frac{100}{1} =$$

$$\overset{1}{\underset{4}{\cancel{\frac{25}{2}}}} \times \frac{1}{100} = \frac{1}{8}$$

$$\begin{array}{r} 0.125 \\ 8\overline{)1.000} \\ \underline{8} \\ 20 \\ \underline{16} \\ 40 \\ \underline{40} \end{array}$$

$$12\frac{1}{2}\% = 0.125$$

Example: $3\frac{3}{4}\%$

$$\frac{15}{4} \div \frac{100}{1} =$$

$$\overset{3}{\underset{20}{\cancel{\frac{15}{4}}}} \times \frac{1}{100} = \frac{3}{80}$$

$$\begin{array}{r} 0.0375 \\ 80\overline{)3.0000} \\ \underline{2\,40} \\ 600 \\ \underline{560} \\ 400 \\ \underline{400} \end{array}$$

$$3\frac{3}{4}\% = 0.0375$$

Finding What Percent One Number Is of Another

1. Write the number following the word *of* as the denominator of a fraction.
2. Write the other number as the numerator of the fraction.
3. Divide the numerator by the denominator, extending the decimal fraction four places to the right of the decimal point.
4. Multiply by 100.
5. Add the % sign.

Example: What percent of 24 is 9?

$$\frac{9}{24} = \frac{3}{8}$$

$$\begin{array}{r} 0.375 \\ 8\overline{)3.000} \\ \underline{2\,4} \\ 60 \\ \underline{56} \\ 40 \\ \underline{40} \end{array}$$

$$0.375 \times 100 = 37.5$$

$$37.5 + \% \text{ sign} = 37.5\%$$

Example: What percent of 5.4 is 1.2?

$$\frac{1.2}{5.4} = 5.4\,\overset{\displaystyle 0.2222}{\overline{)1.2\,0000}}$$

$$\begin{array}{r} 1\,0\,8 \\ 1\,20 \\ \underline{1\,08} \\ 120 \\ \underline{108} \\ 120 \\ \underline{108} \end{array}$$

$$0.2222 \times 100 = 22.22$$

$$22.22 + \% \text{ sign} = 22.22\%$$

Example: What percent of 2 is ¼?

$$¼/2$$

$$\frac{1}{4} \div 2 =$$

$$\frac{1}{4} \div \frac{2}{1} =$$

$$\frac{1}{4} \times \frac{1}{2} = \frac{1}{8}$$

$$\underset{2}{\overset{25}{\frac{1}{\cancel{8}}}} \times \frac{\cancel{100}}{1} = \frac{25}{2} = 12.5$$

$$12.5 + \% \text{ sign} = 12.5\%$$

Example: What percent of 8.7 is 3½?

$$\frac{3½}{8.7} = \frac{3.5}{8.7}$$

$$\begin{array}{r} 0.402 \\ 8.7\,\overline{)3.5\,000} \\ \underline{3\ 4\ 8} \\ 20 \\ \underline{00} \\ 200 \\ \underline{174} \end{array}$$

$$0.402 \times 100 = 40.2$$

$$40.2 + \% \text{ sign} = 40.2\%$$

Finding the Given Percent of a Number

1. Write the percent as a decimal number.
2. Multiply by the other number.

Example: What is 40% of 180?

$$\frac{40}{100} = \begin{array}{r} 0.4 \\ 100\,\overline{)40.0} \\ \underline{40\ 0} \end{array}$$

$$\begin{array}{r} 180 \\ \times\ 0.4 \\ \hline 72.0 \end{array}$$

$$40\% \text{ of } 180 = 72$$

Example: What is ³⁄₁₀% of 52?

$$\frac{\frac{3}{10}}{100} = \frac{3}{10} \div \frac{100}{1} =$$

$$\frac{3}{10} \times \frac{1}{100} = \frac{3}{1000}$$

$$\frac{3}{1000} = 0.003$$

$$\begin{array}{r} 0.003 \\ \times\ \ \ \ 52 \\ \hline 0\ 006 \\ 00\ 15 \\ \hline 00.156 \end{array}$$

$$³⁄₁₀\% \text{ of } 52 = 0.156$$

Study the introductory material on percents. The processes for the calculation of percent problems are listed in steps. Memorize the steps for each calculation before beginning the work sheet. Complete the following work sheet, which provides for extensive practice in the manipulation of percents. Check your answers. If you have any difficulty, go back and review the steps for that type of calculation. When you feel ready to evaluate your learning, take the first posttest. Check your answers. An acceptable score as indicated on the posttest signifies that you are ready for the next chapter. An unacceptable score signifies a need for further study before taking the second posttest.

WORK SHEET

Directions: Change each of the following proper fractions to a percent.

1. $^3/_4$ _____

2. $^1/_2$ _____

3. $^3/_8$ _____

4. $^4/_5$ _____

5. $^8/_{25}$ _____

6. $^3/_{1000}$ _____

7. $^7/_{200}$ _____

8. $^2/_3$ _____

9. $^5/_{12}$ _____

10. $^7/_{30}$ _____

11. $^9/_{400}$ _____

12. $^{27}/_{32}$ _____

13. $^3/_{20}$ _____

14. $^{12}/_{17}$ _____

15. $^5/_{22}$ _____

16. $^9/_{150}$ _____

17. $^{11}/_{16}$ _____

18. $^3/_{14}$ _____

19. $^8/_{21}$ _____

20. $^5/_6$ _____

21. $^{75}/_{10,000}$ _____   **22.** $^2/_{15}$ _____   **23.** $^4/_9$ _____   **24.** $^7/_8$ _____

Directions: Change each of the following decimals to a percent.

1. 0.402 _____   **2.** 0.0367 _____   **3.** 4.31 _____   **4.** 0.163 _____

5. 6.22 _____   **6.** 0.98 _____   **7.** 0.3276 _____   **8.** 0.3 _____

9. 1.3397 _____   **10.** 0.145 _____   **11.** 0.2824 _____   **12.** 0.67 _____

13. 0.7 _____   **14.** 0.62240 _____   **15.** 0.42 _____   **16.** 0.6337 _____

17. 6.2 _____   **18.** 0.159 _____   **19.** 2.9014 _____   **20.** 0.673 _____

21. 0.405 _____   **22.** 0.3712 _____   **23.** 7.234 _____   **24.** 2.2 _____

Directions: Change each of the following percents to a mixed number or a proper fraction.

1. 3.5% _____   **2.** ¾% _____   **3.** 40.6% _____   **4.** 0.125% _____

5. 10% _____   **6.** ⅔% _____   **7.** ⅙% _____   **8.** 0.35% _____

9. 45% _____   **10.** 20.2% _____   **11.** ⅝% _____   **12.** 4½% _____

13. 12% _____   **14.** 0.25% _____   **15.** 2⅜% _____   **16.** 58% _____

17. 8% _____   **18.** 6¼% _____   **19.** 2.1% _____   **20.** 0.15% _____

21. 0.5% _____   **22.** 32.4% _____   **23.** 66⅔% _____   **24.** 1.8% _____

Directions: Change each of the following percents to a decimal.

1. 37.5% _____   **2.** 3% _____   **3.** 1⁷⁄₁₀% _____   **4.** 6¾% _____

5. 0.42% _____   **6.** ¼% _____   **7.** 40% _____   **8.** 1.35% _____

9. 2½% _____   **10.** ⅜% _____   **11.** 5% _____   **12.** 80% _____

13. 0.23% _____   **14.** 72.6% _____   **15.** 16% _____   **16.** 30.64% _____

17. 2.93% _____   **18.** ⁵⁄₁₆% _____   **19.** 87.5% _____   **20.** ½% _____

21. 5¾% _____   **22.** 0.98% _____   **23.** 6⁹⁄₁₀% _____   **24.** ⁷⁄₁₂% _____

Directions: What percent of

1. 40 is 22 _____   **2.** 72 is 12 _____   **3.** 80 is 6.3 _____   **4.** 60 is 30 _____

5. 150 is 70 _____   **6.** 500 is 420 _____   **7.** 22 is 5.4 _____   **8.** 50 is 100 _____

9. 144 is 8.2 _____   **10.** 200 is 4 _____   **11.** 500 is 60 _____   **12.** 20 is 1 _____

13. 24 is 3.6 _____   **14.** 325 is 75 _____   **15.** 163 is 121 _____   **16.** 275 is 55 _____

17. 1000 is 100 _____**18.** 750 is 35.6 _____   **19.** 76 is 8.2 _____   **20.** 800 is 360 _____

21. 25 is ¼ _____   **22.** 250 is 5.2 _____   **23.** 10 is ⅜ _____   **24.** 35 is 7 _____

Directions: What is

1. 25% of 478 _____   **2.** 10% of 34 _____   **3.** 2.8% of 510 _____

4. 75% of 845 _____   **5.** ½% of 28 _____   **6.** 0.25% of 650 _____

7. 85% of 36.2 _____   **8.** 33⅓% of 3000 _____   **9.** 3.5% of 57 _____

10. 1% of 400 _____   **11.** 12% of 96 _____   **12.** ⅕% of 65 _____

13. 2¼% of 26 _____   **14.** ⅜% of 32 _____   **15.** 44.8% of 294 _____

16. 62% of 871 _____

17. ¼% of 68 _____

18. 41% of 27 _____

19. 72% of 234 _____

20. ⅓% of 20 _____

21. 8.4% of 128 _____

22. 150% of 70 _____

23. ³⁄₁₆% of 54 _____

24. 6% of 84.78 _____

Answers on pp. 417-418.

POSTTEST 1

Name _____

Date _____

ACCEPTABLE SCORE __**36**__

YOUR SCORE _____

Directions: Change the following fractions to percents.

1. $4/9$ _____

2. $7/8$ _____

3. $11/20$ _____

4. $8/3$ _____

5. $3/1000$ _____

Directions: Change the following decimals to percents.

6. 0.256 _____

7. 33.3 _____

8. 0.004 _____

9. 1.678 _____

10. 0.9 _____

Directions: Change the following percents to proper fractions.

11. 60% _____

12. 85% _____

13. 0.3% _____

14. ¼% _____

15. 3½% _____

Directions: Change the following percents to decimals.

16. 86.3% _____

17. 4⅝% _____

18. 29.45% _____

19. ⅞% _____

20. 0.36% _____

Directions: What percent of

21. 70 is 7 _____

22. 24 is 1.2 _____

23. 300 is 1 _____

24. 66⅔ is 8 _____

25. 3.5 is 1.5 _____

26. 2.5 is 0.5 _____

27. ¾ is ⅜ _____

28. 160 is 12 _____

29. 65 is 5.5 _____

30. 250 is 20 _____

Directions: What is

31. 65% of 800 _____

32. 90% of 40 _____

33. ⅛% of 72 _____

34. 8.5% of 2000 _____

35. 2¼% of 75 _____

36. 4½% of 940 _____

37. 65% of 450 _____

38. ¼% of 60 _____

39. 4.3% of 56 _____

40. 0.52% of 88 _____

Answers on p. 418.

POSTTEST 2

Name _____

Date _____

ACCEPTABLE SCORE __**36**__

YOUR SCORE _____

Directions: Change the following fractions to percents.

1. $\frac{1}{8}$ _____

2. $\frac{2}{5}$ _____

3. $\frac{1}{6}$ _____

4. $\frac{19}{20}$ _____

5. $\frac{11}{9}$ _____

Directions: Change the following decimals to percents.

6. 0.065 _____

7. 0.005 _____

8. 4.346 _____

9. 0.57 _____

10. 0.2 _____

Directions: Change the following percents to proper fractions.

11. 0.3% _____

12. 16½% _____

13. ⅗% _____

14. 1.75% _____

15. 0.25% _____

Directions: Change the following percents to decimals.

16. 0.4% _____

17. 3¾% _____

18. 7% _____

19. 5.55% _____

20. 65% _____

Directions: What percent of

21. 5.4 is 1.2 _____

22. ¼ is ⅛ _____

23. 250 is 6 _____

24. 40 is 32 _____

25. 160 is 12 _____

26. 500 is 50 _____

27. 5¾ is 2⅜ _____

28. 120 is 15 _____

29. 8.7 is 3½ _____

30. ⁹⁄₁₆ is ⁵⁄₇ _____

Directions: What is

31. 35% of 650 _____

32. ¼% of 116 _____

33. 4½% of 940 _____

34. 11% of 88 _____

35. 16% of 90 _____

36. 7.5% of 261 _____

37. 45% of 24.27 _____

38. ⅞% of 64 _____

39. ³⁄₁₀% of 52 _____

40. 82.4% of 118 _____

Answers on p. 419.

PRETEST

Name _____

Date _____

ACCEPTABLE SCORE __27__

YOUR SCORE _____

Directions: Convert to equivalents.

	Ratio	Fraction	Decimal	Percent
1.	17 : 51			
2.			0.715	
3.		8/20		
4.				12½%
5.	21 : 420			
6.		5/32		
7.			0.286	
8.				71³⁄₇%
9.				16¼%
10.			0.462	

Answers on p. 419.

Chapter 4 | *Ratios*

Learning Objectives

On the completion of the materials provided in this chapter, you will be able to perform computations by mastering the following mathematical concepts:

1 | Changing a proper fraction, decimal fraction, and percent to a ratio reduced to lowest terms

2 | Changing a ratio to a proper fraction, a decimal fraction, and a percent

---

A **ratio** is another way of indicating a relationship between two numbers. In other words, it is another way to express a fraction. A ratio indicates *division*.

Example 1: ¾ written as a ratio is 3 : 4
In reading a ratio the colon is read as "is to." The example would then be read as "three is to four."

Example 2: 7 written as a ratio is 7 : 1
To express any whole number as a ratio, the number following the colon is *always* 1. The example would be read as "seven is to one."

Changing a Proper Fraction to a Ratio Reduced to Lowest Terms

1. Reduce to lowest terms.
2. Write the numerator of the fraction as the first number of the ratio.
3. Place a colon after the first number.
4. Write the denominator of the fraction as the second number of the ratio.

Example 1: ⁴⁄₁₂
⁴⁄₁₂ reduced to lowest terms equals ⅓
⅓ written as a ratio would be 1 : 3

Example 2: ¹⁄₁₀₀₀/¹⁄₁₀

$$\frac{1}{1000} \div \frac{1}{10} =$$

$$\frac{1}{\underset{100}{1000}} \times \frac{\cancel{10}}{1} = \frac{1}{100}$$

¹⁄₁₀₀₀/¹⁄₁₀ reduced to lowest terms equals ¹⁄₁₀₀
¹⁄₁₀₀ written as a ratio would be 1 : 100

Changing a Decimal Fraction to a Ratio Reduced to Lowest Terms

1. Express the decimal fraction as a proper fraction reduced to lowest terms.
2. Write the numerator of the fraction as the first number of the ratio.
3. Place a colon after the first number.
4. Write the denominator of the fraction as the second number of the ratio.

Example 1:   0.85

$$\frac{85}{100} = \frac{17}{20} \text{ (reduced to lowest terms)}$$

$\frac{17}{20}$ written as a ratio would be   17 : 20

Example 2:   0.125

$$\frac{125}{1000} = \frac{1}{8} \text{ (reduced to lowest terms)}$$

$\frac{1}{8}$ written as a ratio would be   1 : 8

Changing a Percent to a Ratio Reduced to Lowest Terms

1. Express the percent as a proper fraction reduced to lowest terms.
2. Write the numerator of the fraction as the first number of the ratio.
3. Place a colon after the first number.
4. Write the denominator of the fraction as the second number of the ratio.

Example 1:   30%

$$\frac{30}{100} = \frac{3}{10} \text{ (reduced to lowest terms)}$$

$\frac{3}{10}$ written as a ratio would be   3 : 10

Example 2:   ½%

$$\frac{\frac{1}{2}}{100} =$$

$$\frac{1}{2} \div \frac{100}{1} =$$

$$\frac{1}{2} \times \frac{1}{100} = \frac{1}{200}$$

$\frac{1}{200}$ written as a ratio would be   1 : 200

Example 3: $3\frac{9}{10}\%$

$$\frac{3\frac{9}{10}}{100} =$$

$$\frac{39}{10} \div \frac{100}{1} =$$

$$\frac{39}{10} \times \frac{1}{100} = \frac{39}{1000}$$

$\frac{39}{1000}$ written as a ratio would be $39 : 1000$

Changing a Ratio to a Proper Fraction Reduced to Lowest Terms

1. Write the first number of the ratio as a numerator.
2. Write the second number of the ratio as the denominator.
3. Reduce to lowest terms.

Example 1: $9 : 15$

$\frac{9}{15} = \frac{3}{5}$ (reduced to lowest terms)

Example 2: $11 : 22$

$\frac{11}{22} = \frac{1}{2}$ (reduced to lowest terms)

Changing a Ratio to a Decimal Fraction

1. Divide the first number of the ratio by the second number of the ratio, using long division.

Example 1: $4 : 5$

$$\begin{array}{r} 0.8 \\ 5)\overline{4.0} \\ \underline{4\ 0} \end{array}$$

$4 : 5$ written as a decimal is 0.8

Example 2: $3\frac{1}{2} : 2\frac{1}{4}$

$3.5 : 2.25$

$$\begin{array}{r} 1.555 \\ 2.25\wedge)\overline{3.50\wedge\ 000} \\ \underline{2\ 25} \\ 1\ 25\ \ 0 \\ \underline{1\ 12\ \ 5} \\ 12\ \ 50 \\ \underline{11\ \ 25} \\ 1\ \ 250 \\ 1\ \ 125 \end{array}$$

$3\frac{1}{2} : 2\frac{1}{4}$ written as a decimal is 1.555

Changing a Ratio to a Percent

1. Express the ratio as a proper fraction or a decimal fraction, whichever you prefer to work with.
2. Multiply by 100.
3. Add the percent sign (%).

Example 1: $3 : 5$

Changing to a proper fraction:

$$\frac{3}{5} \times \frac{\overset{20}{\cancel{100}}}{1} = \frac{60}{1}$$

$$60 + \% = 60\%$$

Changing to a decimal fraction:

$$\begin{array}{r} 0.6 \\ 5\overline{)3.0} \\ 3\,0 \\ \hline \end{array}$$

$$0.6 \times 100 = 60$$

$$60 + \% = 60\%$$

Example 2: $60 : 180$

Changing to a proper fraction:

$$\frac{60}{180} = \frac{1}{3}$$

$$\frac{1}{3} \times \frac{100}{1} = \frac{100}{3} = 33\tfrac{1}{3}$$

$$33\tfrac{1}{3} + \% = 33\tfrac{1}{3}\%$$

Changing to a decimal fraction:

$$\begin{array}{r} 0.333 \\ 180\overline{)60.000} \\ 54\,0 \\ \hline 6\,00 \\ 5\,40 \\ \hline 600 \\ 540 \\ \hline 600 \\ 540 \\ \hline 60 \end{array}$$

$$0.333 \times 100 = 33.3$$

$$33.3 + \% = 33.3\%$$

   Study the introductory material on ratios. The processes for the calculation of ratio problems are listed in steps. Memorize the steps for each calculation before beginning the work sheet. Review previous chapters on fractions, decimals, and percents as necessary. Complete the following work sheet that provides for extensive practice in the manipulation of ratios. Check your answers. If you have difficulties, go back and review the steps for that type of calculation. When you feel ready to evaluate your learning, take the first posttest. Check your answers. An acceptable score as indicated on the posttest signifies that you are ready for the next chapter. An unacceptable score signifies a need for further study before taking the second posttest.

WORK SHEET

Directions: Change the following fractions to ratios reduced to lowest terms.

1. $\frac{3}{4}$ _____

2. $\frac{1}{3}$ _____

3. $\frac{9}{12}$ _____

4. $\frac{4}{6}$ _____

5. $\frac{3}{10}$ _____

6. $\frac{11}{22}$ _____

7. $\frac{6}{9}$ _____

8. $\frac{56}{100}$ _____

9. $\frac{6}{24}$ _____

10. $\frac{20}{50}$ _____

11. $\frac{310}{1000}$ _____

12. $\frac{17}{34}$ _____

13. $\frac{10}{16}$ _____

14. $\frac{3}{8} / \frac{1}{4}$ _____

15. $2\frac{1}{2} / 1\frac{3}{4}$ _____

16. $\frac{5}{6}/3\frac{1}{3}$ _____

17. $4\frac{3}{16}/\frac{7}{8}$ _____

18. $1\frac{3}{5}/2\frac{7}{10}$ _____

19. $\frac{1}{10}/\frac{1}{100}$ _____

20. $\frac{14}{30}/2$ _____

21. $\frac{3}{67}$ _____

22. $1\frac{24}{38}/2\frac{4}{10}$ _____

23. $3\frac{1}{3}/3\frac{1}{3}$ _____

24. $\frac{5}{8}/2\frac{4}{5}$ _____

Directions: Change the following decimal fractions to ratios reduced to lowest terms.

1. 0.896 _____

2. 0.96 _____

3. 0.6738 _____

4. 0.06 _____

5. 0.756 _____

6. 0.6 _____

7. 0.4032 _____

8. 0.821 _____

9. 0.74 _____

10. 0.166 _____

11. 0.4376 _____

12. 0.26 _____

13. 0.492 _____

14. 0.33 _____

15. 0.820 _____

16. 0.95 _____

17. 0.2 _____

18. 0.235 _____

19. 0.67 _____

20. 0.5355 _____

21. 0.846 _____

22. 0.172 _____

23. 0.9 _____

24. 0.4752 _____

Directions: Change the following percents to ratios reduced to lowest terms.

1. 10% _____

2. 2½% _____

3. 33⅓% _____

4. ⅜% _____

5. 25% _____

6. 2⁷⁄₁₀% _____

7. 44% _____

8. 15.7% _____

9. 4⁴⁄₅% _____

10. 55.62% _____

11. 7¾% _____

12. 35% _____

13. 2.5% _____

14. 0.44% _____

15. 0.05% _____

16. 7.8% _____

17. 1% _____

18. 6¾% _____

19. 9⅝% _____

20. 0.14% _____

21. ⅗% _____

22. 12⅑% _____

23. 3³/₇% _____

24. 8.2% _____

Directions: Change the following ratios to fractions reduced to lowest terms.

1. 1 : 2 _____

2. 3 : 4 _____

3. 4 : 64 _____

4. 8 : 10 _____

5. 4 : 800 _____

6. 3 : 150 _____

7. 9 : 300 _____

8. ⅜ : ¼ _____

9. 9 : 27 _____

10. ⁴/₇ : ⅖ _____

11. ⁸/₁₂ : ⅔ _____

12. 2½ : 7½ _____

13. ⅘ : ¼ _____

14. ¹/₁₀ : ⁴/₂₀ _____

15. 12 : 60 _____

16. $^4/_{75}$: $^3/_{10}$ _____

17. $1^5/_{21}$: $2^3/_7$ _____

18. $0.25 : 0.75$ _____

19. $0.68 : 0.44$ _____

20. $1.85 : 3.35$ _____

21. $0.4 : 0.126$ _____

22. $0.7 : 42.9$ _____

23. $1.64 : 2.54$ _____

24. $1.21 : 8.21$ _____

Directions: Change the following ratios to decimal numbers.

1. $7 : 14$ _____

2. $5 : 20$ _____

3. $3 : 8$ _____

4. $20 : 32$ _____

5. $11 : 33$ _____

6. $^5/_8$: $^1/_{10}$ _____

7. $^1/_{1000}$: $^1/_{500}$ _____

8. $^3/_4$: $^1/_2$ _____

9. $^1/_{75}$: $^3/_{15}$ _____

10. $^3/_{1000} : ^3/_{100}$ _____

11. $2 : 5$ _____

12. $0.105 : 0.232$ _____

13. $6^1/_2 : 12^3/_4$ _____

14. $^1/_2 : ^5/_9$ _____

15. $^1/_6 : ^5/_8$ _____

16. $2^5/_{16} : 4^5/_{12}$ _____

17. $7 : 259$ _____

18. $0.42 : 0.88$ _____

19. $0.91 : 2.34$ _____

20. $62.4 : 0.01$ _____

21. $3.5 : 1.2$ _____

22. $4.8 : 0.4$ _____

23. $7 : 9$ _____

24. $1^2/_5 : ^{12}/_{30}$ _____

Directions: Change the following ratios to percents.

1. $2 : 4$ _____

2. $7 : 231$ _____

3. $25 : 250$ _____

4. 30 : 150 _____

5. ⁶⁄₇ : ²⁄₃ _____

6. ¾ : 1¹⁄₂₀ _____

7. 1¼ : 3⅜ _____

8. 0.35 : 0.2 _____

9. 1 : 1000 _____

10. 0.15 : 0.6 _____

11. 0.85 : 1.50 _____

12. 5½ : 2⅔ _____

13. ⁵⁄₁₆ : ³⁄₅ _____

14. ³⁄₂₅ : ⁴⁄₇₅ _____

15. 1 : 500 _____

16. 1⁸⁄₁₂ : 2³⁄₆ _____

17. 19 : 20 _____

18. ⁴⁄₁₁ : 1½ _____

19. 2.5 : 4.5 _____

20. 12 : 38 _____

21. 32 : 160 _____

22. 4 : ³⁄₁₆ _____

23. 5.2 : 2.3 _____

24. 13 : 23 _____

Answers on pp. 419-420.

POSTTEST 1

Name _____

Date _____

ACCEPTABLE SCORE __27__

YOUR SCORE _____

Directions: Convert to equivalents.

	Ratio	Fraction	Decimal	Percent
1.	42 : 48			
2.			0.004	
3.		$^{13}/_{20}$		
4.				2¼%
5.			0.35	
6.		$^{6}/_{25}$		
7.	⅜ : ⅝			
8.				0.3%
9.			0.205	
10.		$^{4}/_{11}$		

Answers on p. 420.

POSTTEST 2

Name _____

Date _____

ACCEPTABLE SCORE __**27**__

YOUR SCORE _____

Directions: Convert to equivalents.

	Ratio	Fraction	Decimal	Percent
1.	7 : 10			
2.		⁵⁄₁₆		
3.			0.075	
4.				6%
5.				³⁄₈%
6.		¹⁄₁₅₀		
7.			0.007	
8.	6 : 21			
9.			0.322	
10.				18.2%

Answers on p. 420.

PRETEST

Name _____

Date _____

ACCEPTABLE SCORE ___**18**___

YOUR SCORE _____

Directions: Find the value of x. Show your work.

1. $25 : 75 :: x : 300$ _____

2. $450 : 15 :: 225 : x$ _____

3. $x : \frac{1}{4}\% :: 8 : 12$ _____

4. $12 : 3 :: x : 0.8$ _____

5. $0.6 : 2.4 :: 32 : x$ _____

6. $150 : x :: 75 : 2$ _____

7. $\frac{1}{8} : \frac{2}{3} :: 75 : x$ _____

8. $\frac{1}{200} : 8 :: x : 800$ _____

9. $x : \frac{1}{2} :: \frac{3}{4} : \frac{7}{8}$ _____

10. $16 : x :: 24 : 12$ _____

11. $\frac{2}{3} : \frac{1}{5} :: x : 24$ _____

12. $x : 9 :: \frac{2}{3} : 36$ _____

13. $\frac{1}{7} : x :: \frac{1}{2} : 49$ _____

14. $0.8 : 4 :: 9.6 : x$ _____

15. $\frac{4}{5} : x :: \frac{2}{3} : \frac{1}{4}$ _____

16. $40 : 80 :: x : 160$ _____   **17.** $2.5 : x :: 4 : 16$ _____   **18.** $8 : 72 :: 14 : x$ _____

19. $x : \frac{1}{15} :: 50 : 500$ _____   **20.** $5 : 100 :: x : 325$ _____

Answers on p. 420.

Chapter 5 | *Proportions*

Learning Objectives

On completion of the materials provided in this chapter, you will be able to perform computations accurately by mastering the following mathematical concepts:

1   Solving simple proportion problems

2   Solving proportion problems involving fractions, decimals, and percents

---

A proportion consists of two ratios of equal value. The ratios are connected by a double colon (::) which symbolizes the word *as*.

$$2 : 3 :: 4 : 6$$

Read the above proportion : "Two is to three as four is to six."

The first and fourth terms of the proportion are the **extremes.** The second and third terms are the **means.**

$$2 : 3 :: 4 : 6$$

2 and 6 are the extremes
3 and 4 are the means

In a proportion the product of the means equals the product of the extremes because the ratios are of equal value. This principle may be used to verify your answer in a proportion problem.

$$3 \times 4 = 12, \text{means}$$
$$2 \times 6 = \ 12, \text{extremes}$$

If three terms in the proportions are known and one term is unknown, an *x* is inserted in the space for the unknown term.

$$2 : 3 :: 4 : x$$

SOLVING A SIMPLE PROPORTION PROBLEM

1. Multiply the means.
2. Multiply the extremes.
3. Place the product including the *x* on the *left* and the product of the known terms on the *right*.
4. Divide the product of the known terms by the number next to *x*. The quotient will be the value of *x*.

Proportion Problem Involving Whole Numbers

Example: $2 : 3 :: 4 : x$

$$2x = 3 \times 4$$

$$2x = 12$$

$$x = 12 \div 2$$

$$x = \frac{12}{2}$$

$$x = 6$$

Proportion Problem Involving Fractions

Example: $\dfrac{1}{150} : \dfrac{1}{100} :: x : 60$

$$\frac{1}{100x} = \frac{1}{150} \times 60$$

$$\frac{1}{100x} = \frac{2}{5}$$

$$x = \frac{2}{5} \div \frac{1}{100}$$

$$x = \frac{2}{\cancel{5}} \times \frac{\overset{20}{\cancel{100}}}{1}$$
$$\phantom{x = \frac{2}{5}} \underset{1}{}$$

$$x = 40$$

Proportion Problem Involving Decimals

Example: $0.4 : 0.8 :: 0.25 : x$

$$0.4x = 0.8 \times 0.25$$

$$0.4x = 0.2$$

$$x = 0.2 \div 0.4$$

$$x = 0.5$$

Proportion Problem Involving Fractions and Percents

Example: $x : \frac{1}{4}\% :: 9\frac{3}{5} : \frac{1}{200}$

Convert $\frac{1}{4}\%$ to a proper fraction and $9\frac{3}{5}$ to an improper fraction. Then rewrite the proportion using these fractions.

$$x : \frac{1}{400} :: \frac{48}{5} : \frac{1}{200}$$

$$\frac{1}{200x} = \frac{1}{400} \times \frac{48}{5}$$

$$\frac{1}{200x} = \frac{1}{\underset{25}{\cancel{400}}} \times \frac{\overset{3}{\cancel{48}}}{5}$$

$$\frac{1}{200x} = \frac{3}{125}$$

$$x = \frac{3}{125} \div \frac{1}{200}$$

$$x = \frac{3}{\underset{5}{\cancel{125}}} \times \frac{\overset{8}{\cancel{200}}}{1}$$

$$x = \frac{24}{5}$$

$$x = 4\frac{4}{5}$$

Proportion Problem Involving Decimals and Percents

Example: $0.3\% : 1.8 :: x : 14.4$

Convert 0.3% to a decimal

$$0.003 : 1.8 = x : 14.4$$

$$1.8x = 0.003 \times 14.4$$

$$1.8x = 0.0432$$

$$x = 0.0432 \div 1.8$$

$$x = 0.024$$

Proportion Problem Involving Numerous Zeros

Example: $250{,}000 : x :: 500{,}000 : 4$

$$500{,}000x = 250{,}000 \times 4$$

$$500{,}000x = 1{,}000{,}000$$

$$x = 1{,}000{,}000 \div 500{,}000$$

$$x = \frac{1{,}000{,}000}{500{,}000}$$

$$x = 2$$

Most problems concerning drug dosage can be solved by a proportion problem, whether it involves fractions, decimals, or percents. If a proportion problem contains any combination of fractions, decimals, or percents, all forms within the problem must be converted to either fractions or decimals.

Study the introductory material on proportions. The process for the calculation of proportion problems is listed in steps. Memorize the steps before beginning the work sheet. Complete the following work sheet, which provides for extensive practice in the manipulation of proportions. Check your answers. If you have difficulties, go back and review the necessary steps. When you feel ready to evaluate your learning, take the first posttest. Check your answers. An acceptable score as indicated on the posttest signifies that you are ready for the next chapter. An unacceptable score signifies a need for further study before taking the second posttest.

WORK SHEET

Directions: Find the value of x. Show your work.

1. $20 : 400 :: x : 1680$ _____

2. $100 : x :: 64 : 384$ _____

3. $0.9 : 2.4 :: x : 75$ _____

4. $5/6 : x :: 5/9 : 4/5$ _____

5. $3 : 90 :: 1\frac{3}{4} : x$ _____

6. $2 : 3 :: 18 : x$ _____

7. $1/300 : 4 :: 6 : x$ _____

8. $75 : x :: 100 : 2$ _____

9. $1/6 : 1 :: 1/8 : x$ _____

10. $200,000 : x :: 1,000,000 : 5$ _____

11. $x : \frac{3}{4}\% :: 3\frac{1}{5} : \frac{1}{200}$ _____

12. $84 : x :: 30 : 90$ _____

13. $24 : x :: 6 : 60$ _____

14. $\frac{1}{150} : 1 :: \frac{1}{100} : x$ _____

15. $3 : 150 :: 40 : x$ _____

16. $\frac{1}{8} : x :: 7 : 56$ _____

17. $\frac{1}{200} : 40 :: \frac{1}{100} : x$ _____

18. $x : 5 :: 3 : 15$ _____

19. $9 : x :: 3 : 800$ _____

20. $15 : 60 :: x : 20$ _____

21. $12\frac{1}{2} : x :: 50 : 2400$ _____

22. $\frac{1}{2}\% : \frac{1}{100} :: x : 80$ _____

23. $x : 6.4 :: 0.03 : 6$ _____

24. $15 : 16 :: 120 : x$ _____

25. $0.25 : 1 :: 0.05 : x$ _____

26. $7 : 14 :: x : 16$ _____

27. $x : 8 :: 6 : 96$ _____

28. $1/120 : 2 :: 4 : x$ _____

29. $x : 1/1000 :: 5 : 1/5000$ _____

30. $6 : 15 :: 8 : x$ _____

31. $x : 3 :: 9 : 54$ _____

32. $1.4 : 0.4 :: 4.2 : x$ _____

33. $x : 0.65 :: 9 : 5$ _____

34. $12\frac{1}{2}\% : 5 :: x : 120$ _____

35. $\frac{1}{300} : 6 :: \frac{1}{120} : x$ _____

36. $x : 45 :: 4 : 6$ _____

37. $25 : 75 :: 16 : x$ _____

38. $30 : 90 :: 5 : x$ _____

39. $0.3 : x :: 7 : 21$ _____

40. $20 : 25 :: x : 5$ _____

41. $x : 12 :: 9 : 6$ _____

42. $4 : x :: 12 : 48$ _____

43. $x : 60 :: 900 : 40$ _____

44. $x : 12 :: 2 : 4$ _____

45. $6 : 20 :: x : 120$ _____

46. $\frac{4}{5} : x :: \frac{1}{3} : \frac{5}{9}$ _____

47. $25 : 50 :: 4 : x$ _____

48. $0.6 : x :: 7 : 42$ _____

49. $15 : x :: 20 : 600$ _____

50. $0.6 : x :: 0.4 : 12$ _____

51. $9\% : x :: 11 : 73$ _____

52. $500,000 : 1 :: 300,000 : x$ _____

53. $\frac{1}{6} : \frac{9}{10} :: \frac{1}{2} : x$ _____

54. $2.5 : x :: 0.5 : 400$ _____

55. $2.8 : 12 :: 40 : x$ _____

56. $8 : \frac{8}{100} :: x : 5$ _____

57. $\frac{1}{8}\% : \frac{1}{200} :: x : 40$ _____

58. $x : 25 :: 18 : 36$ _____

59. $0.15 : 0.25 :: x : 400$ _____

60. $\frac{1}{20} : \frac{1}{15} :: x : 25$ _____

61. $800,000 : 5 :: 960,000 : x$ _____

62. $0.50 : 0.40 :: x : 400$ _____

63. $83.25 : 60 :: x : 45$ _____

64. $27 : x :: 9 : 60$ _____

65. $\frac{1}{20} : \frac{1}{5} :: x : 50$ _____

66. $\frac{1}{150} : \frac{1}{200} :: x : 60$ _____

67. $\frac{1}{2}\% : 4 :: x : 25$ _____

68. $0.6 : 1.2 :: x : 200$ _____

69. $500 : 2.5 :: x : 8.1$ _____

70. $x : 80 :: 14 : 56$ _____

Answers on p. 421.

POSTTEST 1

Name _____

Date _____

ACCEPTABLE SCORE __**18**__

YOUR SCORE _____

Directions: Find the value of x. Show your work.

1. $x : 2.5 :: 4 : 5$ _____

2. $\frac{7}{8} : x :: \frac{4}{5} : \frac{2}{3}$ _____

3. $30 : 90 :: 2 : x$ _____

4. $x : 3.5 :: 25 : 14$ _____

5. $\frac{2}{7} : \frac{1}{2} :: x : 56$ _____

6. $\frac{1}{4} : x :: 160 : 320$ _____

7. $x : 7 :: 5 : 14$ _____

8. $3 : x :: 18 : 12$ _____

9. $\frac{1}{5} : 90 :: x : 250$ _____

10. $1.8 : 4.8 :: x : 96$ _____

11. $x : 8 :: 10 : 20$ _____

12. $\frac{2}{3} : x :: 4.5 : 27$ _____

13. $\frac{1}{150} : x :: \frac{1}{200} : 6$ _____

14. $\frac{2}{3}\% : \frac{1}{5} :: 50 : x$ _____

15. $14 : x :: 6 : 18$ _____

16. $x : \frac{2}{3} :: 12 : 18$ _____   **17.** $50 : 250 :: \frac{4}{5} : x$ _____   **18.** $50 : 3 :: x : 6$ _____

19. $\frac{1}{2} : x :: 40 : 80$ _____   **20.** $0.8 : 10 :: x : 40$ _____

Answers on p. 421.

POSTTEST 2

Name _____

Date _____

ACCEPTABLE SCORE __**18**__

YOUR SCORE _____

Directions: Find the value of x. Show your work.

1. $x : 300 :: 9 : 12$ _____

2. $4 : 32\% :: 16 : x$ _____

3. $18 : x :: 6 : 40$ _____

4. $1.8 : 2.5 :: x : 9.5$ _____

5. $x : 30 :: \frac{1}{3} : \frac{3}{4}$ _____

6. $\frac{7}{8} : x :: \frac{5}{8} : 40$ _____

7. $400 : 500 :: \frac{4}{5} : x$ _____

8. $x : 7.6 :: 3 : 6$ _____

9. $\frac{1}{4} : x :: \frac{2}{3} : \frac{2}{5}$ _____

10. $\frac{1}{150} : \frac{1}{100} :: x : 60$ _____

11. $0.6 : x :: 15 : 90$ _____

12. $3.5 : 12 :: x : 360$ _____

13. $\frac{2}{9} : \frac{4}{5} :: \frac{3}{4} : x$ _____

14. $\frac{1}{8} : x :: \frac{1}{7} : \frac{5}{9}$ _____

15. $x : 2.5 :: 16 : 4$ _____

16. $0.6 : 3 :: 72 : x$ _____

17. $20 : x :: 6 : 4.5$ _____

18. $x : \frac{1}{4} :: 96 : \frac{1}{3}$ _____

19. $300 : 5000 :: x : 18$ _____

20. $\frac{1}{3} : x :: \frac{1}{5} : 90$ _____

Answers on p. 421.

POSTTEST

Name _____

Date _____

ACCEPTABLE SCORE __117__

YOUR SCORE _____

Directions: Complete the following definitions and exercises.

1. *Improper fractions* can be reduced to a _____ number or a _____ number.

In the following fractions, circle only those that are *improper fractions*.

$^4/_{12}$ $^7/_6$ $^6/_3$ $^4/_7$ $^9/_9$ $^{14}/_{21}$

2. A *complex fraction* contains a _____ in either its numerator, its denominator, or both.

In the following examples, circle only the *complex fractions*.

$1^2/_3$ $^1/_2/4$ $^{12}/_4$ $^3/_7/^4/_2$ 21% $21/^2/_3$

3. A *ratio* is the _____ between _____ numbers.

Write each of the following numbers as a *ratio*.

$^4/_{12}$ _____

24% _____

0.03 _____

$^{13}/_8$ _____

2.2% _____

1.24 _____

4. The *divisor* of a fraction is known as the _____ .

Division problems can be expressed in different ways. Circle the *divisor* in each of the following examples.

$^2/_3$ $4 \div 8$ $10 : 5$ $4\overline{)12}$ $^{14}/_8$ $6 \div 24$ $42\overline{)7}$ $7 : 10$

5. The number shown in a decimal is the _____ of a fraction. The denominator of this fraction is implied by the number of decimal places shown, and is _____ or some power of _____.

Write the fraction values for the following *decimal fraction* numbers.

0.436 _____ 0.051 _____ 1.0042 _____ 0.9684 _____ 0.0019 _____ 1.02064 _____

Directions: Add and reduce fractions to lowest terms.

6. $5/9 + 2/5 + 2/3 =$ _____

7. $4\frac{1}{4} + 2\frac{5}{6} =$ _____

8. $5\frac{1}{2} + 3/9 =$ _____

9. $3/4 \big/ 5/6 + 4\frac{3}{5} =$ _____

Directions: Add and round answers to hundredths.

10. $4.02 + 3.4 + 1.099 =$ _____

11. $45.009 + 0.076 + 1.2 =$ _____

12. $0.0082 + 0.923 + 234 =$ _____

13. $456 + 3.56 + 0.0029 =$ _____

Directions: Subtract and reduce fractions to lowest terms.

14. $2/4 - 3/9 =$ _____

15. $4/7 \big/ 2/8 - 2/3 =$ _____

16. $3\frac{4}{5} - 2\frac{8}{9} =$ _____

17. $6\frac{1}{2} - 8/9 =$ _____

Directions: Subtract and round answers to tenths.

18. $23.98 - 0.0987 =$ _____

19. $23.191 - 23.099 =$ _____

20. $9.002 - 4.9089 =$ _____

21. $2.009 - 0.9834 =$ _____

Directions: Multiply and reduce fractions to lowest terms.

22. $9 \times {}^{5}\!/_{8} =$ _____

23. $\frac{3}{4} \times {}^{8}\!/_{9} =$ _____

24. $4{}^{8}\!/_{9} \times 1{}^{5}\!/_{6} =$ _____

25. $3{}^{4}\!/_{5} \times 7 =$ _____

Directions: Multiply and round answers to hundredths.

26. $3.45 \times 0.56 =$ _____

27. $21.4 \times 0.092 =$ _____

28. $0.0452 \times 99.1 =$ _____

29. $739 \times 0.246 =$ _____

Directions: Divide and reduce fractions to lowest terms.

30. ${}^{7}\!/_{8} \div {}^{4}\!/_{9} =$ _____

31. ${}^{2}\!/_{5} \div {}^{7}\!/_{9} =$ _____

32. ${}^{1}\!/_{300} \div {}^{3}\!/_{4} =$ _____

33. $4{}^{7}\!/_{9} \div 5{}^{9}\!/_{11} =$ _____

Directions: Divide and round answers to thousandths.

34. $52.014 \div 9.2 =$ _____

35. $0.0982 \div 75 =$ _____

36. $3200 \div 0.04 =$ _____

37. $78.09 \div 4.501 =$ _____

Directions: Number the following decimal numbers in order from *lesser to greater value.*

38. 0.45 _____ 1.46 _____ 0.407 _____ 2.401 _____ 0.048 _____ 0.014 _____

39. 0.15 _____ 0.015 _____ 1.015 _____ 1.15 _____ 0.155 _____ 1.0015 _____

40. 9.09 _____ 0.99 _____ 0.090 _____ 0.90 _____ 90.90 _____ 9.009 _____

41. 0.6 _____ 0.4 _____ 0.7 _____ 0.52 _____ 0.44 _____ 0.24 _____

42. 0.21 _____ 0.191 _____ 0.021 _____ 0.1091 _____ 0.201 _____ 0.2 _____

Directions: Change the following fractions to decimals, and round the answers to hundredths.

43. $5/6$ _____   **44.** $5/9$ _____

45. $9/16$ _____   **46.** $1/150$ _____

Directions: Change the following decimals to fractions, and reduce to lowest terms.

47. 0.225 _____   **48.** 0.465 _____

49. 0.06 _____   **50.** 0.372 _____

Directions: Calculate the following problems.

51. Express 0.275 as a percent. _____   **52.** Express $3/8$ as a percent. _____

53. Express 42% as a proper fraction and reduce to the lowest terms. _____

54. Express 0.62% as a ratio. _____   **55.** What percent of 3.2 is 0.4? _____

56. What percent of $5/7$ is $5/28$? _____   **57.** What percent of 240 is 36? _____

58. What is ½% of 48? _____

59. What is 6½% of 840? _____

60. What is 46% of 325? _____

Directions: Change the following fractions and decimals to ratios reduced to lowest terms.

61. $^{10}/_{45}$ _____

62. $1¾/4⅔$ _____

63. 0.584 _____

64. $^{250}/_{375}$ _____

65. 0.48 _____

Directions: Find the value of x and round decimal answers to hundredths.

66. $8 : ⁴/_{45} :: x : 3$ _____

67. $x : 34 :: 4 : 81$ _____

68. $4.6 : 3 :: 20 : x$ _____

69. $x : ½\% :: 4.5 : ¹/_{50}$ _____

70. $¹/_{300} : ¹/_{150} :: x : 300$ _____

71. $22 : x :: 4 : 88$ _____

72. $0.35 : 0.75 :: x : 425$ _____

73. $400 : x :: ¹/_{300} : ¹/_{225}$ _____

74. $x : 54 :: 4 : 8$ _____

75. $½/¾ : 8 :: x : 45$ _____

Answers on pp. 421-422.

Part II Units and Measurements for the Calculation of Drug Dosages

PRETEST

Name _____

Date _____

ACCEPTABLE SCORE __**27**__

YOUR SCORE _____

Directions: Change to equivalent metric measurements. Solve each problem by using a proportion. Show your work.

1. 800,000 mcg = _____ g

2. 3 mg = _____ mcg

3. 255 mg = _____ g

4. 3 Tbsp = _____ ml

5. 3000 mcg = _____ mg

6. 0.68 g = _____ mg

7. 326 ml = _____ L

8. 33 kg = _____ lb

9. 2.1 kl = _____ L

10. 3000 g = _____ kg

11. 0.1 L = _____ ml

12. 2½ tsp = _____ ml

13. 5 ml = _____ cc

14. 0.8 kg = _____ g

15. 250 L = _____ kl

16. 1¼ glass = _____ ml

17. 22 lb = _____ g

18. 0.63 L = _____ ml

19. 733 g = _____ kg

20. 1.25 g = _____ mcg

21. 60 gtt = _____ ml

22. 0.25 mg = _____ mcg

23. 0.6 kl = _____ L

24. 45 lb = _____ kg

25. 10,000 mcg = _____ g   **26.** 1.2 kg = _____ g   **27.** 1⅔ c = _____ ml

28. 0.71 g = _____ mg   **29.** 480 ml = _____ L   **30.** 650 g = _____ lb

Answers on p. 422.

Chapter 6

Metric and Household Measurements

Learning Objectives

On completion of the materials provided in this chapter, you will be able to perform computations accurately by mastering the following mathematical concepts:

1   Recall of the metric measures of weight, volume, and length

2   Computation of equivalents within the metric system by using a proportion

3   Recall of approximate equivalents between metric and household measures

4   Computation of equivalents between the metric and household systems of measure by using a proportion

METRIC MEASUREMENTS

The metric system has become the system of choice when dealing with the weights and measures involved in the calculation of drug dosages. This is a result of its accuracy and simplicity because it is based on the decimal system. The use of decimals tends to eliminate errors made when working with fractions. Therefore all answers within the metric system need to be expressed as a decimal, not as a fraction.

Example: 0.5 not ½

0.75 not ¾

0.007 not ⁷⁄₁₀₀₀

Certain prefixes identify the multiples of 10 that are being used. The three most commonly used prefixes of the metric system involved with the calculation of drug dosages are the following:

micro = 0.000001 or one millionth

milli = 0.001 or one thousandth

kilo = 1000 or one thousand

These prefixes may be used with any of the base units of weight (gram), volume (liter), or length (meter). The nurse most often uses the following list of metric measures. Memorize all the entries in the list.

Metric measure of weight
1,000,000 micrograms (mcg) = 1 gram (g)
1000 micrograms (mcg) = 1 milligram (mg)
1000 milligrams (mg) = 1 gram (g)
1000 grams (g) = 1 kilogram (kg)

Metric measure of volume
1000 milliliters (ml) = 1 liter (L)
1000 liters (L) = 1 kiloliter (kl)
1 cubic centimeter (cc) = 1 milliliter (ml)*

Metric measure of length
1 meter (m) = 1000 mm or 100 cm
1 centimeter (cm) = 10 mm or 0.01 m
1 millimeter (mm) = 0.1 cm or 0.001 m

*The abbreviations (cc) and (ml) are used interchangeably. However, in this book, milliliter is used exclusively. Milliliter (ml) should only be used for liquids, whereas cubic centimeter (cc) should be used only for solids and gases.

Sometimes, to compute drug dosages, the nurse must convert a metric measure to an equivalent measure within the system. This may be done easily by using a proportion.

Example: 300 mg equals how many grams?

a. On the left side of the proportion place what you know to be an equivalent between milligrams and grams. From the preceding chart we know that there are 1000 mg in 1 g. Therefore the left side of the proportion would be

$$1000 \text{ mg} : 1 \text{ g} ::$$

b. The right side of the proportion is determined by the problem and by the abbreviations used on the left side of the proportion. Only *two* different abbreviations may be used in a single proportion. The abbreviations must also be in the same position on the right as they are on the left.

$$1000 \text{ mg} : 1 \text{ g} :: \underline{\hspace{1cm}} \text{ mg} : \underline{\hspace{1cm}} \text{ g}$$

From the problem we know we have 300 mg

$$1000 \text{ mg} : 1 \text{ g} :: 300 \text{ mg} : \underline{\hspace{1cm}} \text{ g}$$

We need to find the number of grams 300 mg equals, so we use the symbol x to represent the unknown. Therefore the full proportion would be

$$1000 \text{ mg} : 1 \text{ g} :: 300 \text{ mg} : x \text{ g}$$

c. Rewrite the proportion without using the abbreviations.

$$1000 : 1 :: 300 : x$$

d. Solve for x, writing the answer as a decimal, since the metric system is based on decimals.

$$1000x = 300$$

$$x = \frac{300}{1000}$$

$$x = 0.3$$

Label your answer, as determined by the abbreviation placed next to x in the original proportion.

$$300 \text{ mg} = 0.3 \text{ g}$$

Example 1: 2.5 L equals how many milliliters?

    a. 1000 ml : 1 L ::

    b. 1000 ml : 1 L :: _____ ml : _____ L

       1000 ml : 1 L :: x ml : 2.5 L

    c. 1000 : 1 :: x : 2.5

    d. $1x = 2500$

       $x = 2500$

    e. 2.5 L equals 2500 ml

Example 2: 180 mcg equals how many grams?

    a. 1,000,000 mcg : 1 g ::

    b. 1,000,000 mcg : 1 g :: _____ mcg : _____ g

       1,000,000 mcg : 1 g :: 180 mcg : x g

    c. 1,000,000 : 1 :: 180 : x

    d. $1,000,000x = 180$

$$x = \frac{180}{1,000,000}$$

       $x = 0.00018$

    e. 180 mcg equals 0.00018 g

Example 3: 15 mm equals how many centimeters?

    a. 1 cm : 10 mm

    b. 1 cm : 10 mm :: _____ cm : _____ mm

       1 cm : 10 mm :: x cm : 15 mm

    c. 1 : 10 :: x : 15

    d. $10x = 1 \times 15$

       $10x = 15$

$$x = \frac{15}{10}$$

       $x = 1.5$

    e. 15 mm equals 1.5 cm

HOUSEHOLD MEASUREMENTS

Household measures are not accurate enough for the nurse to use in the calculation of drug dosages in the hospital. However, their metric equivalents are used in keeping a written record of a patient's "I" and "O," or intake and output.

Memorize the following list of approximate equivalents between metric and household measurements.

Metric measure   Household measure
1 milliliter (ml) = 15 drops (gtt)
5 milliliters = 1 teaspoon (tsp)
15 milliliters = 1 tablespoon (Tbsp)
180 milliliters = 1 cup (c)
240 milliliters = 1 glass
1 kilogram (kg) or 1000 grams (g) = 2.2 pounds (lb)
2.5 cm = 1 inch

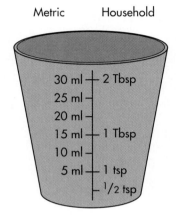

Conversion of measures between the metric and household systems of measure may also be done by using a proportion, as has been illustrated.

Example 1:   1½ c equals how many ml?

a. 1 c : 180 ml ::
b. 1 c : 180 ml :: _____ c : _____ ml
   1 c : 180 ml :: 1½ c : x ml
c. 1 : 180 :: 1½ : x
d. $x = \dfrac{180}{1} \times \dfrac{3}{2}$

   $x = \dfrac{540}{2} = 270$ ml

e. 1½ c equals 270 ml

Example 2:   35 kg equals how many pounds?

a. 1 kg : 2.2 lb ::
b. 1 kg : 2.2 lb :: _____ kg : _____ lb
   1 kg : 2.2 lb :: 35 kg : x lb
c. 1 : 2.2 :: 35 : x
d. $1x = 2.2 \times 35$
   $x = 77$
e. 35 kg equals 77 lbs

Memorize the tables of metric and household measurements. Study the material on forming proportions for the calculation of problems relating to the metric and household systems of measure. Complete the following work sheet, which provides for extensive practice in the manipulation of measurements within the metric and household systems. Check your answers. If you have difficulties, go back and review the necessary material. When you feel ready to evaluate your learning, take the first posttest. Check your answers. An acceptable score as indicated on the posttest signifies that you are ready for the next chapter. An unacceptable score signifies a need for further study before taking the second posttest.

WORK SHEET

Directions: Change to equivalents within the metric system. Solve the problems by using a proportion. Show your work.

1. 230 mcg = _____ g

2. 5 mg = _____ mcg

3. 2.5 g = _____ mcg

4. 4000 mcg = _____ mg

5. 0.33 g = _____ mg

6. 6 kg = _____ g

7. 725 ml = _____ L

8. 2000 mcg = _____ g

9. 3 cm = _____ mm

10. 620 g = _____ kg

11. 36 cc = _____ ml

12. 460 ml = _____ L

13. 0.66 mg = _____ mcg   **14.** 0.5 g = _____ mcg   **15.** 474 L = _____ kl

16. 350,000 mcg = _____ g   **17.** 25 mg = _____ g   **18.** 1.46 L = _____ ml

19. 2.5 kg = _____ g   **20.** 12 mg = _____ mcg   **21.** 3.4 kg = _____ g

22. 920 mcg = _____ g   **23.** 25 mm = _____ cm   **24.** 300 mcg = _____ mg

25. 0.16 L = _____ ml   **26.** 0.01 g = _____ mg   **27.** 500 mcg = _____ mg

28. 360 mg = _____ g

29. 3.25 kl = _____ L

30. 0.45 g = _____ mg

31. 240 ml = _____ L

32. 10 cc = _____ ml

Directions: Change the following household measurements into the approximate equivalents within the metric system. Solve the problems by using a proportion. Show your work.

33. 30 gtt = _____ ml

34. 3 in = _____ cm

35. 2¼ c = _____ ml

36. 1⅖ Tbsp = _____ ml

37. 1⅓ glass = _____ ml

38. 4 Tbsp = _____ ml

39. ⅔ glass = _____ ml

40. 75 gtt = _____ ml

41. 1½ c = _____ ml

42. 3 tsp = _____ ml

43. 8 kg = _____ lb

44. 3825 g = _____ lb

45. 7 in = _____ cm   **46.** 3 lb = _____ kg   **47.** 12 kg = _____ lb

48. 1400 g = _____ lb   **49.** 24 lb = _____ g   **50.** 150 lb = _____ kg

Answers on pp. 422-423.

POSTTEST 1

Name _____

Date _____

ACCEPTABLE SCORE __**27**__

YOUR SCORE _____

Directions: Change to equivalent metric measurements. Solve each problem by using a proportion. Show your work.

1. 5000 mcg = _____ g

2. 10 mg = _____ mcg

3. 0.81 L = _____ ml

4. 35 mg = _____ g

5. 1¾ tsp = _____ ml

6. 0.12 g = _____ mcg

7. 16 kg = _____ lb

8. 280 ml = _____ L

9. 0.4 kg = _____ g

10. 45 gtt = _____ ml

11. 28 lb = _____ g

12. 4 in = _____ cm

13. 500,000 mcg = _____ g   **14.** 37 ml = _____ L   **15.** 20 ml = _____ cc

16. 1⅕ c = _____ ml   **17.** 2.5 g = _____ mg   **18.** 12 cc = _____ ml

19. 6700 g = _____ kg   **20.** 0.3 kl = _____ L   **21.** 4 mg = _____ mcg

22. 2600 g = _____ lb   **23.** 1½ glass = _____ ml   **24.** 0.2 L = _____ ml

25. 533 L = _____ kl   **26.** 1.5 g = _____ mcg   **27.** 620 mg = _____ g

28. 2.3 kg = _____ g   **29.** 6 Tbsp = _____ ml   **30.** 7 lb = _____ kg

Answers on p. 423.

POSTTEST 2

Name _____

Date _____

ACCEPTABLE SCORE __27__

YOUR SCORE _____

Directions: Change to equivalent metric measurements. Solve each problem by using a proportion. Show your work.

1. 4000 mcg = _____ mg

2. 150 g = _____ kg

3. 2½ c = _____ ml

4. 800 g = _____ lb

5. 44 kg = _____ lb

6. 760 mg = _____ g

7. 0.55 L = _____ ml

8. 35 mm = _____ cm

9. ⅓ glass = _____ ml

10. 2⅛ lb = _____ g

11. 0.1 kl = _____ L

12. 32 mg = _____ mcg

13. 618 ml = _____ L

14. 100,000 mcg = _____ g

15. 90 gtt = _____ ml

16. 714 ml = _____ L   **17.** 350 L = _____ kl   **18.** 250,000 mcg = _____ g

19. 0.87 g = _____ mg   **20.** 7 mg = _____ mcg   **21.** 3¼ tsp = _____ ml

22. 1.4 kl = _____ L   **23.** 0.78 g = _____ mg   **24.** 225 mcg = _____ mg

25. 4500 g = _____ kg   **26.** 0.2 L = _____ ml   **27.** 2 Tbsp = _____ ml

28. 40 cc = _____ ml   **29.** 2.6 g = _____ mcg   **30.** 73 lb = _____ kg

Answers on p. 423.

PRETEST

Name _____

Date _____

ACCEPTABLE SCORE __**18**__

YOUR SCORE _____

Directions: Change to equivalents within the apothecaries' system. Solve by using proportions. Show your work.

1. 360 gr = _____ ℥ = _____ ʒ

2. 72 ʒ = _____ ℥ = _____ gr

3. 12½ fl. ʒ = _____ fl. ℥ = _____ ℳ

4. 160 fl. ʒ = _____ fl. ℥ = _____ pt
= _____ qt = _____ gal

5. 5 pt = _____ fl. ℥ = _____ fl. ʒ
= _____ qt

6. 7 qt = _____ gal = _____ fl. ℥
= _____ pt

Directions: Change the following household measurements into approximate equivalents within the apothecaries' system. Solve the problems by using proportions. Show your work.

7. 3 glasses = _____ fl. ℥

8. 1½ Tbsp = _____ fl. ℥

9. 1¾ tsp = _____ fl. ℥

10. 2½ c = _____ fl. ℥

Answers on p. 423.

Chapter 7

Apothecaries' and Household Measurements

Learning Objectives

On completion of the materials provided in this chapter, you will be able to perform computations accurately by mastering the following mathematical concepts:

1   Addition and subtraction of Roman numerals

2   Conversion of Roman numerals to Arabic numerals

3   Conversion of Arabic numerals to Roman numerals

4   Recall of the apothecaries' measures of weights and liquids

5   Computation of equivalents within the apothecaries' system by using a proportion

6   Recall of approximate equivalents between apothecaries' and household measures

7   Computation of equivalents between the apothecaries' and household measurement systems by the use of a proportion

---

The apothecaries' system of measure is a very old English system. It has slowly been replaced by the metric system. When writing orders in the apothecaries' system, physicians often use Roman numerals. All parts of a whole are expressed as a fraction except the fraction one half, which is commonly represented as s̅s̅ or ss.

Following is a list of the more commonly used Roman numerals and their Arabic equivalents. Memorize the list.

Roman numeral	Arabic numeral
i	1
v	5
x	10
l	50
c	100

Only addition and subtraction may be performed in the Roman numeral system.

155

Addition of Roman Numerals

1. Addition is performed when a smaller numeral follows a larger numeral.

Examples: xi = 11   xv = 15   li = 51

2. Addition is performed when a numeral is repeated. However, a numeral is *never* repeated more than three times.

Examples: viii = 8   xii = 12   ccxi = 211

Subtraction of Roman Numerals

1. Subtraction is performed when a smaller numeral is placed before a larger numeral.

Examples: ix = 9   iv = 4   ic = 99

2. Subtraction is performed when a smaller numeral is placed between two larger numerals. The smaller numeral is subtracted from the larger numeral following the smaller numeral.

Examples: xiv = 14   xxiv = 24   cxc = 190

Apothecaries' Measurements

It is still important for a nurse to be knowledgeable about the apothecary system. Some of the older medications are still ordered with the apothecary unit of measure.

Example: aspirin gr x*

Some pharmaceutical companies label a drug using both the apothecary and the metric systems of measure.

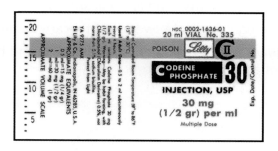

---

*Note: In the apothecary system, the symbol of measure precedes the number.

A nurse is already familiar with many of the units of measure in the apothecaries' system because they are used every day. A nurse most commonly uses the following list of apothecaries' system units of measure. Memorize all entries in the list.

Apothecaries' measure of weight
60 grains (gr) = 1 dram (ʒ)
8 drams (ʒ) = 1 ounce (℥)

Apothecaries' measure of liquid
60 minims (♏︎) = 1 fluidram (fl. ʒ)
8 fluidrams (fl. ʒ) = 1 fluidounce (fl. ℥)
16 fluidounces (fl. ℥) = 1 pint (pt)
32 fluidounces (fl. ℥) = 2 pints (pt) or 1 quart (qt)
4 quarts (qt) = 1 gallon (gal)

Apothecary

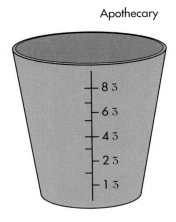

Sometimes, to compute drug dosages, the nurse must convert an apothecaries' measure to an equivalent measure within the same system. This may be done easily by using a proportion.

Example 1:   3 fl. ℥ equals how many fl. ʒ?

    a. On the left side of the proportion, place what you know to be an equivalent between fluidrams and fluidounces. From the preceding chart you know that there are 8 fl. ʒ in 1 fl. ℥. Thus the left side of the proportion would be

$$8 \text{ fl. ʒ} : 1 \text{ fl. ℥} ::$$

    b. The right side of the proportion is determined by the problem and by the abbreviations used on the left side of the proportion. Only *two* different abbreviations may be used in a single proportion. The abbreviations must also be in the same position on the right as they are on the left.

$$8 \text{ fl. ʒ} : 1 \text{ fl. ℥} :: \underline{\hspace{1cm}} \text{ fl. ʒ}: \underline{\hspace{1cm}} \text{ fl. ℥}$$

From the problem, we know we have 3 fl. ℥.

$$8 \text{ fl. ʒ} : 1 \text{ fl. ℥} :: \underline{\hspace{1cm}} \text{ fl. ʒ} : 3 \text{ fl. ℥}$$

We need to find the number of fluidrams that 3 fl. ℥ equals, so we use the symbol x to represent the unknown. Therefore the full proportion would be written as follows:

$$8 \text{ fl. ʒ} : 1 \text{ fl. ℥} :: x \text{ fl. ʒ} : 3 \text{ fl. ℥}$$

    c. Rewrite the proportion without using the abbreviations.

$$8 : 1 :: x : 3$$

    d. Solve for x.

$$1x = 8 \times 3$$
$$x = 24$$

    e. Label your answer, as determined by the abbreviation placed next to x in the original proportion.

$$3 \text{ fl. } ℨ = 24 \text{ fl. } ℨ$$

Example 2:   12 fl. ℨ equals how many pints?

    a. 16 fl. ℨ : 1 pt ::
    b. 16 fl. ℨ : 1 pt :: _____ fl. ℨ : _____ pt
       16 fl. ℨ : 1 pt :: 12 fl. ℨ : x pt
    c. 16 : 1 :: 12 : x
    d. $16x = 12$

$$x = \frac{12}{16} = \frac{3}{4}$$

    e. 12 fl. ℨ equals ¾ pt
Note that fractions (not decimals) are used when working with the apothecaries' system.

Example 3:   1½ fl. ℨ = _____ ♏

    a. 60 ♏ : 1 fl. ℨ ::
    b. 60 ♏ : 1 fl. ℨ :: _____ ♏ : _____ fl. ℨ
       60 ♏ : 1 fl. ℨ :: x ♏ : 1½ fl. ℨ
    c. 60 : 1 :: x : 1½
    d. $1x = 60 \times 1½$

$$x = \frac{\overset{30}{\cancel{60}}}{1} \times \frac{3}{\underset{1}{\cancel{2}}}$$

       $x = 90$
    e. 1½ fl. ℨ = 90 ♏

Household Measurements

    Household measures are not accurate enough to be used by nurses in the calculation of drug dosages in the hospital. It is sometimes necessary to compute their approximate equivalents with the apothecaries' system of measure, especially when sending medicines home from the hospital.

    Memorize the following list of approximate equivalents.

Apothecaries' measures	*Household measures*
1 minim (♏)	= 1 drop (gtt)
1 fluidram (fl. ℨ)	= 1 teaspoon (tsp)
4 fluidrams (fl. ℨ)	= 1 tablespoon (Tbsp)
6 fluidounces (fl. ℥)	= 1 teacup (c)
8 fluidounces (fl. ℥)	= 1 glass

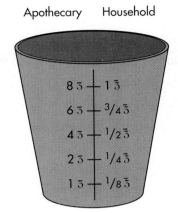

Apothecary   Household

$8\,\text{ʒ}$ — $1\,\text{ʒ}$
$6\,\text{ʒ}$ — $^3/_4\,\text{ʒ}$
$4\,\text{ʒ}$ — $^1/_2\,\text{ʒ}$
$2\,\text{ʒ}$ — $^1/_4\,\text{ʒ}$
$1\,\text{ʒ}$ — $^1/_8\,\text{ʒ}$

Conversion of measures between the apothecaries' and household systems of measure may also be made by using a proportion, as has been illustrated.

Example 1: 1½ c equals how many fl. ʒ?

    a. 6 fl. ʒ : 1 c ::
    b. 6 fl. ʒ : 1 c :: _____ fl. ʒ : _____ c
       6 fl. ʒ : 1 c :: x fl. ʒ : 1½ c
    c. $6 : 1 :: x : 1½$
    d. $x = 6 \times 1½$

$$x = \frac{\overset{3}{\cancel{6}}}{1} \times \frac{3}{\underset{1}{\cancel{2}}}$$

$$x = \frac{9}{1} = 9$$

    e. 1½ c = 9 fl. ʒ

Example 2: 2 tsp = _____ fl. ʒ

    a. 1 fl. ʒ : 1 tsp ::
    b. 1 fl. ʒ : 1 tsp :: _____ fl. ʒ : _____ tsp
       1 fl. ʒ : 1 tsp :: x fl. ʒ : 2 tsp
    c. $1 : 1 :: x : 2$
    d. $1x = 2$
       $x = 2$
    e. 2 tsp = 2 fl. ʒ

Memorize the tables for the apothecaries' and household measurements. Study the material on forming proportions for the calculation of problems relating to the apothecaries' and household systems of measure. Complete the following work sheet, which provides for extensive practice in the manipulation of measurements within the apothecaries' and household systems. Check your answers. If you have difficulties, go back and review the necessary material. When you feel ready to evaluate your learning, take the first posttest. Check your answers. An acceptable score as indicated on the posttest signifies that you are ready for the next chapter. An unacceptable score signifies a need for further study before taking the second posttest.

WORK SHEET

Directions: Express the following Arabic numerals as Roman numerals.

1. 22 _____   **2.** 9 _____   **3.** 3 _____   **4.** 30 _____

5. 14 _____   **6.** 6 _____   **7.** 15 _____   **8.** 12 _____

Directions: Express the following Roman numerals as Arabic numerals.

1. xxix _____   **2.** vii _____   **3.** xx _____   **4.** vi _____

5. xvi _____   **6.** iv _____   **7.** xxv _____   **8.** ccxl _____

Directions: Change to equivalents within the apothecaries' system. Solve by using proportions. Show your work.

1. 30 gr = _____ ℥

2. 180 gr = _____ ℥ = _____ ℨ

3. ⅕ ℥ = _____ gr

4. 16 ℥ = _____ ℨ = _____ gr

5. 90 ♏ = _____ fl. ℥ = _____ fl. ℨ

6. 20 fl. ℥ = _____ fl. ℨ = _____ pt
= _____ ♏

7. 120 fl. ʒ = _____ fl. ʒ = _____ pt

= _____ qt

8. 4 pt = _____ fl. ʒ = _____ fl. ʒ

= _____ qt

9. 2½ pt = _____ fl. ʒ = _____ fl. ʒ

= _____ ♏

10. 8 pt = _____ qt = _____ gal

11. ½ pt = _____ ♏ = _____ fl. ʒ

= _____ fl. ʒ

12. 3 qt = _____ gal = _____ fl. ʒ

= _____ pt

13. 10 qt = _____ pt = _____ fl. ʒ

= _____ gal

14. 1½ gal = _____ qt = _____ pt

= _____ fl. ʒ

Directions: Change the following household measurements into appropriate equivalents within the apothecaries' system. Solve the problems by using proportions. Show your work.

15. 3 Tbsp = _____ fl. ʒ = _____ fl. ʒ

16. 2 glasses = _____ fl. ʒ

17. ½ c = _____ fl. ʒ = _____ fl. ʒ

18. 3¼ glasses = _____ fl. ʒ = _____ fl. ʒ

Answers on pp. 423-424.

POSTTEST 1

Name _____

Date _____

ACCEPTABLE SCORE __**18**__

YOUR SCORE _____

Directions: Change to equivalents within the apothecaries' system. Solve by using proportions. Show your work.

1. 240 gr = _____ ʒ = _____ ℥

2. 4 ℥ = _____ gr = _____ ʒ

3. 40 fl. ʒ = _____ fl. ℥ = _____ ♏
    = _____ pt

4. 10 fl. ℥ = _____ fl. ʒ = _____ pt

5. 5 qt = _____ gal = _____ pt
    = _____ fl. ℥ = _____ fl. ʒ

6. 1¾ gal = _____ qt = _____ pt
    = _____ fl. ℥

Directions: Change the following household measurements into approximate equivalents within the apothecaries' system. Solve the problems by using proportions. Show your work.

7. 1½ glasses = _____ fl. ℥

8. ¾ c = _____ fl. ℥

9. 3 Tbsp = _____ fl. ʒ

10. 2½ tsp = _____ fl. ʒ

Answers on p. 424.

POSTTEST 2

Name _____

Date _____

ACCEPTABLE SCORE __**18**__

YOUR SCORE _____

Directions: Change to equivalents within the apothecaries' system. Solve by using proportions. Show your work.

1. 300 gr = _____ ʒ = _____ ӡ

2. 480 ʒ = _____ ӡ = _____ gr

3. 210 fl. ʒ = _____ fl. ӡ = _____ pt
= _____ qt

4. 72 fl. ӡ = _____ fl. ʒ = _____ pt
= _____ qt

5. 6 qt = _____ gal = _____ fl. ӡ

6. 2½ gal = _____ qt = _____ pt
= _____ fl. ӡ

Directions: Change the following household measurements into approximate equivalents within the apothecaries' system. Solve the problems by using proportions. Show your work.

7. 5 Tbsp = _____ fl. ӡ

8. 2¼ c = _____ fl. ӡ = _____ pt

9. ½ glass = _____ fl. ӡ

10. 3 tsp = _____ Tbsp

Answers on p. 424.

PRETEST

Name _____

Date _____

ACCEPTABLE SCORE __**32**__

YOUR SCORE _____

Directions: Change to approximate equivalents as indicated. Solve the problems by using proportions. Show your work.

1. 180 ♏ = _____ ml

2. 7 fl. ℥ = _____ ml

3. 36 kg = _____ lb

4. 5¼ qt = _____ ml

5. 90 ml = _____ fl. ℥

6. 1¾ qt = _____ L

7. 90 gr = _____ g

8. 4.5 ml = _____ ♏

9. 8⅗ lb = _____ g

10. 2¼ pt = _____ ml

11. 7 fl. ℥ = _____ ml

12. 10 gr = _____ g

13. 5.5 L = _____ qt

14. 5 ♏ = _____ ml

15. 4 gr = _____ mg

16. 360 ml = _____ fl. ʒ

17. 600 ml = _____ pt

18. 5500 g = _____ lb

19. 20 ml = _____ fl. ʒ

20. 12 mg = _____ gr

21. 1/300 gr = _____ mg

22. 85 lb = _____ kg

23. 0.4 mg = _____ gr

24. 2.4 ml = _____ ℳ

25. 4200 ml = _____ qt

26. 1½ fl. ʒ = _____ ml

27. 1/5 gr = _____ mg

28. 4.6 g = _____ gr

29. 98.8° F = _____ ° C

30. 41° C = _____ ° F

31. 97.6° F = _____ ° C

32. 38.5° C = _____ ° F

33. 99.8° F = _____ ° C

34. 39.6° C = _____ ° F

35. 102.6° F = _____ ° C

36. 40.2° C = _____ ° F

Answers on p. 424.

Chapter 8

Equivalents between Apothecaries' and Metric Measurements

Learning Objectives

On completion of the materials provided in this chapter, you will be able to perform computations accurately by mastering the following mathematical concepts:

1 Recall equivalent apothecary and metric measures

2 Compute equivalents between the apothecaries' and metric systems by using a proportion

3 Convert the Fahrenheit scale to the Celsius scale

4 Convert the Celsius scale to the Fahrenheit scale

One of a nurse's many responsibilities is the administration of medication. Two different systems of measurements are used in the calculation of drug dosages: the apothecaries' system and the metric system. Because hospitals and physicians use both systems, nurses must be able to use both systems and know the approximate equivalents between the two systems. Remember, equivalents are not exact—there may be slight discrepancies.

Approximate Equivalents between Apothecaries' and Metric Measurements

A list of the most commonly used equivalents between apothecaries' and metric systems of measure is provided on the next page. Memorize these equivalents.

Apothecaries' measures   Metric measures
15 minims (m) = 1 milliliter (ml)
1 fluidram (fl. ʒ) = 4 ml
1 fluidounce (fl. ʒ) = 30 ml
6 fluidounces (fl. ʒ) = 180 ml
8 fluidounces (fl. ʒ) = 240 ml
16 fluidounces (fl. ʒ) or 1 pint (pt) = 500 ml
32 fluidounces (fl. ʒ) or 1 quart (qt) = 1000 ml or 1 liter (l)
1 grain (gr) = 60 milligrams (mg)
15 grains (gr) = 1 gram (g)
2.2 pounds (lb) = 1000 grams (g) or 1 kilogram (kg)

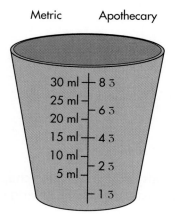

Metric   Apothecary

Sometimes a nurse will have to convert a medication order from one system to the other. This can be done by using a proportion.

Example 1:   3 fl. ʒ equals how many ml?

a. On the left side of the proportion place what you know to be an equivalent between fluidrams and milliliters. In this example the most appropriate equivalent is 1 fl. ʒ = 4 ml. So the left side of the proportion would be

$$1 \text{ fl. ʒ} : 4 \text{ ml} ::$$

b. The right side of the proportion is determined by the problem and by the abbreviations used on the left side. Only *two* different abbreviations may be used in a single proportion. The abbreviations must be in the same position on the right as they are on the left.

$$1 \text{ fl. ʒ} : 4 \text{ ml} :: \underline{\hspace{1cm}} \text{ fl. ʒ} : \underline{\hspace{1cm}} \text{ ml}$$

From the problem we know we have 3 fl. ʒ.

$$1 \text{ fl. ʒ} : 4 \text{ ml} :: 3 \text{ fl. ʒ} : \underline{\hspace{1cm}} \text{ ml}$$

We need to find the number of milliliters in 3 fl. ʒ, so we use the symbol *x* to represent the unknown. Therefore the full proportion would be

$$1 \text{ fl. ʒ} : 4 \text{ ml} :: 3 \text{ fl. ʒ} : x \text{ ml}$$

    c. Rewrite the proportion without using the abbreviations.

$$1 : 4 :: 3 : x$$

    d. Solve for x.

$$1x = 4 \times 3$$
$$x = 12$$

    e. Label your answer, as determined by the abbreviation placed next to x in the original proportion.

$$3 \text{ fl. } \mathfrak{Z} = 12 \text{ ml}$$

Example 2: 150 ml equals how many fl. $\mathfrak{Z}$?

    a. 6 fl. $\mathfrak{Z}$: 180 ml ::
    b. 6 fl. $\mathfrak{Z}$: 180 ml :: _____ fl. $\mathfrak{Z}$: _____ ml
       6 fl. $\mathfrak{Z}$: 180 ml :: x fl. $\mathfrak{Z}$ :: 150 ml
    c. 6 : 180 :: x : 150
    d. $180x = 900$

$$x = \frac{900}{180} = 5$$

    e. 150 ml equals 5 fl. $\mathfrak{Z}$

Example 3: 45 mg equals how many grains?

    a. 1 gr : 60 mg ::
    b. 1 gr : 60 mg :: _____ gr: _____ mg
       1 gr : 60 mg :: x gr : 45 mg
    c. 1 : 60 :: x : 45
    d. $60x = 1 \times 45$
       $60x = 45$

$$x = \frac{45}{60}$$
$$x = \frac{3}{4}$$

    e. 45 mg equals ¾ gr, or 0.75 gr

Example 4: 18 $\mathfrak{m}$ equals how many milliliters?

    a. 15 $\mathfrak{m}$: 1 ml ::
    b. 15 $\mathfrak{m}$: 1 ml :: _____ $\mathfrak{m}$: _____ ml
       15 $\mathfrak{m}$: 1 ml :: 18 $\mathfrak{m}$: x ml
    c. 15 : 1 :: 18 : x
    d. $15x = 18$

$$x = \frac{18}{15}$$
$$x = 1.2$$

    e. 18 $\mathfrak{m}$ equals 1.2 ml

Approximate Equivalents between Celsius and Fahrenheit Measurements

Many hospitals and health care centers use the metric system of measurement, including thermometers calibrated in the Celsius scale. It may be necessary for the nurse to convert the Celsius, or centigrade scale, to the Fahrenheit scale for patient or family information. Because not everyone concerned with patient care uses one scale, it is also important for the nurse to be able to convert the Fahrenheit scale to the Celsius scale.

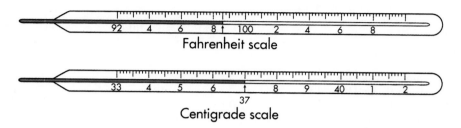

Fahrenheit scale

Centigrade scale

To convert one scale to another, the following proportion may be used:

$$\text{Celsius} : \text{Fahrenheit} - 32 :: 5 : 9$$
$$C : F - 32 :: 5 : 9$$

C or F will be the unknown.
Extend the decimal to hundredths, round to tenths.
Another means of converting Celsius and Fahrenheit temperatures to equivalents is to follow the rules listed in the box below.

Fahrenheit to Celsius	*Celsius to Fahrenheit*
Subtract 32	Multiply by 1.8
Divide by 1.8	Add 32

The following examples illustrate each method:

Example 1:   100.6° F equals _____ ° C.

$$C : F - 32 :: 5 : 9$$

$$C : 100.6 - 32 :: 5 : 9$$

$$9C = (100.6 - 32) \times 5$$
$$9C = 68.6 \times 5$$
$$9C = 343$$
$$C = \frac{343}{9}$$
$$C = 38.11$$

$$100.6 - 32 = 68.6$$

$$68.6 \div 1.8 = 38.111 \ldots$$
or 38.1° C

100.6° F equals 38.1° C.

Example 2: 37.6° C equals _____ ° F.

$$C : F - 32 :: 5 : 9 \qquad\qquad 37.6 \times 1.8 = 67.68$$

$$37.6 : F - 32 :: 5 : 9 \qquad\qquad 67.68 + 32 = 99.68$$
$$5(F - 32) = 9 \times 37.6 \qquad\qquad \text{or } 99.7° \text{ F}$$
$$5F - 160 = 338.4$$

$$5F - 160 + 160 = 338.4 + 160$$

$$5F = 498.4$$
$$F = \frac{498.4}{5}$$
$$F = 99.68$$

37.8° C equals 99.7° F.

Memorize the table of approximate equivalents between the apothecaries' and the metric systems of measure. Study the material on forming proportions for the calculations of problems converting between the apothecaries' and metric systems. Complete the following work sheet, which provides for extensive practice in the manipulation of measurements between the apothecaries' and metric systems. Check your answers. If you have difficulties, go back and review the necessary material. When you feel ready to evaluate your learning, take the first posttest. Check your answers. An acceptable score as indicated on the posttest signifies that you are ready for the next chapter. An unacceptable score signifies a need for further study before taking the second posttest.

WORK SHEET

Directions: Change to approximate equivalents as indicated. Solve the problems by using a proportion. Show your work.

1. 200 mg = _____ gr

2. 240 ℳ = _____ ml

3. 24 fl. ʒ = _____ ml

4. 60 gr = _____ g

5. 300 ml = _____ fl. ʒ

6. 150 gr = _____ g

7. 1¾ qt = _____ ml

8. 210 ml = _____ fl. ʒ

9. 40 ℳ = _____ ml

10. 10 kg = _____ lb

11. 1750 ml = _____ pt

12. ½ fl. ʒ = _____ ml

13. 4½ gr = _____ mg

14. 4200 g = _____ lb

15. 420 mg = _____ gr

16. 5 ml = _____ ℳ

17. 6 pt = _____ ml

18. 3500 ml = _____ qt

19. 5 gr = _____ mg

20. 150 ml = _____ fl. ʒ

21. 30 ℳ = _____ ml

22. 6 fl. ʒ = _____ ml

23. 3.3 g = _____ gr

24. 6⅘ lb = _____ g

25. 12 ml = _____ ℳ

26. ⅜ fl. ʒ = _____ ml

27. 2¾ gr = _____ mg

28. 7 g = _____ gr

29. 5 lb = _____ kg

30. 2700 ml = _____ pt

31. 18 fl. ℥ = _____ ml

32. 340 mg = _____ gr

33. 2½ qt = _____ L

34. 3650 g = _____ lb

35. 6000 ml = _____ qt

36. 8 fl. ℥ = _____ ml

37. 8 ml = _____ ♏

38. 45 gr = _____ g

39. 45 ♏ = _____ ml

40. 4 fl. ℥ = _____ ml

41. 12 lb = _____ g

42. 75 ml = _____ fl. ℥

43. 3 ml = _____ ♏

44. 75 lb = _____ kg

45. 2⅛ qt = _____ ml

46. 100 mg = _____ gr

47. 3.5 L = _____ qt

48. 1½ gr = _____ mg

49. 3 pt = _____ ml

50. 25 kg = _____ lb

51. 99.6° F = _____ ° C

52. 101.8° F = _____ ° C

53. 104.2° F = _____ ° C

54. 97.4° F = _____ ° C

55. 40.4° C = _____ ° F

56. 35.4° C = _____ ° F

57. 36.8° C = _____ ° F

58. 39.2° C = _____ ° F

59. 33° C = _____ ° F

60. 98.4° F = _____ ° C

61. 41.2° C = _____ ° F

62. 103.6° F = _____ ° C

63. 40.6° C = _____ ° F

64. 102.2° F = _____ ° C

65. 37.4° C = _____ ° F

66. 100.4° F = _____ ° C

Answers on p. 425.

POSTTEST 1

Name _____

Date _____

ACCEPTABLE SCORE __**32**__

YOUR SCORE _____

Directions: Change to approximate equivalents as indicated. Solve the problems by using proportions. Show your work.

1. 3 gr = _____ mg

2. 12 ℥ = _____ ml

3. 5 fl. ʒ = _____ ml

4. 75 gr = _____ g

5. 3 fl. ʒ = _____ ml

6. 1½ pt = _____ ml

7. 15 mg = _____ gr

8. 1500 ml = _____ qt

9. 7½ lb = _____ g

10. 260 ℥ = _____ ml

11. 1.7 L = _____ qt

12. 5 gr = _____ g

13. 8 ml = _____ fl. ℨ

14. 20 lb = _____ kg

15. ⅙ gr = _____ mg

16. 1000 ml = _____ pt

17. 2 ml = _____ ♏

18. 0.3 mg = _____ gr

19. 3 g = _____ gr

20. 60 ml = _____ fl. ℨ

21. 2700 g = _____ lb

22. 5 fl. ℥ = _____ ml

23. 32 kg = _____ lb

24. 0.5 mg = _____ gr

25. 1.5 ml = _____ ♏

26. 80 gr = _____ g

27. 2¾ qt = _____ L

28. 540 ml = _____ fl. ℥

29. 95.4° F = _____ ° C

30. 35.6° C = _____ ° F

31. 103.2° F = _____ ° C

32. 40.8° C = _____ ° F

33. 104.2° F = _____ ° C

34. 37.2° C = _____ ° F

35. 99.4° F = _____ ° C

36. 33.8° C = _____ ° F

Answers on p. 425.

POSTTEST 2

Name _____

Date _____

ACCEPTABLE SCORE __**32**__

YOUR SCORE _____

Directions: Change to approximate equivalents as indicated. Solve the problems by using proportions. Show your work.

1. 4.3 ml = _____ ℥

2. 60 lb = _____ kg

3. 2500 ml = _____ qt

4. 4 gr = _____ g

5. 1¼ pt = _____ ml

6. ¼ gr = _____ mg

7. 1.25 L = _____ qt

8. 20 mg = _____ gr

9. 22½ ℥ = _____ ml

10. 20 lb = _____ g

11. ¾ pt = _____ ml

12. 2⅜ qt = _____ ml

13. 3 g = _____ gr

14. $^1/_{120}$ gr = _____ mg

15. 10 fl. ℥ = _____ ml

16. 7 gr = _____ g

17. 3½ qt = _____ L

18. 1500 ml = _____ pt

19. 1200 g = _____ lb

20. 10 ♏ = _____ ml

21. 0.8 mg = _____ gr

22. 42 kg = _____ lb

23. 12 fl. ℥ = _____ ml

24. $^1/_{20}$ gr = _____ mg

25. 1.4 ml = _____ ♏

26. 1.3 g = _____ gr

27. 3½ lb = _____ g

28. 10 ml = _____ fl. ℥

29. 96.2° F = _____ ° C

30. 38.2° C = _____ ° F

31. 36.8° C = _____ ° F

32. 97.8° F = _____ ° C

33. 40.4° C = _____ ° F

34. 100.8° F = _____ ° C

35. 41.4° C = _____ ° F

36. 103.2° F = _____ ° C

Answers on p. 425.

Part III | *Calculation of Drug Dosages*

Chapter 9

Interpretation of the Physician's Orders

Learning Objectives

On completion of the materials provided in this chapter, you will be able to successfully complete a patient's medication administration record based on a physician's order.

Administration of medications is one of the most important responsibilities of the nurse. For medications to be administered safely and effectively, the nurse must know how to interpret the physician's medication orders.

Written Orders

The physician prescribes medications. In hospitals and health care centers, the physician uses a physician's order sheet, which is part of the patient's hospital chart or record. The orders are written for a drug to be given until a stated date and time, until a certain amount of the medication has been given, or until the order is changed or discontinued.

The physician's order requires the date the order was written, the name and dosage of the drug, the route and frequency of administration, and any special instructions. For drugs ordered as needed (p.r.n.), the purpose for administration is also added. The physician's signature is required each time orders are written. In many institutions the time that the order is written is also encouraged. However, if the time is not included, the order is still valid.

To interpret the medication order, the nurse must know the terminology, abbreviations, and symbols used in writing medical prescriptions and orders for medications. A list of the most frequently used abbreviations and symbols relating to medications is listed in Table 9-1. Memorize this list. Refer to the Glossary for help with unfamiliar terms.

Verbal Orders

Although verbal orders are discouraged as routine policy, certain situations or emergencies may require telephone orders. Such orders are generally initiated by the nurse. The order must include the same information as the written order: the date the order is recorded, the name and dosage of the drug, the route and frequency of administration, and any special instructions. After the nurse has recorded the orders on the patient's chart, the orders must be repeated to the physician for verification. The physician's name, notation that this is a telephone order, and the nurse's signature are required. The physician should sign the verbal orders as soon as possible.

Example: 1/18/94   Demerol 100 mg I.M. q.4 h. p.r.n. for pain
             1400   T.O. Dr. James T. Smith/Helen Alexander, R.N.

Scheduling the Administration of Medications

The physician's orders provide guidelines for the nurse when planning when each medication will be given to the patient. The purpose for prescribing the medication, drug interactions, absorption of the drug, or side effects caused by the drug may determine when the drug is given. The prescribed order may be very specific or may give the nurse latitude in scheduling.

Most hospitals and health care centers have routine times for administering medications. These times may differ from one hospital to another, but the guidelines assist the nurse in planning a medication routine that is safe for the patient. Table 9-1 will assist in planning times for administering each medication.

TABLE 9-1   *Recommended Times for Administering Medications*

Abbreviations	Definition	Recommended times of administration
a.c.*	Before meals	7:30-11:30-5:30
A.M.	Morning, before noon	9 A.M.
b.i.d.	Twice a day	9-9
h.s.	At bedtime	9 P.M.
p.c.*	After meals	8:30-11:30-6:30
p.r.n.	As needed	
q.d.	Once a day	9 A.M.
q.h.	Every hour	8-9-10-etc.
q.2 h.	Every 2 hours	8-10-12-etc.
q.3 h.	Every 3 hours	9-12-3-etc.
q.4 h.	Every 4 hours	8-12-4-etc.
q.6 h.	Every 6 hours	9-3-9-3
q.8 h.	Every 8 hours	8-4-12
q.12 h.	Every 12 hours	9-9
q.i.d.	Four times a day	8-12-4-8
q.o.d.	Every other day	
q.o.h.	Every other hour	8-10-12-2-4-6-etc.
s.o.s.	Once if necessary	
STAT	Immediately	
t.i.d.	Three times a day	9-1-5

*Providing that meals are served at 8:00 A.M., 12:00 noon, and 6:00 P.M.

Many hospitals use military time rather than ante meridiem (A.M.) and post meridiem (P.M.) time. Table 9-2 will assist in conversion from military time. Military time can be computed quickly by adding 12 to P.M. time—for example, 12 + 3 = 1500 hours.

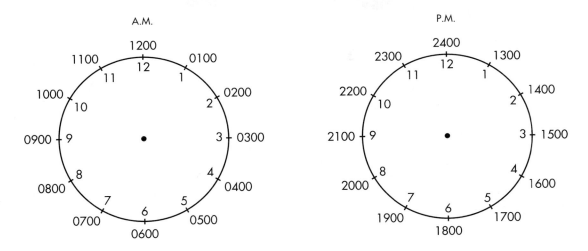

TABLE 9-2   *Conversion from Military Time to* A.M.–P.M. *Time*

0100—1:00 A.M.	0900—9:00 A.M.	1700—5:00 P.M.
0200—2:00 A.M.	1000—10:00 A.M.	1800—6:00 P.M.
0300—3:00 A.M.	1100—11:00 A.M.	1900—7:00 P.M.
0400—4:00 A.M.	1200—12:00 noon	2000—8:00 P.M.
0500—5:00 A.M.	1300—1:00 P.M.	2100—9:00 P.M.
0600—6:00 A.M.	1400—2:00 P.M.	2200—10:00 P.M.
0700—7:00 A.M.	1500—3:00 P.M.	2300—11:00 P.M.
0800—8:00 A.M.	1600—4:00 P.M.	2400—12:00 midnight

Introduction to Drug Dosages

The nurse obtains the medication from the pharmacy or from an available supply on the clinical unit, prepares the dosage, and administers the medication. Unit dosages are prepared in individual doses by the manufacturer and are ready for the nurse to administer.

Most medications are secured in the required dosage. However, problems of drug calculation arise when a drug is not manufactured in the strength required by the patient, the drug is not available in the strength ordered, or the drug is ordered in one system of measurement but is available only in another system of measurement.

When you change from one system of measurement to another, you have an equivalent measure that may or may not be exact. Therefore the answer to your problem may vary according to the system of measurement used. For example, if you change the required dosage to the available dosage, the equivalent dosage may be different than if you changed the available dosage to the required dosage. All problems in this book are calculated by changing the required dosage to the available dosage. The answers reflect this method of calculation. This is good practice because you have the medication on hand in the dosage provided.

The nurse is ethically and legally responsible for the medications administered to the patient. Even though the physician writes the order for the medication to be given to the patient, or even if the pharmacy prepares the wrong medication, the nurse who administers the medication is responsible for the error. Before preparing the drug, the nurse *must know* the maximum and minimum dosages, and the actions and contraindications for each administered drug. In addition, the nurse should consult the patient and the patient's medical record for any known allergies.

The Five Rights of Medication Administration

Because the nurse is legally responsible for ensuring that medications are correctly administered, the following five rights of medication administration listed in the box must be assiduously checked.

1. Drug
2. Dose
3. Patient
4. Route
5. Time

A sixth right, the right documentation, might also be included. Anytime these rights are not checked in the preparation and administration of medications, an error may occur for which the nurse is legally responsible.

When preparing medications for administration, the information on the medication profile sheet or drug card should be checked *three* times:
1. As the medicine is taken from the drawer or shelf
2. As the medicine is prepared
3. As the medicine is replaced

If unit doses are used, the label should be checked three times. It is critical that all calculations are done accurately and checked. It is especially important to check computations involving fractions and decimals. Many nurses use calculators. In some institutions certain medications (for example, heparin and insulin) are to be checked by another nurse before administering the medicine to the patient. Always use the appropriate measuring devices.

When administering the medication, *ALWAYS* call the patient by his or her name, and *ALWAYS* check the patient's identification armband.

Medications can be ordered by various routes. However, they must be administered only by the route included in the physician's order. Never assume the route by which the medication is to be given. If the route has not been included in the order, the physician must be notified to clarify the route requested.

Timing is very important—both the time of day and the interval between doses. With all medications, judgment and assessment by the nurse are required as to whether the medication should be given or held.

Medication Administration Record: Documentation has become more and more important for legal purposes. Remember that documentation of medications administered must include the five components of drug, dose, patient, route, and time. It is also necessary to document if a medication has been held or refused. Each facility has its own policy concerning the full documentation of medications. The official medication administration record (commonly called the patient's MAR) varies in format from one institution to another. It is mandatory that all documentation be legible, and it usually is written in blue or black ink.

In most institutions, personnel other than nurses perform the transcription of the physician's orders to the patient's MAR. Nurses are then required to verify the transcription against the physician's order and to place their initials on the form indicating the transcription was correctly completed.

Figure 9-1 represents examples of *A*, a physician's order, and *B*, a patient's MAR. Notice that the appropriate drug interpretations for the MAR include the patient's name, the medication name, the date, the drug dosage, the medication route, and the medication schedule.

PHYSICIAN'S ORDERS

Patient, James A.

1. ADDRESSOGRAPH BEFORE PLACING IN PATIENT'S CHART ▶
2. INITIAL AND DETACH COPY EACH TIME PHYSICIAN WRITES ORDERS
3. TRANSMIT COPY TO PHARMACY
4. ORDERS MUST BE DATED AND TIMED

DATE	ORDERS			TRANS BY
	Diagnosis:	Weight:	Height:	
	Sensitivities/Drug Allergies:			
1/12/99	0900	Lasix 80 mg. p.o. b.i.d.		
		Digoxin 0.125 mg. p.o. q.d.		
		Slow-K 10 mEq. p.o. b.i.d.		
		A. Physician, M.D.		

Do Not Write Orders If No Copies Remain; Begin New Form   Copies ——— Remaining

MEDICAL RECORDS COPY	**PHYSICIAN'S ORDERS**								**T-5**
B-CLIN. NOTES	E-LAB	G-X-RAY	K-DIAGNOSTIC	M-SURGERY	Q-THERAPY	T-ORDERS	W-NURSING	Y-MISC.	

A

Transcription of Med Sheet by: _____

Reviewed by: _____   Page _____ of _____

Patient, James A.

Initials	Signature
NJ	N. Jones R.N.
AN	A. Nurse R.N.

Allergies: ☑ NKDA

Injection Sites:
A = RUE E = Abdomen
B = LUE F = R Glut
C = RLE G = L Glut
D = LLE

Special Notes:

☐ Inpatient   ☐ Outpatient

See Legend on Back

DATE	DRUG				08 09 10 11	12 13 14 15	16 17 18 19	20 21 22 23	24 01 02 03	04 05 06 07	1/12/99	1/13/99	1/15/99	1/16/99	1/17/99
1 1/12	Lasix										09 AN 21 AN	09 NJ 21 NJ			
	80 mg dose	p.o. route	b.i.d. interval		09		21								
2 1/12	Digoxin										09 AN	09 NJ			
	0.125 mg dose	p.o. route	q.d. interval		09										
3 1/12	Slow-K										09 AN 21 AN	09 NJ 21 NJ			
	10 mEq dose	p.o. route	b.i.d. interval		09		21								
4															
	dose	route	interval												
5															
	dose	route	interval												

MEDICATION PROFILE

B-CLIN. NOTES	E-LAB	G-X-RAY	K-DIAGNOSTIC	M-SURGERY	Q-THERAPY	T-ORDERS	W-NURSING	Y-MISC.

B

FIGURE 9-1
Examples of physician's orders **(A)** and patient's medication administration record **(B)** with appropriate drug interpretations. (Forms courtesy Clarian Health—Indiana University.)

POSTTEST

Name _____

Date _____

ACCEPTABLE SCORE ___**17**___

YOUR SCORE _____

Directions: Copy the following physician's orders onto the medication record sheet below. Be sure to schedule the times for each drug administration.

PHYSICIAN'S ORDERS

Patient, James A.

1. ADDRESSOGRAPH BEFORE PLACING IN PATIENT'S CHART ▶

2. INITIAL AND DETACH COPY EACH TIME PHYSICIAN WRITES ORDERS

3. TRANSMIT COPY TO PHARMACY

4. ORDERS MUST BE DATED AND TIMED

DATE	ORDERS			TRANS BY
	Diagnosis:	Weight:	Height:	
	Sensitivities/Drug Allergies:			
1/12/99	0800 Cefuroxime $\frac{.}{1}$ Gm. IV q. 8 hours			
	Lasix 40 mg. p.o. b.i.d.			
	Slow-K 10 mEq. p.o. b.i.d.			
	A. Physician, M.D.			

Transcription of Med Sheet by: _____

Reviewed by: _____ Page _____ of _____

Patient, James A.

Initials   Signature

_____ _____

_____ _____

_____ _____

_____ _____

_____ _____

_____ _____

Allergies:	☐ NKDA	Injection Sites:
		A = RUE
		B = LUE E = Abdomen
		C = RLE F = R Glut
		D = LLE G = L Glut

Special Notes:

See Legend on Back

☐ Inpatient ☐ Outpatient

DATE	DRUG	08 09 10 11	12 13 14 15	16 17 18 19	20 21 22 23	24 01 02 03	04 05 06 07	DATES									
1 /	dose route interval																
2 /	dose route interval																
3 /	dose route interval																
4 /	dose route interval																
5 /	dose route interval																

Answers on p. 426.

Chapter 10 | *How to Read Drug Labels*

Learning Objectives

On completion of the materials provided in this chapter, you will be able to identify the following parts of each drug label:

1 | Trade name of medication

2 | Generic name of medication

3 | Strength of the medication dosage

4 | Form in which the medication is provided

5 | Route of administration

6 | Total amount or volume of medication provided in container

7 | Directions for mixing of medication if required

The safe administration of medications to patients begins with the nurse accurately reading and interpreting the drug label. Thus it is important for the nurse to be familiar and comfortable with the information that is found on the drug label.

Parts of a Drug Label

1. TRADE NAME. Trade names are usually capitalized and written in bold print. They are the first name written on the label. The trade name is always followed by the ® registration symbol. Different manufacturers market the same medication under different trade names.

2. GENERIC NAME. The generic name is the official name of the drug. Each drug has only *one* generic name. This name appears directly under the trade name, usually in smaller or different type letters. Physicians may order a patient's medication by generic or trade name. Nurses need to be familiar with both names and cross-check references as needed. Occasionally, only the generic name will appear on the label.

3. DOSAGE STRENGTH. The strength indicates the amount or weight of the medication that is supplied in the specific unit of measure. This amount may be per capsule, tablet, or milliliter.

4. FORM. The form indicates how the drug is supplied. Examples of various forms are tablets, capsules, liquids, suppositories, or ointments.

5. ROUTE. The label will indicate how the drug is to be administered. The route can be oral, topical, injection, or intravenous.

6. AMOUNT. The total amount of volume of the medication may be indicated. Some examples are 250 milliliters of oral suspension, or a bottle that contains 50 capsules.

7. DIRECTIONS. Some medications must be mixed before use. The amounts and types of diluent required will be listed along with the resulting strengths of the medication.

Other information may be found on drug labels: the name of the manufacturer, expiration date, special instructions for storage, and an NDC (National Drug Code) number.

Examples of Reading Drug Labels

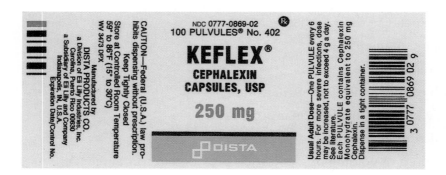

1. Trade name ....Keflex
2. Generic name............................cephalexin
3. Dosage strength........................250 mg
4. Form ....capsules
5. Amount.....................................100
6. Directions.................................Keep tightly closed. Store at controlled room temperature 59°
   to 86° F (15° to 30° C).
7. NDC number...........................0777-0869-02
8. Manufacturer...........................DISTA

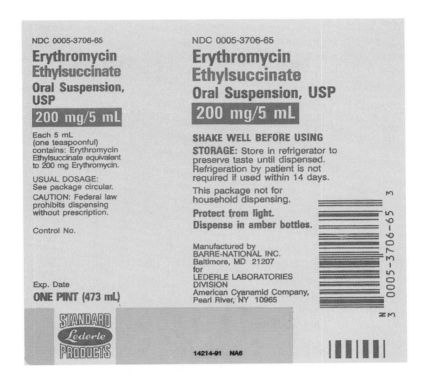

1. Trade name......................Erythromycin
2. Generic name ....erythromycin ethylsuccinate
3. Dosage strength ....200 mg/5 ml
4. Form...............................suspension
5. Route..............................oral
6. Amount...........................1 pint or 473 ml
7. Directions ....Shake well before using. Storage: Store in refrigerator to preserve taste until dispensed. Refrigeration by patient is not required if used within 14 days. Protect from light. Dispense in amber bottles.
8. NDC number 0005-3706-65
9. Manufacturer ....Barre-National Inc. for Lederle Laboratories Division

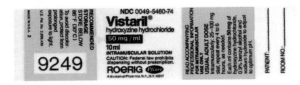

1. Trade name...............................Vistaril
2. Generic name ....hydroxyzine hydrochloride
3. Dosage strength/form...............50 mg/ml
4. Route.......................................intramuscular injection
5. Amount....................................total amount of 10 ml in vial
6. Directions ....Recommended storage directions listed.
7. NDC..0049-5460-74

Occasionally a drug label will only have one name listed. The one name is the generic name. These are drugs that have been in use for many years and are very well known. The drug companies do not market under a different trade name. They all simply use the generic name.

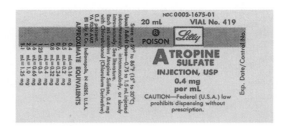

1. Trade name ....none
2. Generic name ....atropine sulfate
3. Dosage strength ....0.4 mg per ml
4. Form..................................milliliters
5. Route.................................injection
6. Amount.............................20 ml
7. NDC number 0002-1675-01

Study the material and examples of reading drug labels. When you feel ready to evaluate your learning, take the first posttest. Check your answers. An acceptable score as indicated on the posttest signifies that you are ready for the next chapter. An unacceptable score signifies a need for further study before taking the second posttest.

POSTTEST 1

Name _____

Date _____

ACCEPTABLE SCORE __**18**__

YOUR SCORE _____

Directions: Identify the requested part of each of the following medication labels.

NDC 0028-0023-61 FSC 2503

Lioresal® **10**mg

baclofen

100 tablets—Unit Dose

Caution: Federal law prohibits dispensing without prescription.

Geigy

1. Trade name _____
   Generic name _____
   Dosage strength _____
   Form _____
   Amount _____

NDC 0663-3940-71

250 Tablets

6505-00-817-2279

Diabinese®

chlorpropamide

250 mg

CAUTION: Federal law prohibits dispensing without prescription.

Pfizer Distributed by LABORATORIES DIVISION
New York, N.Y. 10017

2. Trade name _____
   Generic name _____
   Dosage strength _____
   Form _____
   Amount _____

To open—Cut seal along dotted line

Exp.

Lot

NDC 0031-7890-95

Twenty-Five **2 ml** Single Dose Vials

Robinul®Injectable

Brand of

Glycopyrrolate Injection, USP

0.4 mg/2 ml

(0.2 mg/ml)

Water for Injection, USP q.s./Benzyl Alcohol, NF (preservative) 0.9%.

pH adjusted, when necessary, with hydrochloric acid and/or sodium hydroxide.

For I.M. or I.V. administration.

For dosage and other directions for use, consult accompanying product literature.

Store at Controlled Room Temperature, Between 15°C and 30°C (59°F and 86°F).

CAUTION: Federal law prohibits dispensing without prescription.

MANUFACTURED FOR PHARMACEUTICAL DIVISION
A. H. ROBINS COMPANY, RICHMOND, VA. 23220
by ELKINS-SINN, INC., CHERRY HILL, N.J. 08034
a subsidiary of A.H. Robins Company   10.81

A·H·ROBINS

3. Trade name _____

Generic name _____

Dosage strength _____

Form _____

Route _____

100 ml

75 ml

50 ml

25 ml

APPROX VOLUME SCALE

PHARMACY BULK PACKAGE

Add Sterile Water for Injection –shake well

Amount of Diluent	Concentration of Solution
95ml	100 mg/ml

Reconstitute by adding 95 ml of Sterile Water for Injection in two separate aliquots. Add 45 ml, shake to dissolve and add 50 ml, shake for final solution. The resulting solution will contain 100 mg/ml of cefoperazone. Transfer individual doses to appropriate intravenous infusion solutions. Discard unused solution from bulk package within 24 hours after initial entry. After reconstitution, no significant loss of potency occurs for 24 hours at room temperature and for 5 days if refrigerated. Discard unused transferred solutions held longer than these time periods.

MADE IN U.S.A.   05-4482-77-2

NDC 0049-1219-28

Cefobid®

sterile cefoperazone sodium, USP

PHARMACY BULK PACKAGE NOT FOR DIRECT INFUSION

equivalent to

10g

of cefoperazone

10

For Intravenous Use

CAUTION: Federal law prohibits dispensing without prescription.

ROERIG *Pfizer*

A division of Pfizer Inc. N.Y. N.Y. 10017

Reconstituted bulk solution should not be used for direct infusion.

RECOMMENDED STORAGE IN DRY FORM

STORE BELOW 77°F (25°C) PROTECT FROM LIGHT

READ ACCOMPANYING PACKAGE INSERT FOR PROFESSIONAL INFORMATION INCLUDING DILUTION, DOSAGE AND ADMINISTRATION, AND THE USE OF PHARMACY BULK PACKAGE.

DATE PREPARED _____

TIME _____

25 ml

50 ml

75 ml

100 ml

APPROX VOLUME SCALE

4. Trade name _____

Generic name _____

Dosage strength _____

Form _____

Route _____

Answers on p. 426.

POSTTEST 2

Name _____

Date _____

ACCEPTABLE SCORE __**18**__

YOUR SCORE _____

Directions: Identify the requested parts of each of the following medication's labels.

NDC 0149-0735-15
LIST 73515

5 mg/ml

Furadantin®
(nitrofurantoin)
oral suspension

Store below 86°F (30°C).
Protect from freezing.
SHAKE VIGOROUSLY TO
BREAK GEL.

URINARY TRACT ANTIBACTERIAL

60 ml

CAUTION: Federal law prohibits dispensing without prescription.

USUAL ADULT DOSE: 50 to 100 mg q.i.d. with meals and with food or milk on retiring.
CHILDREN: 2.2 to 3.2 mg per lb of body weight per 24 hours.
Each teaspoonful (5 ml) contains 25 mg Furadantin, brand of nitrofurantoin.

Manufactured by   73515-L9
Eaton Laboratories, Inc.   © 1984
Manati, Puerto Rico 00701   NEPI
Distributed by
Norwich Eaton Pharmaceuticals, Inc.
Norwich, New York 13815
A Procter & Gamble Company

Norwich Eaton

1. Trade name _____
   Generic name _____
   Dosage strength _____
   Form _____
   Route _____
   Amount _____

USUAL ADULT DOSAGE:
See accompanying circular.

Dispense in a well-closed container.

CAUTION: Federal (USA) law prohibits dispensing without prescription.

50 | No. 7638   7605309

MSD   NDC 0006-0095-50

50 TABLETS

Decadron®
(Dexamethasone, MSD)

DECADRON

1.5 mg

MERCK SHARP & DOHME
DIVISION OF MERCK & CO., INC.
WEST POINT, PA 19486, USA

Lot   Exp.

2. Trade name _____
   Generic name _____
   Dosage strength _____
   Form _____

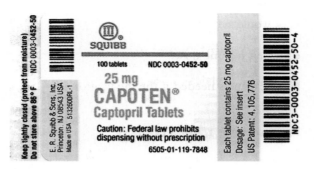

3. Trade name _____
    Generic name _____
    Dosage strength _____
    Form _____
    Amount _____

NDC 0002-1497-01
VIAL No. 767
℞   *Lilly*
KEFZOL®
STERILE
CEFAZOLIN
SODIUM, USP
Equiv. to
500 mg
Cefazolin

4. Trade name _____
    Generic name _____
    Dosage strength _____
    Form _____
    Route _____

Answers on p. 426.

Chapter 11 | *Oral Dosages*

Learning Objectives

On completion of the materials provided in this chapter, you will be able to perform computations accurately by mastering the following mathematical concepts:

1. Convert all measures within the problem to equivalent measures in one system of measurement

2. Use a proportion to solve problems of oral dosage involving tablets, capsules, or liquid medications

3. Use a proportion to solve problems of oral dosages of medications measured in milliequivalents

4. Use the stated formula as an alternative method of solving oral-drug dosage problems

Oral drugs are the preferred choice for administration of medications because they are easy to take and convenient for the patient. Oral medications are safe because they can be taken through the gastrointestinal tract; therefore the skin is not interrupted. Oral medications may be more economical because the production cost is usually lower than for other forms of medication.

Oral medications are absorbed primarily in the small intestine. Because of the differences in absorption factors, they might not be as effective as other forms of medication. Some oral medications are irritating to the alimentary canal and must be given with meals or a snack. Others may be harmful to the teeth and should be taken through a straw or feeding tube.

Oral medications are supplied in a variety of forms (Figure 11-1). The most common form is a tablet. Tablets come in many colors, sizes, and shapes. A tablet is produced from a drug powder. The tablet may be grooved for ease in administering only a fraction of the whole tablet. Some tablets are scored into halves and others are divided into fourths.

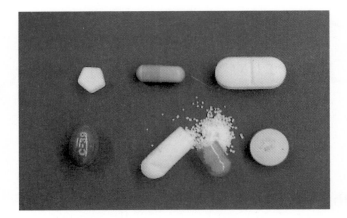

FIGURE 11-1
Forms of solid oral medication. *(From Elkin M, Perry A, Potter P:* Nursing interventions and clinical skills, *St Louis, 1996, Mosby.)*

Oral medications also may be supplied in capsule form. A capsule is a hard or soft gelatin that houses a powder, liquid, or granular form of a specific medicine(s). Capsules are produced in a variety of sizes and colors (Figure 11-2). Capsules cannot be divided or crushed.

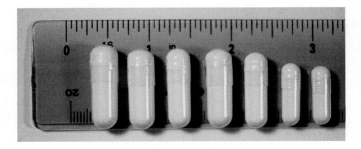

FIGURE 11-2
Various sizes and numbers of gelatin capsules (actual size).

Oral medications also may be administered in liquid form such as an elixir or an oral suspension. Oral liquid medications can be measured with a syringe, dropper, or medication cup (Figures 11-3 and 11-4).

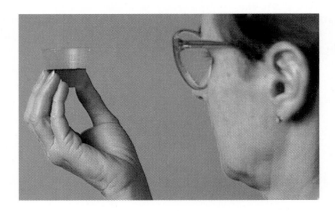

FIGURE 11-3
Oral liquid medication measured with a medication cup. *(From Potter P:* Fundamentals of nursing, *ed 4, St Louis, 1997, Mosby.)*

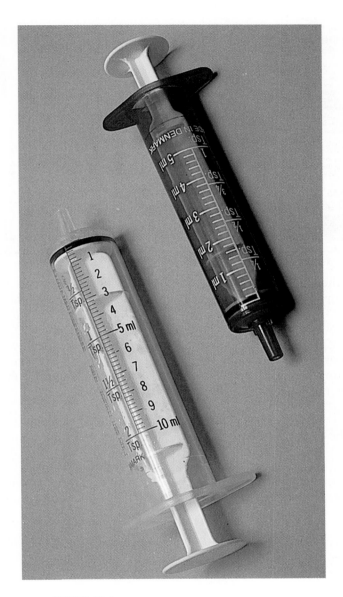

FIGURE 11-4
Plastic oral syringe. *(Courtesy Chuck Dresner.)*

Oral Dosages Involving Capsules and Tablets

Example: ASA gr xx p.o. q.i.d. ASA tablets gr v are available. Give _____ .

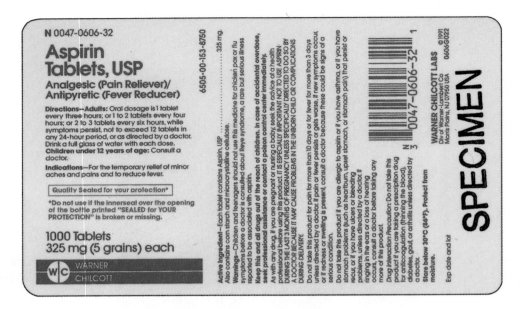

a. On the left side of the proportion place what you know or have available. In this example, each tablet contains 5 grains. So the left side of the proportion would be

1 tablet : 5 gr ::

b. The right side of the proportion is determined by the physician's order and the abbreviations used on the left side of the proportion. Only *two* different abbreviations may be used in a single proportion. The abbreviations must be in the same position on the right as they are on the left.

1 tablet : 5 gr :: _____ tablet : _____ gr

In the example, the physician has ordered gr xx or 20 grains.

1 tablet : 5 gr :: _____ tablet : 20 gr

We need to find the number of tablets to be given, so we use the symbol x to represent the unknown. Therefore the full proportion would be

1 tablet : 5 gr :: x tablet : 20 gr

c. Rewrite the proportion without using the abbreviations.

1 : 5 :: x : 20

d. Solve for x.

$$5x = 1 \times 20$$
$$5x = 20$$
$$x = \frac{20}{5}$$
$$x = 4$$

e. Label your answer, as determined by the abbreviation placed next to x in the original proportion.

20 gr = 4 tablets

Sometimes the physician's order is in one system of measurement, and the drug is supplied in another system of measurement. It is therefore necessary to convert one of the measurements so that they are both in either the apothecaries' or the metric system of measurement. After this is done, another proportion will be written to calculate the actual drug dosage.

Example: Ampicillin 0.5 g p.o. q.i.d. The drug is supplied in 250 mg capsules.
            Give _____ .

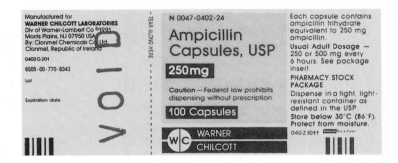

The physician's order is in grams and the drug is supplied in milligrams. The order and the supplied drug must be in the same metric measurement because only two different abbreviations can be used in each proportion. Therefore first convert 0.5 g to milligrams.

$$1000 \text{ mg} : 1 \text{ g} :: x \text{ mg} : 0.5 \text{ g}$$

$$1000 : 1 :: x : 0.5$$

$$1x = 1000 \times 0.5$$

$$x = 500 \text{ mg}$$

$$0.5 \text{ g} = 500 \text{ mg}$$

Now that the order and the supplied drug are in the same metric measurement, a proportion may be written to calculate the amount of the drug to be given.

a. 250 mg : 1 capsule ::

b. 250 mg : 1 capsule :: _____ mg : _____ capsule
    250 mg : 1 capsule :: 500 mg : x capsule

c. $250 : 1 :: 500 : x$

d. $250x = 1 \times 500$

   $250x = 500$

   $x = \dfrac{500}{250}$

   $x = 2$

e. $x = 2$ capsules. Therefore 2 capsules, or 0.5 g, of the medication ordered would be given to the patient.

How many capsules will be given in 1 day? _____

The drug is to be given q.i.d., or four times a day.

a. 2 capsules : 1 dose ::

b. 2 capsules : 1 dose :: _____ capsules : _____ dose
    2 capsules : 1 dose :: x capsules : 4 doses

c. $2 : 1 :: x : 4$

d. $1x = 2 \times 4$

   $x = 8$

e. 8 capsules will be given each day.

Oral Dosages Involving Liquids

Example: Phenobarbital gr ¾ p.o. b.i.d. Phenobarbital elixir 20 mg per 5 ml is available. Give _____ .

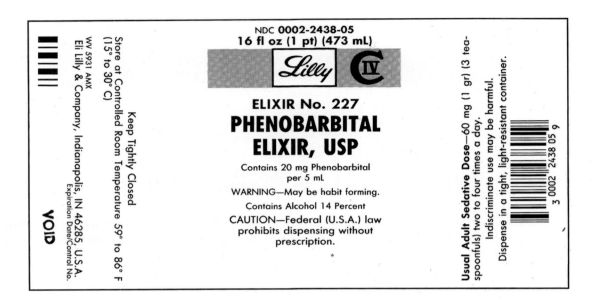

The physician's order is in the apothecaries' system and the drug is available in the metric system. Both the order and the available drug must be in the same system of measurement. Therefore convert gr ¾ to milligrams.

$$60 \text{ mg} : 1 \text{ gr} :: x \text{ mg} : \text{¾ gr}$$

$$60 : 1 :: x : \text{¾}$$

$$x = \frac{\overset{15}{\cancel{60}}}{1} \times \frac{3}{\underset{1}{\cancel{4}}}$$

$$x = \frac{15 \times 3}{1 \times 1}$$

$$x = \frac{45}{1}$$

$$x = 45 \text{ mg}$$

$$\text{gr ¾} = 45 \text{ mg}$$

Now that the order and available drug are in the same system of measurement, a proportion may be written to calculate the actual amount of the drug to be administered.

    a. 20 mg : 5 ml ::

    b. 20 mg : 5 ml :: _____ mg : _____ ml

       20 mg : 5 ml :: 45 mg : x ml

    c. 20 : 5 :: 45 : x

d. $20x = 5 \times 45$

$20x = 225$

$x = \dfrac{225}{20}$

$x = 11.25$

e. $x = 11.25$ ml. Therefore 11.25 ml is the amount of each individual dose b.i.d.

Example: Thorazine 20 mg p.o. q.4 h. The drug is available in ℥ iv bottles of Thorazine syrup containing 10 mg per 5 ml. Give _____ . How many doses are available in ℥ iv? _____ .

1. a. 10 mg : 5 ml ::
   b. 10 mg : 5 ml :: _____ mg : _____ ml
      10 mg : 5 ml :: 20 mg : x ml
   c. 10 : 5 :: 20 : x
   d. $10x = 5 \times 20$

   $10x = 100$

   $x = \dfrac{100}{10}$

   $x = 10$

   e. $x = 10$ ml. Therefore 10 ml is the amount of each individual dose q.4 h.

2. The physician's order is in the metric system and the drug is supplied in the apothecaries' system. Both the order and the available drug must be in the same system of measurement. Therefore convert 10 ml to ℥, or the ℥ iv to ml, whichever is easier.

$$30 \text{ ml} : 1 \text{ fl. } ℥ :: x \text{ ml} : 4 \text{ fl. } ℥$$

$$30 : 1 :: x : 4$$

$$x = 120$$

$$℥ \text{ iv bottle} = 120 \text{ ml}$$

Now that the order and available drug are in the same system of measurement, a proportion may be written to calculate the number of doses in a ℥ iv bottle.

a. 10 ml : 1 dose ::
b. 10 ml : 1 dose :: _____ ml : _____ dose
   10 ml : 1 dose :: 120 ml : x dose
c. 10 : 1 :: 120 : x
d. $10x = 120$

$x = \dfrac{120}{10}$

$x = 12$

e. $x = 12$ doses. Therefore each ℥ iv bottle contains 12 doses.

Oral Dosages Involving Milliequivalents

Example: KCl 60 mEq. KCl 40 mEq per 30 ml is available. Give _____ .

A **milliequivalent** is the number of grams of a solute contained in one milliliter of a normal solution. The milliequivalent is used in a drug dosage proportion, the same as a form of measurement in the apothecary or metric systems.

a. 40 mEq : 30 ml ::
b. 40 mEq : 30 ml :: _____ mEq : _____ ml
   40 mEq : 30 ml :: 60 mEq : x ml
c. 40 : 30 :: 60 : x
d. $40x = 30 \times 60$

$$40x = 1800$$

$$x = \frac{1800}{40}$$

$$x = 45$$

e. $x = 45$ ml

Alternative Formula Method of Oral Drug Dosage Calculation

There is a formula that has been used for many years in the calculation of drug dosages by nurses. I believe that the proportion method is the easiest method for new students to learn and use, allowing fewer mistakes to occur. However, the formula method may be the method that some students learned first in an earlier nursing role (e.g., a licensed practical nurse). If this is the case and the student accurately uses the formula method, I do not recommend changing to the proportion method. However, if calculations frequently have been difficult or incorrect, we recommend using the proportion method. Remember, choose the method that you feel is best for you and consistently use the chosen method. I do not recommend switching back and forth between the formula and proportion method.

$$\text{Formula: } \frac{D}{A} \times Q = x$$

Where
   D represents the desired amount of the medication that has been ordered by the physician

   A represents the strength of the medication that is available

   Q represents the quantity or amount of the medication that contains the available strength (*Note: When the medication is a solid such as a tablet, capsule, or caplet, the quantity will always be 1. If the medication is in liquid form, the number will vary. Remember from the math review, the denominator of a whole number is always one.* $\frac{1}{1}, \frac{2}{1}, \frac{3}{1},$ *etc.*)

   x represents the dosage that is unknown

This formula can be read as:

Desired over available multiplied by the quantity available equals x
or the amount to be given to the patient.

Let's go back to our first example in this chapter and use the formula method to calculate the drug dosage.

Example: ASA gr xx p.o. q.i.d. ASA tablets gr v are available.

$$\frac{D}{A} \times Q = x$$

a. The desired amount of ASA is gr xx or 20 grains. The available amount or strength the ASA supplied is gr v or 5 grains.

$$\frac{20}{5}$$

b. The quantity of the medication for gr v is 1 tablet.

$$\frac{20}{5} \times \frac{1}{1}$$

c. We can now solve for x.

$$x = \frac{20}{5} \times \frac{1}{1}$$

$$x = \frac{20 \times 1}{5 \times 1}$$

$$x = \frac{20}{5}$$

$$x = 4$$

d. Label your answer as determined by the quantity.

20 grains = 4 tablets

If the physician's order is in one system of measurement and the drug is supplied in another system of measurement, it will still be necessary to convert one of the measurements so that both are expressed in the same system. After this is done, the formula may be used to calculate the drug dosage to be administered.

Example: Ampicillin 0.5 g p.o. q.i.d. The drug is supplied in 250 mg capsules.

The physician's order is expressed in grams and the drug is supplied in milligrams. Therefore convert the order to milligrams as outlined in Chapter 8.

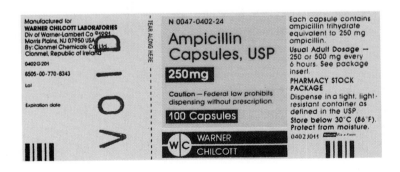

$$1000 \text{ mg} : 1 \text{ g} :: x \text{ mg} : 0.5 \text{ g}$$

$$1000 : 1 :: x : 0.5$$

$$1x = 1000 \times 0.5$$

$$x = 500 \text{ mg}$$

Now the numbers may be filled into the formula $\dfrac{D}{A} \times Q = x$.

   a. The desired amount of ampicillin is 500 mg. The available amount of strength of ampicillin supplied is 250 mg.

$$\frac{500}{250}$$

   b. The quantity available is in capsule form or 1.

$$\frac{500}{250} \times \frac{1}{1}$$

   c. Solve for x.

$$x = \frac{500}{250} \times \frac{1}{1}$$

$$x = \frac{500 \times 1}{250 \times 1}$$

$$x = \frac{500}{250}$$

$$x = 2$$

   d. Label your answer as determined by the quantity.

$$500 \text{ mg} = 2 \text{ capsules}$$

Formula Involving Liquids

Example: Phenobarbital gr ¾ p.o. b.i.d. Phenobarbital elixir 20 mg per 5 ml is available. Give _____ .

The physician's order is in the apothecaries' system and the drug is available in the metric system. Change the order to an equivalent within the metric system of measure as outlined in Chapter 8.

$$60 \text{ mg} : 1 \text{ gr} :: x \text{ mg} : \text{¾ gr}$$

$$60 : 1 :: x : \text{¾}$$

$$x = \frac{\overset{15}{\cancel{60}}}{1} \times \frac{3}{\underset{1}{\cancel{4}}}$$

$$x = 45$$

$$\text{gr ¾} = 45 \text{ mg}$$

Now the numbers may be filled into the formula $\frac{D}{A} \times Q = x$.

    a. The desired amount is 45 mg. The available amount or strength of phenobarbital is 20 mg.

$$\frac{45}{20}$$

    b. The quantity available is 5 ml.

$$\frac{45}{20} \times \frac{5}{1}$$

    c. Solve for x

$$x = \frac{45}{20} \times \frac{5}{1}$$

$$x = \frac{45}{\overset{}{\underset{4}{20}}} \times \frac{\overset{1}{\cancel{5}}}{1}$$

$$x = \frac{45 \times 1}{4 \times 1}$$

$$x = \frac{45}{4}$$

$$x = 11.25$$

    d. Label your answer as determined by the quantity.

$$45 \text{ mg} = 11.25 \text{ ml}$$

Complete the following work sheet, which provides for extensive practice in the calculation of oral dosage problems. Use either the proportion or formula method. Check your answers. It is sometimes impossible to administer the exact amount ordered. All capsules and those tablets not grooved are impossible to divide accurately. If the exact answer contains a fraction less than one half, drop the fraction and give the number of capsules or tablets indicated by the whole number. If the fraction is one half or more, round off to the nearest whole number to determine the number of tablets or capsules to be given. Note that in actual practice the physician would need to be notified and the order for the amount of medication changed to allow for giving more than the original prescribed amount. If you have difficulties, go back and review the necessary material. When you feel ready to evaluate your learning, take the first posttest. Check your answers. An acceptable score as indicated on the posttest signifies that you are ready for the next chapter. An unacceptable score signifies a need for further study before taking the second posttest.

WORK SHEET

Directions: The medication order is listed at the beginning of each problem. Calculate the oral dosages. Show your work. Shade each medicine cup when provided to indicate the correct dosage.

1.   The physician orders Minipress 2 mg p.o. b.i.d. for Mr. Shaw's high blood pressure. Give _____ .

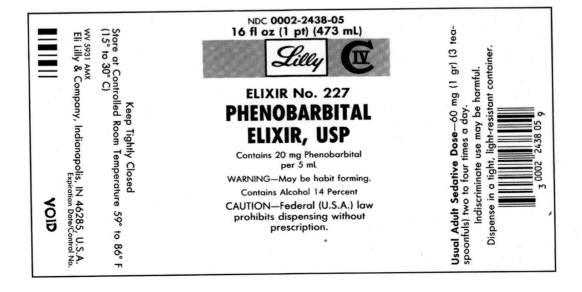

NDC 0663-4310-71

250 Capsules

Minipress®

prazosin hydrochloride

1 mg †

CAUTION: Federal law prohibits dispensing without prescription.

Distributed by **Pfizer** LABORATORIES DIVISION New York, N.Y. 10017

4444

6505-01-039-6320

RECOMMENDED STORAGE STORE BELOW 86° F (30° C) Dispense in tight, light resistant containers (USP).

†Each capsule contains prazosin hydrochloride equivalent to 1 mg of prazosin.

Manufactured by Pfizer Pharmaceuticals, Inc., Barceloneta, P.R. 00617

READ ACCOMPANYING PROFESSIONAL INFORMATION

DOSAGE: See accompanying prescribing information.

IMPORTANT: This closure is not child-resistant.

2.   Mrs. Taylor has a long history of seizures. Elixir of phenobarbital 30 mg p.o. q.12 h. is ordered. Give _____ .

NDC 0002-2438-05
16 fl oz (1 pt) (473 mL)

Lilly   C IV

ELIXIR No. 227
PHENOBARBITAL ELIXIR, USP

Contains 20 mg Phenobarbital per 5 mL

WARNING—May be habit forming.

Contains Alcohol 14 Percent

CAUTION—Federal (U.S.A.) law prohibits dispensing without prescription.

Store at Controlled Room Temperature 59° to 86° F (15° to 30° C)

Keep Tightly Closed

WV 5931 AMX Eli Lilly & Company, Indianapolis, IN 46285, U.S.A. Expiration Date/Control No.

VOID

Usual Adult Sedative Dose—60 mg (1 gr) (3 teaspoonfuls) two to four times a day. Indiscriminate use may be harmful. Dispense in a tight, light-resistant container.

3 0002 2438 05 9

3. Crystodigin 0.2 mg p.o. b.i.d. for 4 days, then 0.15 mg q.d. You have Crystodigin 0.05 mg tablets available. How many tablets would you give for each dose the first 4 days? _____ . How many tablets would you give for each dose thereafter? _____ .

4. The physician orders Thorazine gr ⅙ p.o. q.8 h. for Mr. Hine's nausea. Give _____ .

STORE AT CONTROLLED ROOM TEMPERATURE
DISPENSE IN A TIGHT, LIGHT-RESISTANT CONTAINER

Each tablet contains chlorpromazine hydrochloride, 50 mg.
Dosage: See package insert for dosage information.
Important: Use safety closures when dispensing this product unless otherwise directed by physician or requested by purchaser.

AE, LOT
EXPIRES

100 tablets
NDC 0007-5076-20

50mg.
Thorazine® brand of
chlorpromazine hydrochloride
Tablets
Smith Kline &French Laboratories
Div. of SmithKline Beckman Corporation, Phila., Pa. 19101

SPECIMEN
SK&F

CAUTION—Federal law prohibits dispensing without prescription.

5. Mrs. Clay complains of nausea. Compazine 2.5 mg p.o. t.i.d. is ordered. The stock supply is Compazine syrup 5 mg per 5 ml. Give _____ .

6. Temaril 2.5 mg p.o. q.4 h. The drug is supplied in ℥ iv bottles containing 2.5 mg per 5 ml. How many doses are available in ℥ iv? _____ .

7. Librium 10 mg p.o. q.6 h. has been ordered to treat Mr. Snow's anxiety disorder. You have Librium capsules gr $\frac{1}{12}$. Give _____ .

8. Mandelamine 1 g p.o. q.i.d. is scheduled for Mr. Eaton to treat his urinary tract infection. You have 0.5 g tablets available. Give _____ .

9. Your patient has Noctec ordered for his sleep pattern disturbance 0.5 g p.o. h.s. p.r.n. The drug is available as 500 mg per 5 ml. Give _____ ml.

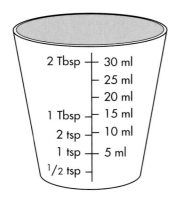

10. Mr. Scott has Parkinson's disease and is to receive Cogentin 1 mg p.o. at 1900. Give _____ .

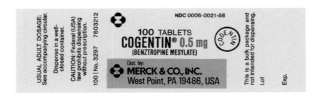

11. Mrs. Martin receives Motrin 300 mg p.o. t.i.d. for arthritis pain. The drug is supplied in gr v tablets. Give _____ .

12. Lithium carbonate 0.6 g p.o. b.i.d. The drug is supplied in 300 mg scored tablets. Give _____ . How many mg will be given each day? _____ .

13. Your patient has Naprosyn 0.25 g p.o. b.i.d. ordered for chronic back pain. You have Naprosyn 500 mg scored tablets available. Give _____ .

14. Mr. Hill is to receive Persantine 25 mg p.o. b.i.d. after valve surgery. Persantine 50 mg tablets are available. Give _____ .

15. The physician has ordered $FeSO_4$ 300 mg p.o. q.d. to treat Mrs. Basey's anemia. You have $FeSO_4$ gr v tablets available. Give _____ .

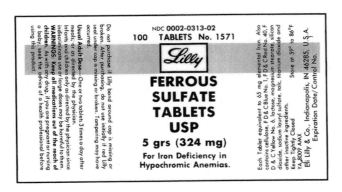

16. Gantrisin 4 g p.o. stat, then 2 g q.6 h. How many tablets are given for the stat dose? _____ . How many tablets are given for each of the 2 g doses? _____ .

17. Chloral hydrate 90 mg p.o. stat is ordered to treat Mr. Ritter's insomnia. Chloral hydrate 500 mg per 10 ml is available. Give _____ .

18. Gaviscon 30 ml p.o. q.i.d. p.c. h.s. Gaviscon is supplied in ℥ xii bottles. Each dose is equal to _____ ℥. How many ℥ would be given in 1 day? _____ .

19. Ms. Evans complains of a rash on her abdomen and has Benadryl 30 mg p.o. t.i.d. ordered. Give _____ .

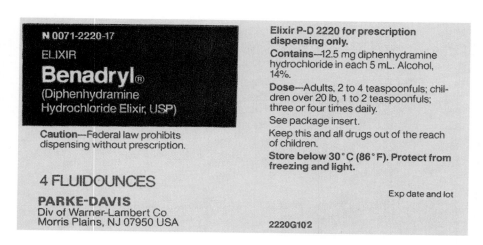

20. Mr. Gifford has had a lumbar laminectomy and requires pain medication. The patient has codeine 60 mg p.o. q.3 h. p.r.n. Give _____ .

21. The physician orders Keflex suspension 5.5 ml p.o. q.6 h. for your tonsillectomy patient. Give _____ mg/6 hours.

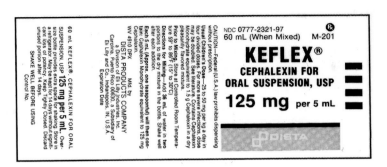

22. Mr. Sawyer is admitted with congestive heart failure. His orders require Lasix 80 mg p.o. q.d. Give _____ .

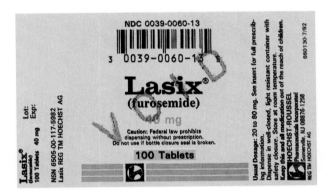

23. Achromycin-V 0.5 g p.o. q.i.d. The drug is available in 250 mg capsules. How many capsules will you give for one dose? _____ . How many capsules will the patient receive in 1 day? _____ .

24. Mr. Koehler suffers from rheumatoid arthritis and has Decadron 1.5 mg p.o. q.12 h. ordered. You have Decadron elixir 0.5 mg per 5 ml. Give _____ ml. Give _____ ʒ.

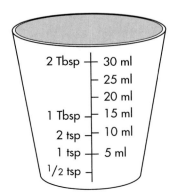

25. Your patient with chronic hiccups has Thorazine 15 mg p.o. q.4 h. ordered. The drug is available in ℥ iv bottles of Thorazine syrup containing 10 mg per 5 ml. Give _____ .

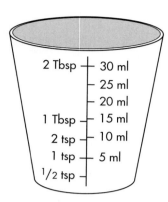

26. Mrs. Turner is admitted with hypertension. Apresoline 25 mg p.o. q.i.d. is ordered. You have 50 mg tablets available. Give _____ .

27. Your patient complains of indigestion during meals. Mylanta 30 ml p.o. p.c. q.i.d. is ordered. Mylanta is supplied in a ℥ xii bottle. There are _____ doses in a one ℥ xii bottle.

28. Thorazine 200 mg p.o. stat. The drug is available in 100 mg tablets. Give _____ .

29. Mr. Bates has a past history of seizure activity. Phenobarbital 15 mg p.o. q.3 h. is ordered. Give _____ .

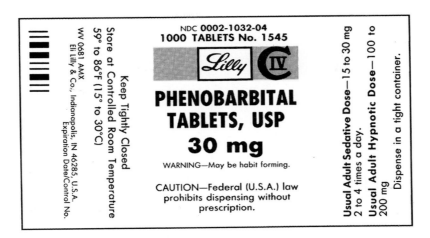

30. Mrs. Turner has chronic sinusitis. Her physician orders amoxicillin 125 mg p.o. q.8 h. Give _____ .

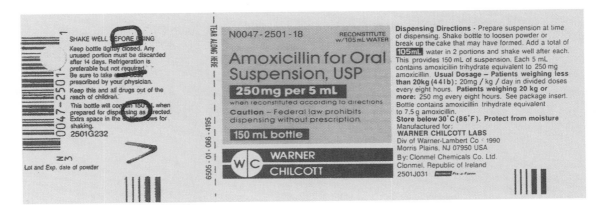

31. The physician prescribes Tenormin 25 mg p.o. q.4 h. for Mr. Hutton's high blood pressure. You have Tenormin 50 mg scored tablets available. Give _____ .

32. Quinidine 0.6 g p.o. q.4 h. Quinidine is supplied in 200 mg tablets. How many tablets would you give for one dose? _____ . How many tablets will be given in 24 hours? _____ .
.

33. Mrs. Farmer has Phenergan 12.5 mg p.o. t.i.d. ordered for nausea. The drug is available in syrup containing 6.25 mg per 5. Give _____ .

34. Your patient has Dalmane 30 mg p.o. h.s. for sleep. You have Dalmane capsules gr ¼ available. Give _____ .

35. Mr. Golden, recovering from a left great toe amputation, has Colace elixir 100 mg p.o. h.s. ordered for constipation. Give _____ .

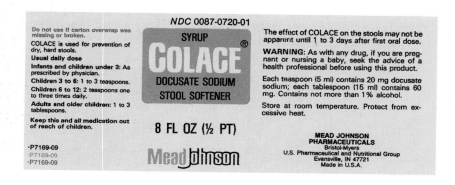

36. Your patient receives KCl 80 mEq p.o. q.d. for hypokalemia. Give _____ .

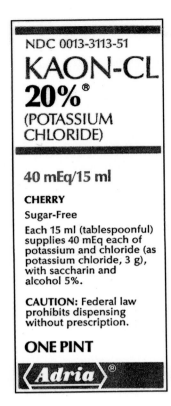

37. Mr. Mikal was admitted for leukemia and receives Deltasone 7.5 mg p.o. t.i.d. as part of his chemotherapy. The drug is available in 2.5 mg tablets. Give _____ .

38. The physician orders Tegretol 0.2 g p.o. t.i.d. for Mr. Pine's epilepsy. Give _____ .

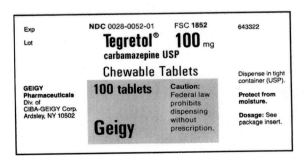

39. Elixir of Tylenol gr v p.o. t.i.d. is ordered for Mrs. Lindl's dysmenorrhea. You have the drug containing 160 mg per 5 ml. Give _____ .

40. Mrs. Cross was admitted with myasthenia crisis. Decadron 0.5 mg p.o. q.12 h. is ordered. Give _____ .

USUAL ADULT DOSAGE:
See accompanying circular.

This is a bulk package and not intended for dispensing.

CAUTION: Federal (USA) law prohibits dispensing without prescription.

100 | No. 7592 7273206

MSD   NDC 0006-0020-68
           100 TABLETS

Decadron
(Dexamethasone, MSD)

0.25 mg

MERCK SHARP & DOHME
DIVISION OF MERCK & CO. INC.
WEST POINT PA 19486 USA

Lot   Exp.

41. Mr. Cook requires medication for nausea. Compazine 10 mg p.o. q.4 h. p.r.n. is ordered. You have Compazine 5 mg tablets available. Give _____ .

42. Mr. Pace receives Atarax 100 mg p.o. h.s. p.r.n. to relieve anxiety. You have 50 mg tablets available. Give _____ .

43. The physician orders thyroid gr ss p.o. q.i.d. for Mrs. Grass's replacement hormone. Give _____ .

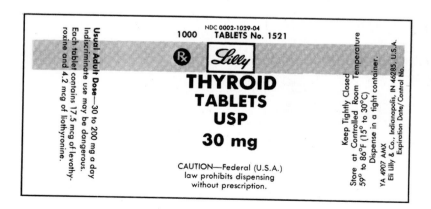

Usual Adult Dose—30 to 200 mg a day Indiscriminate use may be dangerous.
Each tablet contains 17.5 mcg of levothyroxine and 4.2 mcg of liothyronine.

NDC 0002-1029-04
1000   TABLETS No. 1521

Rx   **Lilly**

THYROID TABLETS USP

30 mg

CAUTION—Federal (U.S.A.)
law prohibits dispensing
without prescription.

Keep Tightly Closed
Store at Controlled Room Temperature
59° to 86°F (15° to 30°C)
Dispense in a tight container.
YA 4907 AMX
Eli Lilly & Co., Indianapolis, IN 46285, U.S.A.
Expiration Date/Control No.

44. Mr. Day receives Lanoxin 0.25 mg p.o. q.d. for atrial fibrillation. Give _____ .

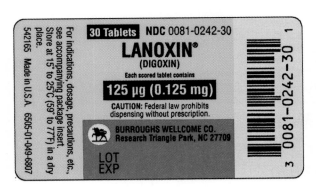

45. Mr. Payne receives Keflex 500 mg p.o. q.i.d. before his dental extraction. Give _____ capsules/dose. Give _____ capsules/day.

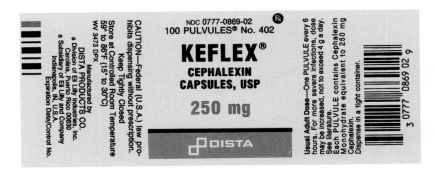

46. Mr. Tune is admitted with pancreatitis and receives Valium 5 mg p.o. q.6 h. p.r.n. for anxiety. You have 10 mg tablets available. Give _____ .

47. Mrs. Graves receives phenobarbital tablets gr i ss p.o. q.3 h. p.r.n. for seizure activity. Give _____ .

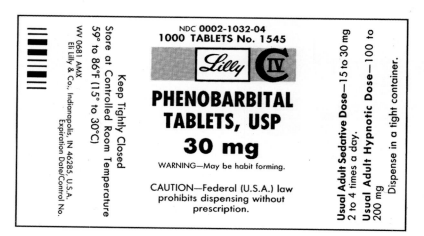

48. The physician prescribes a supplement of KCl 2 mEq p.o. q.8 h. for Mr. Vee, admitted with chronic abdominal pain. Give _____ .

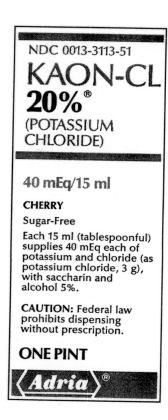

49. Mr. Sahl, recovering from a coronary artery bypass graft, receives aspirin gr x p.o. q.3 h. Give _____ .

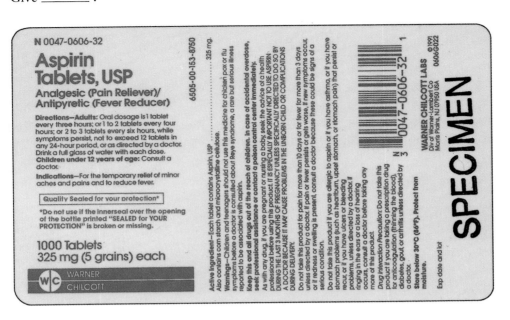

50. Mr. Dale receives terpin hydrate 10 ml p.o. q.4 hours p.r.n. as part of his treatment for pneumonia. Give _____ ℥.

51. Mrs. Line has erythromycin prescribed 1 g p.o. q.6 h. for treatment of her strep throat. You have 250 mg capsules available. Give _____ .

52. The physician prescribes $FeSO_4$ gr v p.o. t.i.d. to supplement Mr. Bay, a cardiac catherization patient. Give _____ . How many mg will be given? _____ .

53. Mr. Jones, admitted with chronic obstructive lung disease, takes Bentyl 20 mg p.o. t.i.d. a.c. The drug is available in 10 mg capsules. Give _____ .

54. Mrs. Tyth suffers pruritic dermatoses. The physician prescribes Atarax 30 mg p.o. b.i.d. as part of her therapy. The drug is supplied in syrup containing 10 mg per teaspoon. Give _____ .

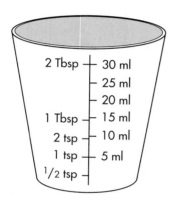

55. Mrs. Gale, admitted for alcohol abuse, is supplemented with ascorbic acid 0.75 g p.o. daily while hospitalized. You have 250 mg tablets available. Give _____ .

56. Your chronic pancreatitis patient has Phenergan 25 mg p.o. q.4 h. p.r.n. nausea. The drug is supplied in 12.5 mg tablets. Give _____ .

57. Mr. Nade, hospitalized for a radical neck dissection, has Vistaril 15 mg p.o. q.i.d. ordered to suppress nausea. You have Vistaril 25 mg per 5 ml available. Give _____ .

58. Terramycin 1.5 g p.o. stat; then give 0.5 g q.i.d. until a total of 9 g is given. Terramycin is supplied in 250 mg capsules. How many capsules will be given stat? _____ . How many capsules will be given for each q.i.d. dose? _____ . How many capsules will be given in 1 day when given q.i.d.? _____ . How many doses in addition to the stat dose will be required to give 9 g of the drug? _____ .

59. Your thyroidectomy patient receives Noctec elixir 250 mg p.o. q. h.s. p.r.n. for insomnia. You have 500 mg per 5 ml available. Give _____ .

60. Mr. Aden requires Chloromycetin 250 mg p.o. q.6 h. for treatment of salmonella. You have Chloromycetin 150 mg per 5 ml available. Give _____ .

61. Mr. Scheottle receives Vibramycin 100 mg p.o. q.12 h. for treatment of inclusion conjunctivitis. Give _____ ml.

Vibramycin®
SYRUP   Calcium
doxycycline calcium
oral suspension
50 mg / 5 ml†
1 PINT (473 ml)
†Each teaspoonful (5 ml) contains
 doxycycline calcium equivalent
 to 50 mg of doxycycline.
USUAL DOSAGE:
Adults: 200 mg on the first day
(100 mg every 12 hours) followed by
a maintenance dose of 100 mg a day.
Children above eight years of age:
Under 100 lbs.—2 mg/lb. of body
weight daily divided in two doses
on the first day, followed by
1 mg/lb. of body weight on
subsequent days in one or two doses.
Over 100 lbs.—See adult dosage.
doxycycline U.S. Pat. No. 3,200,149
READ ACCOMPANYING
PROFESSIONAL INFORMATION
RECOMMENDED STORAGE
STORE BELOW 86°F. (30°C.)
Dispense in tight, light resistant
containers (USP).
CAUTION: Federal law prohibits
dispensing without prescription.

Pfizer LABORATORIES
DIVISION
PFIZER INC.,
NEW YORK, N.Y 10017

MADE IN U.S.A. 2

Pfizer
NDC 0069-0971-93
6188
Vibramycin®
SYRUP   Calcium
doxycycline calcium
oral suspension

50 mg/5ml†

1 PINT
(473 ml)

RASPBERRY/APPLE
FLAVORED

For oral use
only

SHAKE WELL
BEFORE USING

IMPORTANT:
This closure is
not child-resistant.

62. Your patient, admitted for cardiac catheterization, receives HydroDiuril 25 mg p.o. b.i.d. for hypertension. You have 50 mg tablets available. Give _____ .

63. Tylenol 240 mg p.o. q.4 h. for temperature 38.9° C. You have Tylenol 80 mg chewable tablets available. How many tablets will be required for each dose? _____ .

64. The physician prescribes Lanoxin elixir 90 mcg p.o. b.i.d. for your patient with atrial fibrillation. Give _____ .

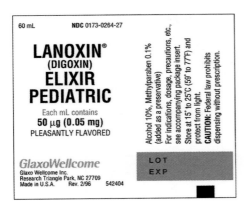

65. Mr. Ceney, admitted for contact dermatitis, receives elixir of Benadryl 10 ml p.o. q.6 h. p.r.n. for itching. The drug is supplied 12.5 mg per 5 ml. Give _____ mg.

66. Orinase 0.5 g p.o. t.i.d. Orinase 500 mg tablets are available. Give _____ .

67. Your patient receives Dilantin gr i ss p.o. t.i.d. for past seizure activity. Give _____ .

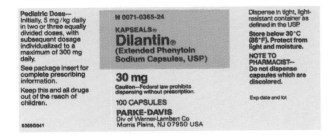

68. Milk of Magnesia 2 Tbsp p.o. h.s. Give _____ ℥, or _____ ʒ.

69. Your patient admitted with a small-bowel obstruction has KCl 10 mEq p.o. q.d. ordered for his low potassium level. The drug is available as a liquid in KCl 20 mEq per 15 ml. Give _____ .

70. Mr. Brown receives Nalfon 300 mg p.o. with meals or a snack for his osteoarthritis. Give _____ .

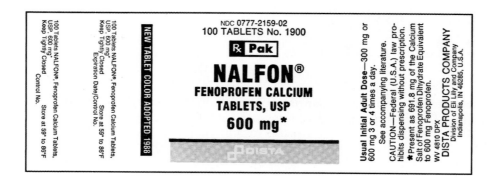

71. Mrs. Roget has been placed on digoxin 0.5 mg p.o. q.d. for her cardiac arrhythmia. The drug is available in 0.25 mg tablets. Give _____ .

72. Acetaminophen 650 mg p.o. q.4 h. is prescribed for a temperature of more than 38.5° C × 24 h. Give _____ ml q.4 h.

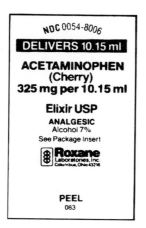

73. The physician prescribes Decadron 0.5 mg p.o. q.12 h. for your patient's keratitis. Give _____ .

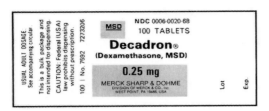

74. Mr. Pein receives Keflex ℥ ss p.o. q.6 h. after his thyroidectomy. Give _____ .

75. Your lumbar laminectomy patient receives Demerol 30 mg p.o. q.4 h. p.r.n. for pain. The drug is supplied 50 mg per 5 ml. Give _____ .

76. Crystodigin gr ¹⁄₂₀₀ p.o. q.d. You have Crystodigin in 0.05, 0.15, and 0.2 mg tablets. The tablet strength of choice is to give _____ tablets of _____ mg.

77. Mr. Zeman was given prednisone 7.5 mg p.o. q.d. for exfoliative dermatitis. Prednisone is supplied in 5 mg grooved tablets. Give _____ .

78. Your patient who has had a partial craniotomy has V-Cillin K suspension 250 mg p.o. q.i.d. ordered. Give _____ .

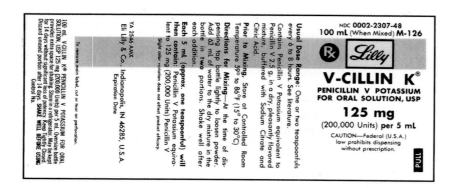

79. Your patient, status post coronary artery bypass graft, receives Surfak 250 mg p.o. q.d. as a stool softener. Give _____ .

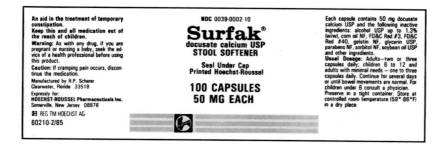

80. Elixir of KCl 15 ml p.o. t.i.d. Elixir of KCl 15 mEq per 11.25 ml is available. How many mEq will be given? _____ .

81. Your epileptic patient receives phenobarbital 55 mg p.o. b.i.d. Give _____ .

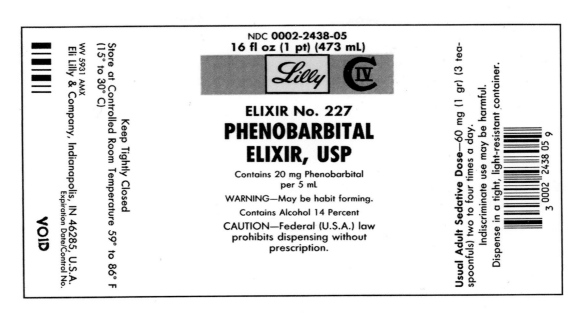

82. Aldomet 250 mg p.o. b.i.d. Give _____ .

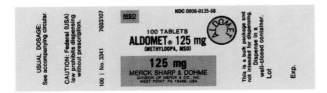

83. Mrs. Richardson, a thyroidectomy patient, receives Synthroid 0.05 mg p.o. q.A.M. Give _____ .

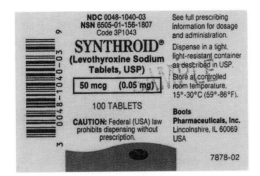

84. Theo-Dur 0.2 g p.o. q.8 h. Theo-Dur is supplied in 100, 200, and 300 mg sustained action tablets. Give _____ tablets of _____ mg. How many mg will be given per day? _____ .

85. Your valve repair patient is started on Coumadin 15 mg p.o. stat. Coumadin 5 mg scored tablets are available. Give _____ .

86. Your status post angioplasty patient receives cimetidine 300 mg p.o. q.i.d. p.c. h.s. Give _____ mg/day.

87. The physician prescribes Restoril 30 mg p.o. h.s. p.r.n. for your presurgery patient for insomnia. Give _____ capsules/h.s.

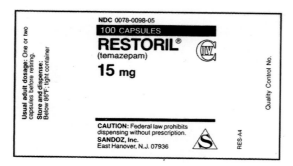

88. Imipramine 50 mg p.o. q.A.M. and h.s. The drug is supplied in 25 mg tablets. Give _____ .

89. Your patient admitted with depression receives Mellaril 40 mg p.o. b.i.d. for his mental condition. Give _____ .

NDC 0078-0001-31

4 fl. oz. (118 ml)

CONCENTRATE

MELLARIL®
(thioridazine) HCl
oral solution, USP

30 mg/ml

Each ml contains:
thioridazine HCl, USP . . . . .30 mg
alcohol, USP . . . . .3.0% by volume
CAUTION: Federal law prohibits
dispensing without prescription.
6505-00-059-3497
Store and dispense: Below 86°F;
tight, amber glass bottle

SANDOZ
PHARMACEUTICALS
CORPORATION
EAST HANOVER, NJ 07936

SPECIMEN

Quality Control No.
Exp.

MEL-A19

2891-41

Dosage: See package insert for dosage information. It is recommended that the Concentrate be used only for severe neuropsychiatric conditions.
Immediately before administration, dilute the dose of Concentrate with distilled water, acidified tap water, or suitable juices.
Suggested Dilution: 25 mg dose in 2 teaspoonfuls of diluent-liquid. For higher doses increase the volume of diluent.

90. Lasix 0.6 ml p.o. b.i.d. with meals. Lasix is available in an oral solution of 10 mg per ml. How many mg will be given? _____ .

91. Mrs. Adams receives Cleocin 150 mg p.o. q.6 h. for her upper respiratory tract infection. Cleocin is supplied in 75 mg capsules. Give _____ .

92. Your patient receives Crystodigin 0.05 mg p.o. q.A.M. for congestive heart failure. Give _____ .

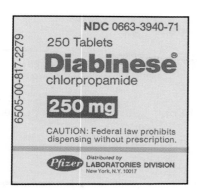

93. Coumadin 10 mg p.o. at 6:00 P.M. today. Give _____ .

COUMADIN®   2½ mg
(Warfarin Sodium Tablets, USP)
Crystalline
DuPont Pharma
Wilmington, Delaware 19880
LOT JJ275A
EXP 8/98

94. Your diabetic patient receives Diabinese 0.25 g p.o. q.A.M. Give _____ .

NDC 0663-3940-71
250 Tablets
Diabinese®
chlorpropamide
250 mg
CAUTION: Federal law prohibits
dispensing without prescription.
Distributed by
Pfizer LABORATORIES DIVISION
New York, N.Y. 10017

6505-00-817-2279

95. The physician prescribes Apresoline 25 mg p.o. b.i.d. for Mr. Yu's hypertension. You have Apresoline tablets gr ⅙ available. Give _____ .

96. Chloral hydrate elixir 600 mg p.o. h.s. p.r.n. Chloral hydrate 500 mg per 5 ml is available. Give _____ .

97. Your patient has been placed on prednisone 15 mg p.o. q.d. for asthma. Prednisone is available in 5 mg tablets. Give _____ .

98. Mr. Gray, status post cervical discectomy, receives Restoril 0.015 g p.o. h.s. for insomnia. Give _____ .

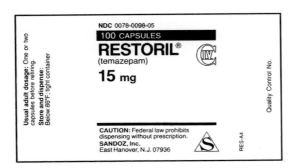

99. KCl elixir 40 mEq p.o. q.i.d. c̄ juice. KCl 20 mEq per 15 ml is available. Give _____ .

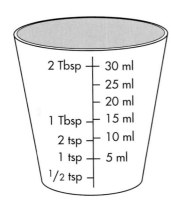

100. Mrs. Endres receives furosemide 20 mg p.o. q.8 h. for congestive heart failure. Give _____ .

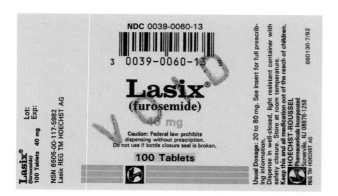

Answers on pp. 426-446.

POSTTEST 1

Name _____

Date _____

ACCEPTABLE SCORE __18__

YOUR SCORE _____

Directions: The medication order is listed at the beginning of each problem. Calculate the oral dosages. Show your work. Shade each medicine cup when provided to indicate the correct dosage.

1. The physician orders ASA gr xv p.o. q.i.d. for your mitral valve repair patient. Give _____ .

N 0047-0606-32

6505-00-153-8750   325 mg.

Aspirin Tablets, USP

Analgesic (Pain Reliever)/ Antipyretic (Fever Reducer)

Directions—Adults: Oral dosage is 1 tablet every three hours; or 1 to 2 tablets every four hours; or 2 to 3 tablets every six hours, while symptoms persist, not to exceed 12 tablets in any 24-hour period, or as directed by a doctor. Drink a full glass of water with each dose. **Children under 12 years of age:** Consult a doctor.

Indications—For the temporary relief of minor aches and pains and to reduce fever.

Quality Sealed for your protection*

***Do not use if the innerseal over the opening of the bottle printed "SEALED for YOUR PROTECTION" is broken or missing.**

1000 Tablets
325 mg (5 grains) each

WC WARNER CHILCOTT

Active Ingredient—Each tablet contains Aspirin, USP . . . . Also contains corn starch and microcrystalline cellulose.

Warnings—Children and teenagers should not use this medicine for chicken pox or flu symptoms before a doctor is consulted about Reye syndrome, a rare but serious illness reported to be associated with aspirin.

Keep this and all drugs out of the reach of children. In case of accidental overdose, seek professional assistance or contact a poison control center immediately.

As with any drug, if you are pregnant or nursing a baby, seek the advice of a health professional before using this product. IT IS ESPECIALLY IMPORTANT NOT TO USE ASPIRIN DURING THE LAST 3 MONTHS OF PREGNANCY UNLESS SPECIFICALLY DIRECTED TO DO SO BY A DOCTOR BECAUSE IT MAY CAUSE PROBLEMS IN THE UNBORN CHILD OR COMPLICATIONS DURING DELIVERY.

Do not take this product for pain for more than 10 days or for fever for more than 3 days unless directed by a doctor. If pain or fever persists or gets worse, if new symptoms occur, or if redness or swelling is present, consult a doctor because these could be signs of a serious condition.

Do not take this product if you are allergic to aspirin or if you have asthma, or if you have stomach problems (such as heartburn, upset stomach, or stomach pain) that persist or recur, or if you have ulcers or bleeding problems, unless directed by a doctor. If ringing in the ears or a loss of hearing occurs, consult a doctor before taking any more of this product.

Drug Interaction Precaution: Do not take this product if you are taking a prescription drug for anticoagulation (thinning the blood), diabetes, gout, or arthritis unless directed by a doctor.

Store below 30°C (86°F). Protect from moisture.

Exp date and lot

WARNER CHILCOTT LABS ©1991
Div of Warner-Lambert Co   0606G022
Morris Plains, NJ 07950 USA

N 3 0047-0606-32 1

SPECIMEN

2. Mr. Clay receives tetracycline 0.5 g p.o. q.i.d. for a gastrointestinal infection. The drug is supplied in 500 mg capsules. Give _____ .

3. The physician orders ampicillin 1 g p.o. q.6 h. for treatment of shigellosis. Give _____ .

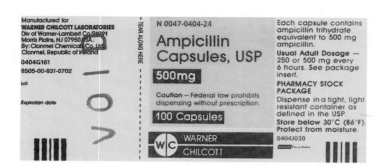

4. The physician prescribes Milk of Magnesia 1 Tbsp. p.o. h.s. for your thyroidectomy patient's complaints of constipation. Give _____ 5.

5. Orinase 500 mg p.o. t.i.d. You have 0.5 g tablets available. Give _____ .

6. Mr. Shen, admitted with psychoneurotic disorder, receives Atarax 25 mg p.o. q.A.M. You have Atarax 10 mg per 5 ml. Give _____ .

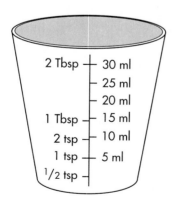

7. Your patient with chronic back pain has Mellaril 30 mg p.o. t.i.d. p.r.n. for muscle relaxation. Mellaril 15 mg tablets are available. Give _____ .

8. The physician prescribes codeine 30 mg p.o. q.3 h. p.r.n. for pain for your total hip replacement patient. Give _____ .

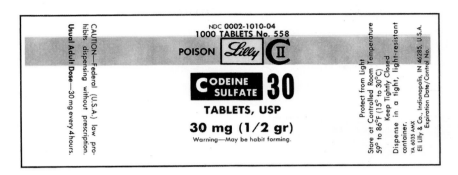

9. Your preop patient receives Vistaril 50 mg p.o. t.i.d. for anxiety. Vistaril oral suspension 25 mg per teaspoon is available. Give _____ .

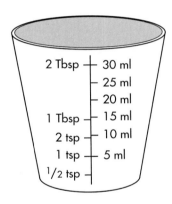

10. Naprosyn 0.25 g p.o. b.i.d. Naprosyn is supplied in 250 mg scored tablets. How many grams will you give each day? _____ .

11. Your patient receives Crystodigin gr $\frac{1}{600}$ p.o. q.d. for an atrial arrhythmia. Crystodigin tablets gr $\frac{1}{300}$ are available. Give _____ .

12. The physician prescribes KCl 20 mEq p.o. b.i.d. for hypokalemia. KCl liquid is supplied 30 mEq per 22.5 ml. Give _____ .

13. Gantrisin 2 g p.o. t.i.d. Give _____ .

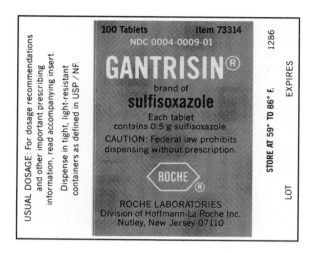

14. Your lumbar laminectomy patient has Benadryl 100 mg p.o. h.s. p.r.n. for insomnia. Give _____ .

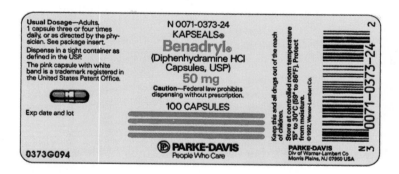

15. Your patient has Lasix 9 mg p.o. q.12 h. ordered for hypercalcemia. You have Lasix 10 mg per ml. Give _____ .

16. Mrs. Cook receives Keflex 100 mg p.o. q.6 h. for a sinus infection. Give _____ .

NDC 0777-2321-97
60 mL (When Mixed)   M-201

KEFLEX®
CEPHALEXIN FOR
ORAL SUSPENSION, USP
125 mg per 5 mL

DISTA

17. Achromycin ʒ ii p.o. q.6 h. You have a ʒ ii bottle of Achromycin syrup containing 125 mg per teaspoon. How many mg will be given? _____ .

18. Mr. Jones receives Inderal 80 mg p.o. b.i.d. for an arrhythmia. You have Inderal 40 mg scored tablets. Give _____ .

19. The physician prescribes Apresoline 20 mg p.o. t.i.d. for your patient's hypertension. You have 10 mg tablets available. Give _____ .

20. Your epileptic patient receives phenobarbital gr i ss p.o. t.i.d. Give _____ tabs/dose. Give _____ tabs/day.

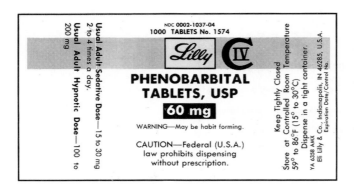

Answers on pp. 446-450.

POSTTEST 2

Name _____

Date _____

ACCEPTABLE SCORE __**18**__

YOUR SCORE _____

Directions: The medication order is listed at the beginning of each problem. Calculate the oral dosages. Show your work. Shade each medicine cup when provided to indicate correct dosage.

1. Your patient receives Feldene 20 mg p.o. q.d. for gouty arthritis. Feldene capsules 10 mg are available. Give _____ .

2. Robitussin ℨ ii p.o. q.4 h. Robitussin is supplied in ℨ iv bottles. How many ℨ ii doses will each bottle provide? _____ .

3. Your cleft palate revision patient requires Tylenol elixir 30 mg p.o. stat. You have Children's Tylenol elixir 160 mg per 5 ml. Give _____ ℳ.

4. The physician prescribes dicumarol 150 mg p.o. stat for your patient with myocardial infarction. Dicumarol is supplied in 50 mg grooved tablets. Give _____ .

5. Your patient being treated for congestive heart failure requires KCl 5 mEq p.o. b.i.d. for hypokalemia. KCl 20 mEq per 30 ml is available. Give _____ .

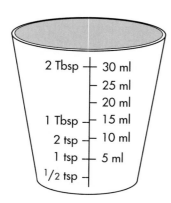

6. Your tonsillectomy patient receives Keflex 250 mg p.o. q.i.d. Give _____ .

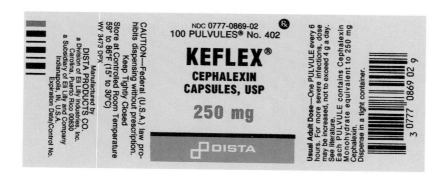

7. Mrs. Pace receives prednisone 7.5 mg p.o. q.i.d. for asthma. Prednisone is supplied as 2.5 mg tablets. Give _____ .

8. Your patient receives Lanoxin 0.05 mg p.o. q.d. for cardiac arrhythmia. Give _____ .

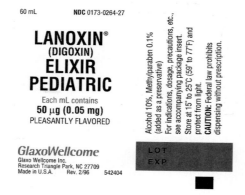

9. Macrodantin 0.1 g p.o. q.i.d. Give _____ .

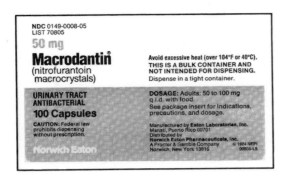

10. Your bilateral turbinate reduction patient receives acetaminophen gr vi p.o. q.4 h. for pain. Acetaminophen is supplied in 325 mg tablets. Give _____ .

11. The physician prescribes Dilantin gr ¾ p.o. b.i.d. for seizure activity in your epileptic patient. Dilantin 50 mg Infatabs are available. Give _____ .

12. Mr. Bales requires Pen-Vee K 250 mg p.o. q.6 h. for bacterial endocarditis. Pen-Vee K solution 125 mg per 5 ml is available. Give _____ .

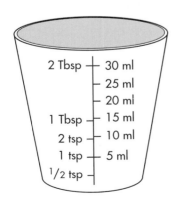

13. Deltasone 20 mg p.o. q.i.d. Deltasone is supplied in 2.5 mg, 5 mg, and 50 mg tablets. Give _____ tablets of _____ mg.

14. Mr. Cy, status post mitral valve repair, receives Lanoxin 0.25 mg p.o. q.d. Give _____ .

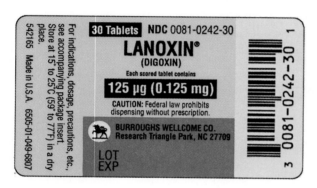

15. Colace elixir 25 ml p.o. p.r.n. for constipation is ordered for your ethmoidectomy patient. Give _____ .

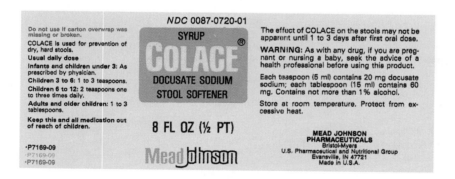

16. Mr. Tate, status post left-leg debridement, receives ASA 0.6 g p.o. q.3 h. p.r.n. for pain. Give _____ .

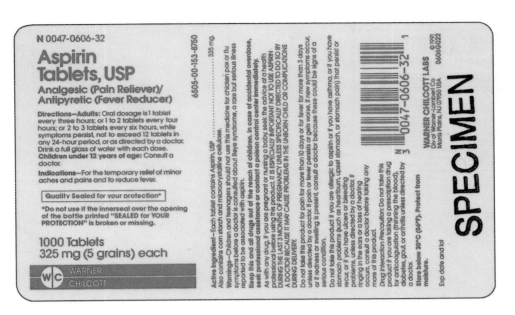

17. Your preop patient has Noctec 500 mg p.o. h.s. ordered for insomnia. You have Noctec syrup gr vii ss per 5. Give _____ .

18. Gantrisin tablets 1.5 g p.o. q.i.d. Give _____ .

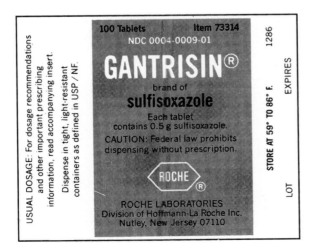

19. Your patient was admitted with seizure activity. The physician orders phenobarbital 30 mg p.o. q.8 h. Give _____ .

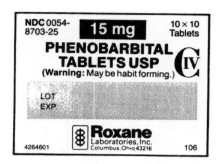

20. The physician orders Flagyl 750 mg p.o. t.i.d. for 5 days for a yeast infection. Flagyl is supplied in 250 mg tablets. Give _____ .

Answers on pp. 450-454.

Chapter *12* | *Parenteral Dosages*

Learning Objectives

On completion of the materials provided in this chapter, you will be able to perform computations accurately by mastering the following mathematical concepts:

1 | Convert the measure within the problem to equivalent measures in one system of measurement

2 | Use a proportion to solve problems of parenteral dosages when medication is in liquid or reconstituted powder form

3 | Use a proportion to solve problems of parenteral dosages of medications measured in milliequivalents

4 | Use the stated formula as an alternative method of solving parenteral drug dosage problems

Parenteral refers to outside the alimentary canal or gastrointestinal tract. Medications may be given parenterally when they cannot be taken by mouth or when a rapid action is desired. Parenteral medications are absorbed directly into the bloodstream; therefore the amount of drug needed can be determined more accurately. This type of administration of medications is necessary for the irrational or unconscious patient, or for a patient who has been designated *NPO* (nothing by mouth). Drugs given parenterally also have the advantage of not upsetting the gastrointestinal system. An advantage of intravenous parenteral medications is that the patient does not have to endure the discomfort of multiple injections, especially when used for pain control.

Parenteral medications are administered by (1) subcutaneous injection—beneath the skin, (2) intramuscular injection—within the muscle, or (3) intradermal injection—within the skin (Figure 12-1). Parenteral medications also may be given intravenously—within the vein (Figure 12-2). Intravenous (I.V.) drugs may be diluted and administered by themselves, in conjunction with existing intravenous fluids, or added to I.V. fluids (Figure 12-3). Any time that the integrity of the skin—the body's prime defense against microorganisms—is threatened, infection may occur. Thus the nurse must use sterile technique when preparing and administering parenteral medications.

Drugs for parenteral use are supplied as liquids or powders. The medications are packaged in a variety of forms. First, a liquid may be contained in an ampule, which is a single-dose container that must be broken at the neck to withdraw the drug (Figures 12-4 and 12-5).

Vials are also used to package parenteral medications in liquid or powder form. A vial is a glass or plastic container that is sealed with a rubber stopper (Figure 12-6). Because vials usually contain more than one dose of a medication, the amount desired is withdrawn by inserting a needle through

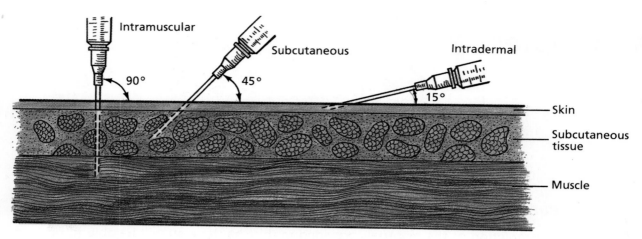

FIGURE 12-1
Intramuscular, subcutaneous, and intradermal injections, with comparison of the angles of insertion. *(From Potter P, Perry A:* Fundamentals of nursing, *ed 4, St Louis, 1997, Mosby.)*

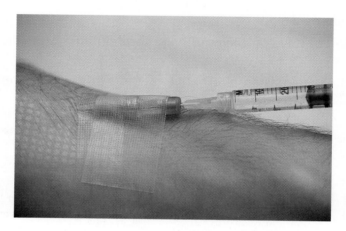

FIGURE 12-2
Intravenous injection. *(From Potter P, Perry A:* Fundamentals of nursing, *ed 4, St Louis, 1997, Mosby.)*

the rubber stopper and removing the required amount (Figure 12-7). If the medication is in powder form, the drug must be reconstituted before withdrawal and administration. The diluent to dissolve the powder is usually sterile water or normal saline. The amount of diluent recommended is normally printed on the vial; however, if it is not, no less than 1 ml is used for a single-dose vial. The powder must be completely dissolved. If one is using a multiple-dose vial, the date and time of mixing should be noted on the vial's label.

Some of the more unstable drugs may be supplied in vials that have a compartment containing the liquid. Pressure applied to the top of the vial releases the stopper between the compartments and allows the drug to be dissolved. These are called Mix-O-Vials (Figure 12-8).

Medications may also be supplied in either prefilled disposable syringes or a plastic syringe with a disposable cartridge and a needle unit. Such units contain a specific amount of medication. If the medication order is less than the amount supplied, discard the unneeded portion before administering the medication to the patient. Figures 12-9 and 12-10 show the Tubex and Carpuject® types of filled syringes.

Text continued on p. 259

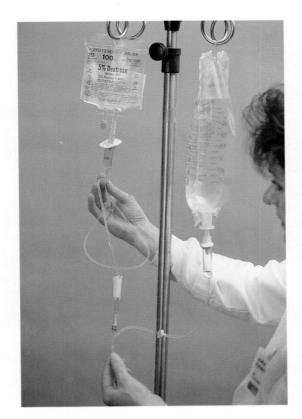

FIGURE 12-3
Intravenous drug administered with existing intravenous fluids. *(From Potter P, Perry A: Fundamentals of nursing, ed 4, St Louis, 1997, Mosby.)*

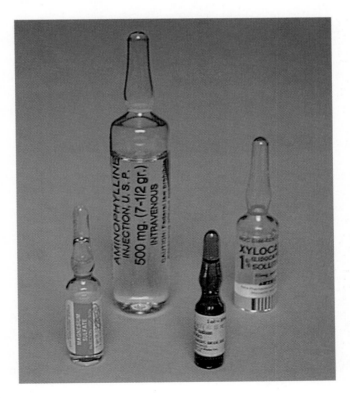

FIGURE 12-4
Examples of ampules. *(From Elkin M, Perry A, Potter P: Nursing interventions and clinical skills, St Louis, 1996, Mosby.)*

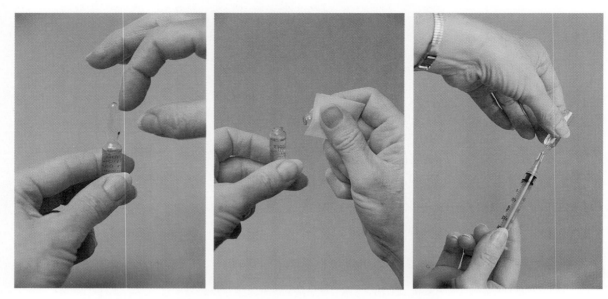

FIGURE 12-5
Breaking the ampule to withdraw the medication. *(From Potter P, Perry A:* Fundamentals of nursing, *ed 4, St Louis, 1997, Mosby.)*

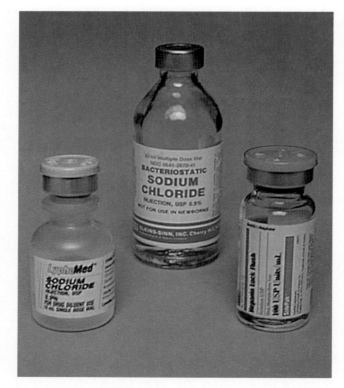

FIGURE 12-6
Examples of vials. *(From Elkin M, Perry A, Potter P:* Nursing interventions and clinical skills, *St Louis, 1996, Mosby.)*

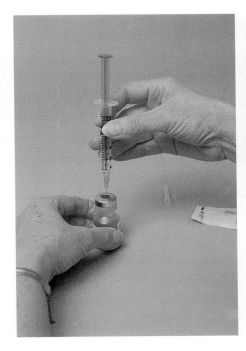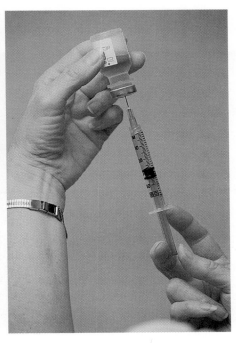

FIGURE 12-7
Withdrawing medication in a vial through the rubber stopper. *(From Potter P, Perry A: Fundamentals of nursing, ed 4, St Louis, 1997, Mosby.)*

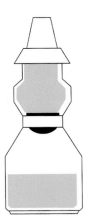

FIGURE 12-8
Example of a Mix-O-Vial.

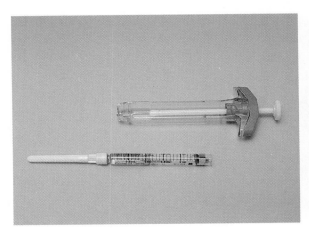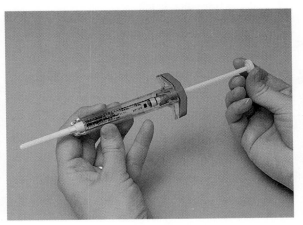

FIGURE 12-9
Directions for use of Carpuject sterile cartridge-needle units with self-contained medication. *(Courtesy Winthrop-Breon Laboratories, New York.)*

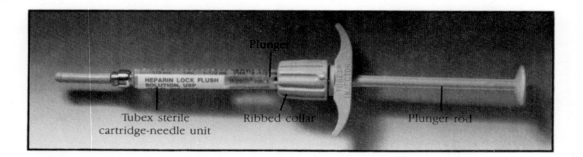

How to load

1. Turn the ribbed collar to the "open" position until it stops.

How to administer

Method of administration is the same as with conventional syringe. Remove needle cover by grasping it securely; twist and pull. Introduce needle into patient, aspirate by pulling back slightly on the plunger, and inject.

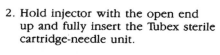

2. Hold injector with the open end up and fully insert the Tubex sterile cartridge-needle unit.

Firmly tighten the ribbed collar in the direction of the "close" arrow.

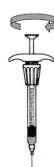

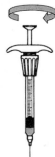

How to unload and discard used unit

1. Do not recap the needle. Disengage the plunger rod.

2. Hold the injector, needle down, over a needle disposal container and loosen the ribbed collar. Tubex cartridge-needle unit will drop into the container.

Discard the needle cover.

The Tubex injector is reusable; do not discard.

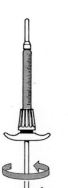

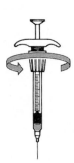

Thread the plunger rod into the plunger of the Tubex sterile cartridge-needle unit until slight resistance is felt.

The injector is now ready for use in the usual manner.

FIGURE 12-10
Directions for use of the Tubex closed-injection system. *(Courtesy Wyeth-Ayerst Laboratories, Philadelphia.)*

Syringes

To accurately measure medications that are to be administered by the parenteral route, a syringe must be used. Each syringe is supplied in a sterile package. Although syringes may be made of glass or plastic, plastic syringes are most commonly used. They are designed to be used only once and then discarded. The syringe that is used to withdraw and measure the medication from its container may also be used to administer the medication to the patient.

Figure 12-11 shows the parts of a syringe.

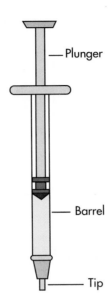

FIGURE 12-11
Parts of a syringe. *(From Clayton B:* Basic pharmacology for nurses, *ed 11, St Louis, 1997, Mosby.)*

1. TIP. The tip is located at the end of the syringe. This is the part that holds the needle.

2. BARREL. This is the outer part of the syringe that holds the medicine. The various calibrations are printed on the outside of the barrel.

3. PLUNGER. This is the interior part of the syringe that slides within the barrel. The plunger is moved backward to withdraw and measure the medication. Then it is pushed forward to inject the medicine into the patient.

   Syringes come in a variety of sizes. The size used depends on the amount and type of medication to be administered. There are three types of syringes: hypodermic, tuberculin, and insulin syringes.

   Hypodermic syringes. Hypodermic syringes vary in size as to the amount of fluid they can measure. The most commonly used sizes are 2, 2½, 3, and 5 cc syringes (Figure 12-12). Hypodermic syringes are also available in 10, 20, 30, and 50 cc sizes. Remember that a cc is equivalent to a ml and that syringes are labeled using both abbreviations. Small hypodermic syringes will also be calibrated in minims (ℳ). It is critical to use syringes with this calibration when the amount of medication to be administered has been calculated in minims.

   Syringes that are smaller capacity may easily be used to measure decimal fractions of a cc/ml. Longer lines mark the ½ and whole number cc/ml, and shorter lines mark the decimal fractions. Each line indicates one tenth of a cc/ml. With larger capacity syringes, each mark may represent 0.2 cc increments, or whole cc increments. The larger-capacity syringes would not be appropriate for measuring smaller quantities of medication for administration.

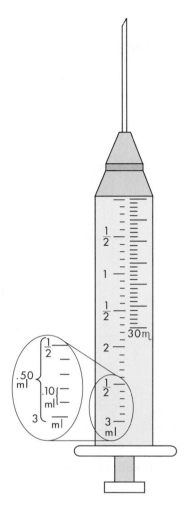

FIGURE 12-12
3 cc syringe. *(From Clayton B:* Basic pharmacology for nurses, *ed 11, St Louis, 1997, Mosby.)*

Tuberculin syringes. A tuberculin syringe is a thin, 1 cc/ml syringe (Figure 12-13). The cc/ml side of the syringe includes markings for hundredths of a cc/ml. The other side of the syringe is calibrated in minims. These syringes are commonly used in pediatrics and also to measure medications given in very small amounts, such as heparin.

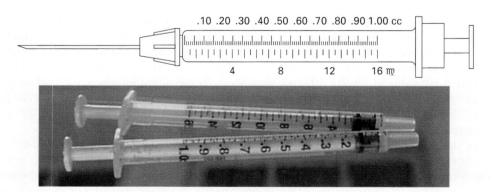

FIGURE 12-13
Tuberculin syringes. *(From Brown M, Mulholland J:* Drug calculations: process and problems for clinical practice, *ed 5, St Louis, 1996, Mosby.)*

Insulin syringes. Insulin syringes were developed specifically for the administration of insulin. They are calibrated in units (U). These syringes were designed to be used with U-100 insulin. There are three types of insulin syringes.

1. The Lo-Dose syringe is used for administration of 50 units or less of insulin. The syringe is marked for each unit, with longer lines for each 5 units (Figure 12-14).

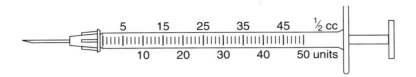

FIGURE 12-14
Lo-Dose insulin syringe. *(From Brown M, Mulholland J:* Drug calculations: process and problems for clinical practice, *ed 5, St Louis, 1996, Mosby.)*

2. The 30 U syringe is used for insulin doses that equal less than 30 units of U-100 insulin only (Figure 12-15).

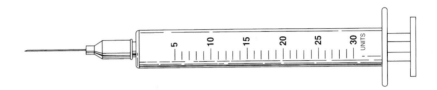

FIGURE 12-15
A 30 U syringe. *(From Brown M, Mulholland J:* Drug calculations: process and problems for clinical practice, *ed 5, St Louis, 1996, Mosby.)*

3. The U-100/1-ml syringe is used for the administration of up to 100 units of U-100 insulin. These syringes may be labeled with odd units on the left and even units on the right (Figure 12-16).

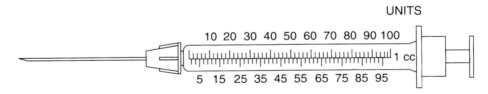

FIGURE 12-16
A 100-unit (U-100) insulin syringe. Measurement in units and cc. *(From Brown M, Mulholland J:* Drug calculations: process and problems for clinical practice, *ed 5, St Louis, 1996, Mosby.)*

Remember, when preparing medication for administration, it is important to choose the correct size of syringe for accurate measurement of the medication.

Calculation of Parenteral Drug Dosages

Parenteral drug dosages may also be calculated by using a proportion. The physician's order and the available medication must be in the same system of measurement to write a proportion for the actual amount of medication to be administered. Examples of parenteral drug dosage problems follow.

Example 1:   Apresoline 30 mg I.M. Apresoline 20 mg per ml is available. Give _____ .

a. On the left side of the proportion, place what you know or have available. In this example, there are 20 mg per 1 ml. Therefore the left side of the proportion would be

$$20 \text{ mg} : 1 \text{ ml} ::$$

b. The right side of the proportion is determined by the physician's order and the abbreviations placed on the left side of the proportion. Remember, only *two* different abbreviations may be used in a single proportion.

$$20 \text{ mg} : 1 \text{ ml} :: _____ \text{ mg} : _____ \text{ ml}$$

The physician ordered 30 mg.

$$20 \text{ mg} : 1 \text{ ml} :: 30 \text{ mg} : _____ \text{ ml}$$

The symbol x is used to represent the unknown number of ml.

$$20 \text{ mg} : 1 \text{ ml} :: 30 \text{ mg} : x \text{ ml}$$

c. Rewrite the proportion without the abbreviations.

$$20 : 1 :: 30 : x$$

d. Solve for x.

$$20 : 1 :: 30 : x$$
$$20x = 30$$
$$x = \frac{30}{20}$$
$$x = 1.5$$

e. Label your answer as determined by the abbreviation placed next to x in the original proportion.

$$1.5 \text{ ml}$$

The patient would receive 1.5 ml of Apresoline containing 30 mg.

Example 2:   Demerol 30 mg I.M. q.4 h. p.r.n. Demerol 25 mg per 0.5 ml is available. Give _____ .

a. On the left side of the proportion, place what you know or have available. In this example, each 0.5 ml contains 25 mg. So the left side of the proportion would be

$$25 \text{ mg} : 0.5 \text{ ml} ::$$

b. The right side of the proportion is determined by the physician's order and the abbreviations on the left side of the proportion. Only *two* different abbreviations may be used in a single proportion. The abbreviations must be in the same position on the right side as they are on the left.

$$25 \text{ mg} : 0.5 \text{ ml} :: _____ \text{ mg} : _____ \text{ ml}$$

In this example the physician ordered 30 mg.

$$25 \text{ mg} : 0.5 \text{ ml} :: 30 \text{ mg} : _____ \text{ ml}$$

We need to find the number of milliliters to be given, so we use the symbol x to represent the unknown.

$$25 \text{ mg} : 0.5 \text{ ml} :: 30 \text{ mg} : x \text{ ml}$$

    c. Rewrite the proportion without using the abbreviations.

$$25 : 0.5 :: 30 : x$$

    d. Solve for x.

$$25x = 0.5 \times 30$$
$$25x = 15$$
$$x = \frac{15}{25}$$
$$x = 0.6$$

    e. Label your answer as determined by the abbreviation placed next to x in the original proportion.

    0.6 ml would be measured in order to administer 30 mg of Demerol.

If the question asks for the answer to be in minims, another proportion must be written and solved using your new knowledge.

    a. 15 ℳ : 1 ml ::
    b. 15 ℳ : 1 ml :: _____ ℳ : _____ ml
       15 ℳ : 1 ml :: x ℳ : 0.6 ml
    c. 15 : 1 :: x : 0.6
    d. $x = 9$
    e. $x = 9$ ℳ

Example 3:   Gentamicin 9 mg IV q.6 h. Gentamicin 20 mg per 2 ml is available. Give _____ .

    a. 20 mg : 2 ml ::
    b. 20 mg : 2 ml :: _____ mg : _____ ml
       20 mg : 2 ml :: 9 mg : x ml
    c. 20 : 2 :: 9 : x
    d. $20x = 18$

$$x = \frac{18}{20}$$
$$x = 0.9$$
$$x = 0.9 \text{ ml}$$

Alternative Formula Method of Parenteral Drug Dosage Calculation

In Chapter 11, the alternative formula was introduced as another method of calculating drug dosages. This formula also may be used when calculating parenteral drug dosages.

Remember, the formula is

$$\frac{D}{A} \times Q = x$$

or

$$\frac{\text{desired}}{\text{available}} \times \text{quantity available} = x \text{ (unknown)}$$

Example 1:   Amikin 150 mg I.M. q.8 h. Amikin 500 mg per 2 ml is available. Give _____ .

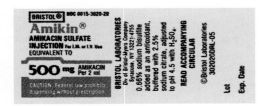

    a. The desired amount of Amikin is 150 mg.

$$150$$

    b. The available amount of Amikin is 500 mg.

$$\frac{150}{500}$$

    c. The quantity of the medication for 500 mg is 2 ml.

$$\frac{150}{500} \times \frac{2}{1} = x$$

    d. We can now solve for x.

$$x = \frac{150}{500} \times \frac{2}{1}$$

$$x = \frac{150 \times \overset{1}{\cancel{2}}}{\underset{250}{\cancel{500}} \times 1} = \frac{150}{250}$$

$$x = \frac{150}{250}$$

$$x = \frac{3}{5} \text{ or } 0.6$$

    e. Label your answer as determined by the quantity.

$$150 \text{ mg} = 0.6 \text{ ml}$$

If the physician's order is in one system of measurement and the drug is supplied in another system of measurement, one of the measurements must be converted so that they are both expressed in the same system. After this is done, the formula may be used to calculate the amount of medication to be administered.

Example 2:   Mr. Davis is to receive atropine gr $\frac{1}{150}$ I.M. stat. Atropine 0.4 mg per ml is available. Give _____ .

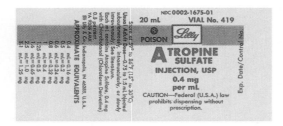

The physician's order is expressed in grains and the drug is supplied in milligrams. Convert the order to milligrams as outlined in Chapter 8.

$$60 \text{ mg} : 1 \text{ gr} :: x \text{ mg} : \tfrac{1}{150} \text{ gr}$$

$$60 : 1 :: x : \tfrac{1}{150}$$

$$x = \frac{60}{1} \times \frac{1}{150}$$

$$x = \frac{\overset{2}{\cancel{60}} \times 1}{1 \times \underset{5}{\cancel{150}}}$$

$$x = \frac{2}{5} \text{ or } 0.4$$

$$x = 0.4 \text{ mg}$$

$$\text{gr } \tfrac{1}{150} = 0.4 \text{ mg}$$

Now the numbers may be filled into the formula.

a. The desired amount is 0.4 mg.

$$0.4$$

b. The available amount or strength of atropine is 0.4 mg.

$$\frac{0.4}{0.4}$$

c. The quantity available is in 1 ml.

$$\frac{0.4}{0.4} \times \frac{1}{1}$$

d. Solve for x

$$x = \frac{0.4 \times 1}{0.4 \times 1}$$

$$x = 1$$

e. Label your answer as determined by the quantity.

$$0.4 \text{ mg} = 1 \text{ ml}$$

Example 3: Mr. Lewis's physician has ordered 60 mg phenobarbital for agitation. Phenobarbital 120 mg per ml is available. Give _____ .

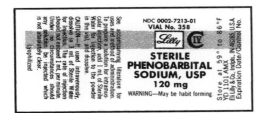

a. The desired amount of phenobarbital is 60 mg.

$$\frac{60}{}$$

b. The available amount or strength is 120 mg.

$$\frac{60}{120}$$

c. The quantity available is 1 ml.

$$\frac{60}{120} \times 1$$

d. Solve for x.

$$x = \frac{60}{120} \times \frac{1}{1}$$

$$x = \frac{60 \times 1}{120 \times 1}$$

$$x = \frac{1}{2}$$

$$x = 0.5$$

e. Label your answer as determined by the quantity.

$$60 \text{ mg} = 0.5 \text{ ml}$$

Complete the following work sheet, which provides for extensive practice in the calculation of parenteral drug dosages. Check your answers. If you have difficulties, go back and review the necessary material. When you feel ready to evaluate your learning, take the first posttest. Check your answers. An acceptable score as indicated on the posttest signifies that you have successfully completed this chapter. An unacceptable score signifies a need for further study before taking the second posttest.

WORK SHEET

Directions: The medication order is listed at the beginning of each problem. Calculate the parenteral dosages. Show your work. Shade the syringe when provided to indicate the correct dosage.

1. The physician orders gentamicin 30 mg I.M. q.8 h. for your patient with a central line infection. Gentamicin 10 mg per ml is available. Give _____ .

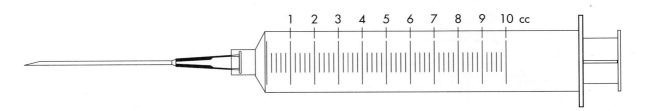

2. Your atrial valve repair patient has Lanoxin 110 mcg I.V. q.12 h. ordered. Give _____ .

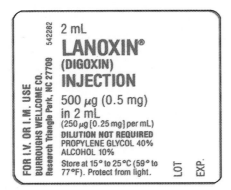

3. Atropine gr ¹⁄₂₀₀ I.M. at 6:15 A.M. Give _____ .

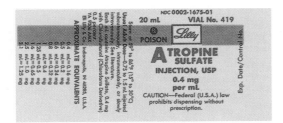

4. Your pacemaker-placement patient complains of nausea and has Compazine 10 mg I.M. q.6 h. ordered. Compazine is supplied in a 10 ml vial containing 5 mg per ml. Give _____ .

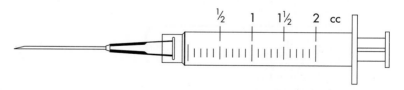

5. Meperidine 45 mg I.M. q.4 h. Give _____ .

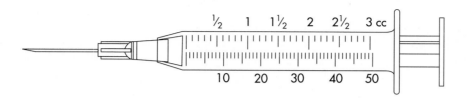

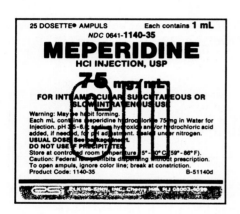

6. The physician orders piperacillin 3 g. I.V. q.8 h. for your septic patient. You have piperacillin 1 g per 2.5 ml available. Give _____ .

7. Morphine 5 mg subq. q.4 h. You have morphine gr ⅙ per ml available. Give _____ .

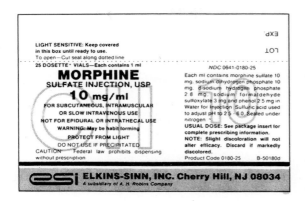

8. The physician orders vancomycin 1 g I.V.S.S. q.12 h. for your right-hand-amputation patient. After reconstitution of the medication, you have vancomycin 500 mg per 6 ml. Give _____ .

9. Your congestive heart failure patient requires Furosemide 30 mg. I.M. stat. Give _____ .

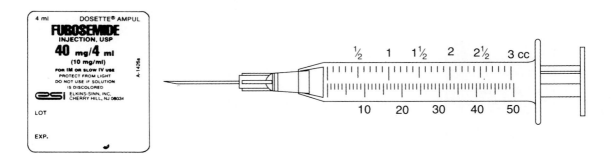

10. Morphine gr ¹⁄₂₄ subq. q.4 h. You have morphine gr ⅛ per 30 ℳ available. Give _____ .

11. D_5W 1000 ml plus $NaHCO_3$ 25.8 mEq at 12 ml per h. $NaHCO_3$ is supplied in a 50 ml ampule containing 44.6 mEq. How many ml of $NaHCO_3$ will be added to the 1000 ml of D_5W? _____ .

12. Your asthma patient requires aminophylline 100 mg I.V. q.6 h. Give _____ .

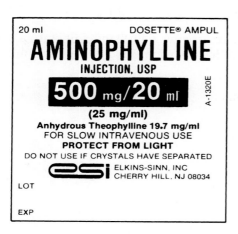

13. Dilaudid gr ¹/₁₅ subq. q.3 h. Give _____ ℳ.

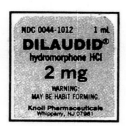

14. Gantrisin gr xv I.V. stat. You have a 5 ml ampule containing 2 g. Prepare _____ .

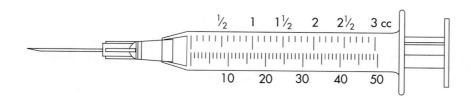

15. The physician orders Solu-Cortef 0.05 g I.M. q.6 h. for your patient with scleroderma. Give _____ .

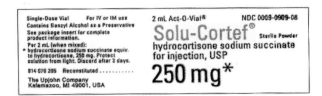

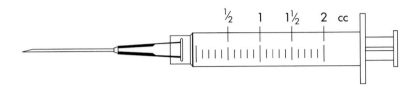

16. Your epileptic patient requires phenobarbital 0.3 g I.M. t.i.d. Give _____ .

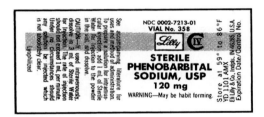

17. Tagamet 300 mg I.V.S.S. q.6 h. The drug is supplied in a single dose vial with 300 mg per 2 ml. Give _____ .

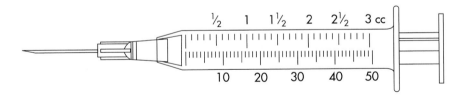

18. Mrs. Andis, status postadrenalectomy, requires hydrocortisone 8 mg I.M. q.d. You have hydrocortisone 100 mg per 2 ml. Give _____ ℳ.

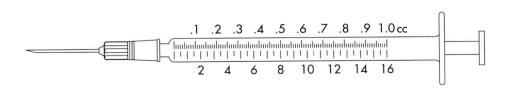

19. The physician orders Stadol 0.5 mg I.M. q.4 h. for Mrs. Switzer after childbirth. Give _____ .

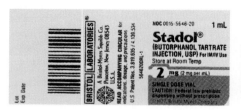

20. Mr. Lewis requires Ativan 1 mg I.M. stat for severe agitation. Ativan is supplied 4 mg per ml. Give _____ .

21. Mrs. Carroll requires Apresoline 10 mg I.M. q.6 h. for high blood pressure. Apresoline is supplied in 1 ml ampules containing 20 mg. Give _____ .

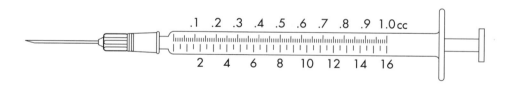

22. D$_5$W 1000 ml plus KCl 30 mEq at 60 ml per h. How many ml of KCl will be added to the 1000 ml of D$_5$W? _____ .

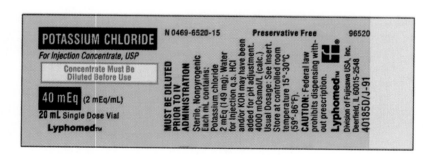

23. The physician orders Valium 10 mg I.M. q.6 h. for your anxious patient. You have Valium 5 mg per ml. Give _____ .

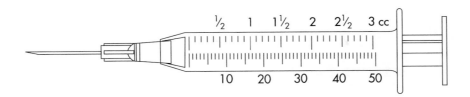

24. Mr. Keesling is diagnosed with an acoustic neuroma and complains of pain. He has codeine gr ¼ I.M. q.3 h. p.r.n. ordered. Give _____ .

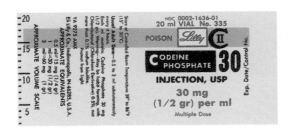

25. AquaMEPHYTON 0.01 g I.M. q.A.M. The drug is supplied in 1 ml ampules containing 10 mg per ml. Give _____ .

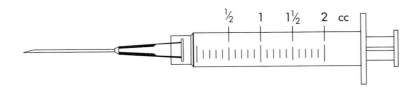

26. Your patient, status postorchiectomy, has carbenicillin 6 g I.V.S.S. q.6 h. ordered. You have carbenicillin 2 g per 6 ml. Give _____ .

27. Mrs. Ring, status posthysterectomy, has morphine 12 mg I.M. q.4 h. p.r.n. for pain. Give _____ .

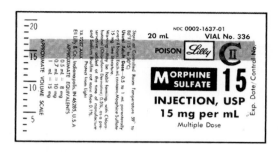

28. Benadryl 100 mg I.M. q.i.d. The drug is supplied in ampules containing 50 mg per ml. Give _____ .

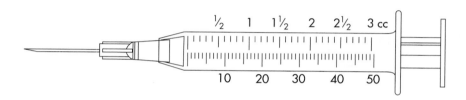

29. Mr. Fields requires digoxin 100 mcg I.M. q.d. for his cardiac arrhythmia. Give _____ .

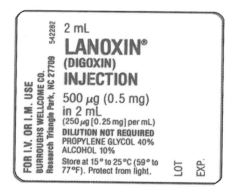

30. Kefzol 500 mg I.V.S.S. q.6 h. × 4 days. Give _____ .

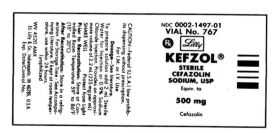

31. Your epileptic patient receives phenobarbital gr v I.M. q.3 h. Give _____ .

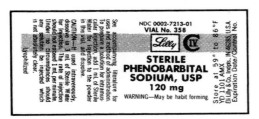

32. The physician orders Solu-Cortef 100 mg I.M. q.8 h. for your patient with severe contact dermatitis. Solu-Cortef 250 mg per 2 ml is available. Give _____ .

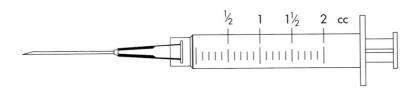

33. D_5W 250 ml plus NaCl 7.5 mEq at 2 ml per h. NaCl is supplied in a 40 ml vial containing 2.5 mEq per ml. How many ml of NaCl will be added to the 250 ml of D_5W? _____ .

34. Your lumbar laminectomy patient receives Vistaril 3 ml I.M. t.i.d. Give _____ mg.

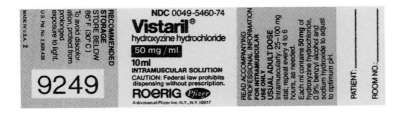

35. The physician orders atropine gr ¹⁄₁₀₀ I.M. stat for your preop patient. Give _____ .

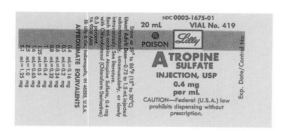

36. Your patient admitted with neuroleptic disorder has Seconal 50 mg I.M. h.s. p.r.n. ordered. Give _____ .

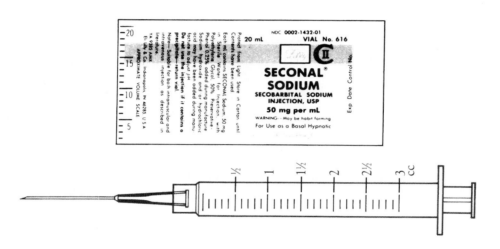

37. Demerol 75 mg I.M. q.4 h. p.r.n. Demerol is supplied in a 2 ml ampule containing 100 mg of the drug. Give _____ .

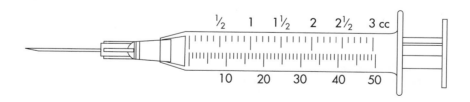

38. Your C.O.P.D. patient receives aminophylline 75 mg q.6 h. Give _____ .

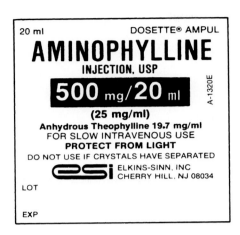

39. The physician orders Librium 75 mg. I.M. stat for your patient with severe depression. Librium 100 mg per 2 ml is available. Give _____ .

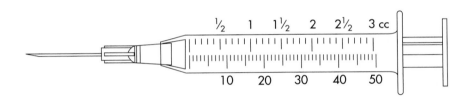

40. Valium 15 mg I.V. stat. Valium is supplied in a 10 ml vial containing 5 mg per ml. Prepare _____ .

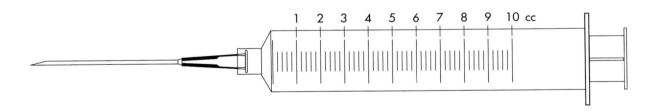

41. Mr. Norcross is suffering from psoriasis and requires hydrocortisone 25 mg I.M. q.d. The drug is available 100 mg per 2 ml. Give _____ .

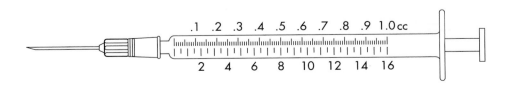

42. Your patient with *Pseudomonas* receives Kantrex 400 mg I.M. q.12 h. Give _____ .

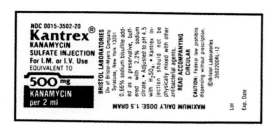

43. The physician orders ascorbic acid 0.25 g I.M. q.d. for your patient admitted with alcohol abuse. You have ascorbic acid 500 mg per ml. Give _____ .

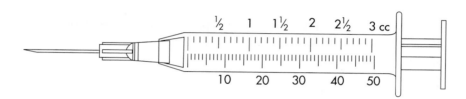

44. D₅W 250 ml plus CaCl₂ 5 mEq at 2 ml per h. CaCl₂ is supplied in a 10 ml ampule containing 13.6 mEq. How many ml of CaCl₂ will be added to the 250 ml of D₅W? _____ .

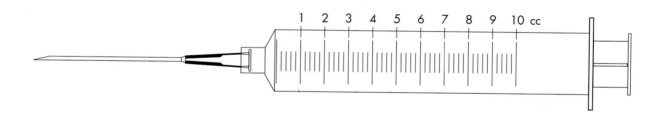

45. The physician orders phenobarbital 70 mg subq. q.8 h. for your epileptic patient. The drug is supplied in a 1 ml ampule containing 65 mg. Give _____ .

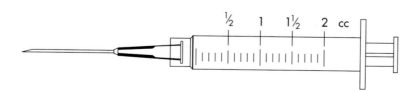

46. Vibramycin 200 mg I.V. q.d. You have Vibramycin 10 mg per ml after reconstitution. Give _____ .

47. Dilaudid gr ¹⁄₃₀ I.M. q.4 h. p.r.n. Give _____ .

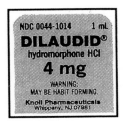

48. Your patient with atrial fibrillation has digoxin 0.2 mg I.M. q.d. ordered. Digoxin is supplied in a 2 ml ampule containing 0.5 mg. Give _____ .

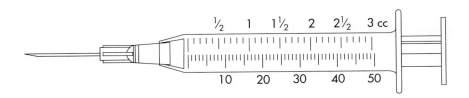

49. Morphine gr ¹⁄₆ subq. q.3 h. Give _____ ℳ.

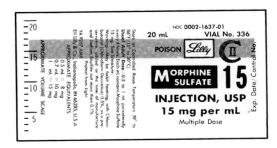

50. Your manic-depressive patient receives Haldol 3 mg I.M. q.i.d. The drug is supplied in a 1 ml ampule containing 5 mg. Give _____ m.

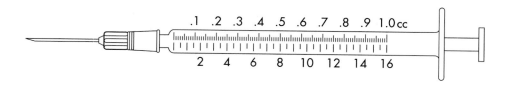

51. Demerol 0.6 ml I.M. q.3 h. p.r.n. Demerol is supplied in a 30 ml vial containing 50 mg per ml. How many mg will you give? _____ .

52. Your preop patient needs atropine 0.9 mg I.M. at 6:15 A.M. Give _____ .

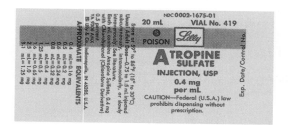

53. The physician orders codeine gr ss subq. q.4 h. for pain in your lumbar laminectomy patient. Give _____ .

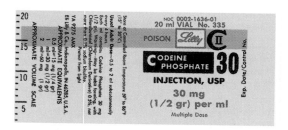

54. The physician orders phenobarbital gr ¼ subq. q.3 h. for your patient with head trauma. Phenobarbital is supplied in 1 ml ampules containing 65 mg. Give _____ ℳ.

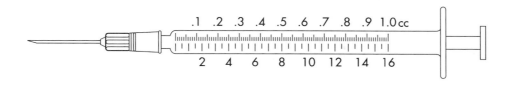

55. D$_5$W 500 ml plus 6 mEq of NaHCO$_3$ at 42 ml per h. NaHCO$_3$ is available in a 10 ml ampule containing 0.89 mEq per ml. How many ml of NaHCO$_3$ will be added to the 500 ml of D$_5$W? _____ .

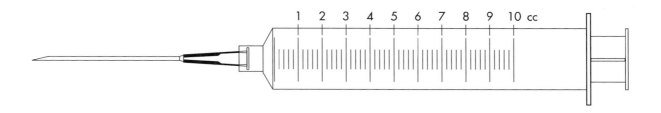

56. Mr. Grey, status post–cervical discectomy, has Garamycin 20 mg I.M. q.8 h. ordered. Give _____ .

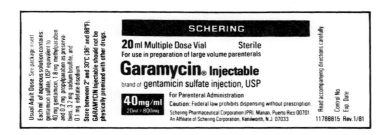

57. Mr. Ali receives Thorazine 0.2 ml I.M. q.4 h. for severe hiccups. Give _____ mg.

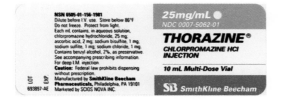

58. Your sinusitis patient receives ampicillin 500 mg I.V.S.S. q.12 h. You have ampicillin 100 mg per ml. Give _____ .

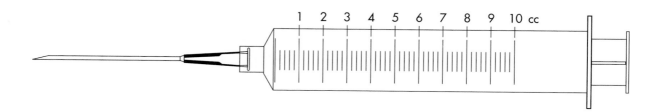

59. Demerol 50 mg I.M. q.4 h. p.r.n. Demerol is supplied in a vial containing 100 mg per ml. Give _____ .

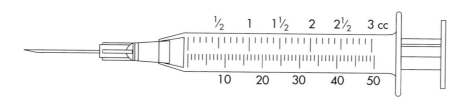

60. The physician orders Ativan 0.5 mg I.M. stat for your patient with severe anxiety. The drug is supplied in a 1 ml vial containing 2 mg per ml. Give _____ .

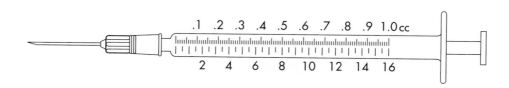

61. Aminophylline 0.2 g I.V. t.i.d. Aminophylline is supplied in a 10 ml ampule containing 0.25 g per 10 ml. Give _____ .

62. Codeine 15 mg I.M. q.4 h. Codeine is available in an ampule containing gr ss per ml. Give _____ .

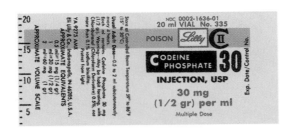

63. Mr. Ciele, status post–partial craniotomy, receives Dilantin 100 mg I.V. q.8 h. You have available Dilantin 50 mg per ml. Give _____ .

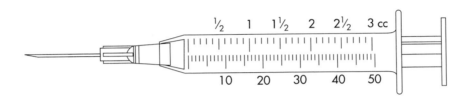

64. The physician orders digoxin 0.25 mg I.V. q.d. for your patient with atrial flutter. Digoxin is supplied in a 2 ml ampule containing 0.5 mg. Give _____ .

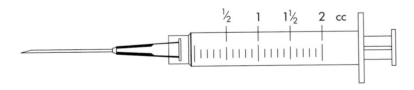

65. Mrs. Peterson needs Demerol 35 mg I.M. q.3 h. for severe pain after a total hip replacement. The drug is supplied in an ampule containing 25 mg per 0.5 ml. Give _____ .

66. D_{7.5}W 250 ml plus calcium gluconate 5 mEq at 2 ml per h. Calcium gluconate is supplied in a 10 ml ampule containing 4.8 mEq. How many ml of calcium gluconate will be added to the 250 ml of $D_{7.5}W$? _____ .

67. Mr. Thompson, admitted with erythrasma, receives Cleocin 50 mg I.V. q.8 h. Give _____ .

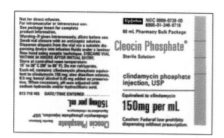

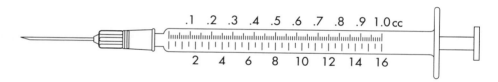

68. Atropine 0.2 mg I.M. at 7:30 A.M. Atropine is supplied in a 1 ml ampule containing 1 mg. Give _____ .

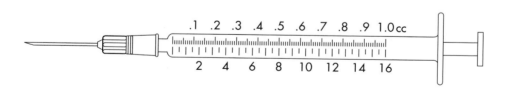

69. Mr. Riley receives tobramycin 55 mg I.V. q.8 h. for sepsis. You have tobramycin 40 mg per ml available. Give _____ .

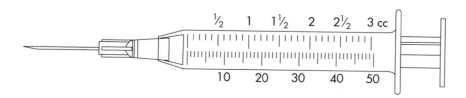

70. Phenobarbital 22 mg I.M. as an anticonvulsant. Phenobarbital is supplied in 1 ml ampules containing 65 mg. Give _____ .

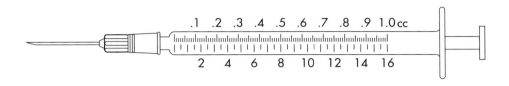

71. Your patient needs morphine gr ⅙ subq. stat for myocardial infarction. Give _____ .

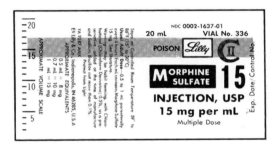

72. Vitamin B$_{12}$ 1 mg I.M. q. Monday. Give _____ .

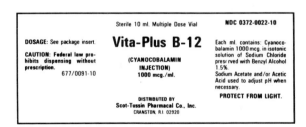

73. Morphine gr ⅟₃₀ I.M. q.3 h. Morphine is available in an ampule containing gr ⅛ per ml. Give _____ ℳ.

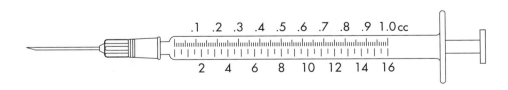

74. Mr. Paley receives Phenergan 6.5 mg I.M. at 9:30 A.M. for nausea after a colonoscopy. Phenergan is supplied in an ampule containing 25 mg per ml. Give _____ .

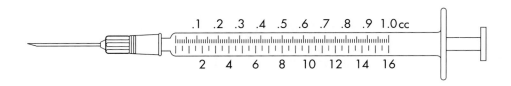

75. Your patient receives Robinul 0.28 mg I.M. at 6:00 A.M. for treatment of trichomonas. Give _____ .

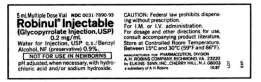

76. Mr. Eli receives Demerol 10 mg I.M. q.6 h. for pain after denervation from a gunshot wound. Demerol is available in an ampule containing 25 mg per ml. Give _____ .

77. D_5W 1000 ml plus NaCl 15 mEq at 30 ml per h. NaCl is supplied in a 40 ml vial containing 100 mEq. How many ml of NaCl will be added to the 1000 ml of D_5W? _____ .

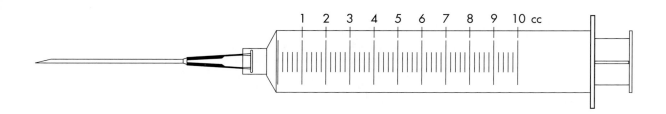

78. Mr. Neal receives Kefzol 250 mg I.V. q.6 h. for 12 doses after an ethmoidectomy. The drug is available in a vial containing 125 mg per ml. Give _____ .

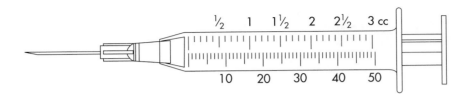

79. Your patient receives the antibiotic Cleocin 300 mg I.V. q.6 h. for treatment of diphtheria. Cleocin is available in a 4 ml ampule containing 600 mg. Give _____ .

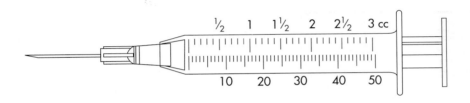

80. Lidocaine 75 mg I.V. stat. Lidocaine is available in a 5 ml vial containing 100 mg per 5 ml. Give _____ m.

81. Your patient receives sodium phenobarbital 20 mg I.M. b.i.d for seizures. The drug is supplied in an ampule containing gr ii per ml. Give _____ .

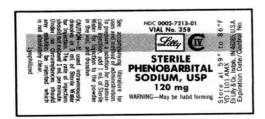

82. Solu-Medrol 100 mg I.V. stat. Give _____ .

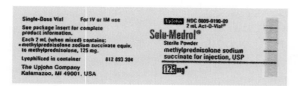

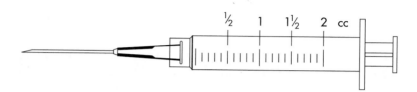

83. Your preop patient receives Demerol 25 mg I.M. on call to the operating room. Demerol is available in an ampule containing 50 mg per ml. Give _____ .

84. Scopolamine gr ¹⁄₁₅₀ at 7 A.M. Give _____ ♏.

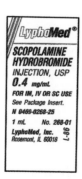

85. Your patient requires Phenergan 0.2 ml I.M. stat for nausea and vomiting. Phenergan is supplied in an ampule containing 25 mg per ml. Give _____ mg.

86. Dilaudid gr ¹⁄₆₀ q.4 h. p.r.n. Give _____ .

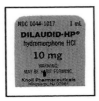

87. Your patient requires Vistaril 50 mg I.M. q.4 h. p.r.n. for severe agitation. Vistaril is supplied in a 2 ml vial containing 100 mg. Give _____ .

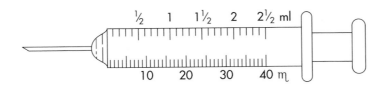

88. D₅W 500 ml plus KCl 10.8 mEq at 42 ml per h. How many ml of KCl will be added to the 500 ml of D₅W? _____ .

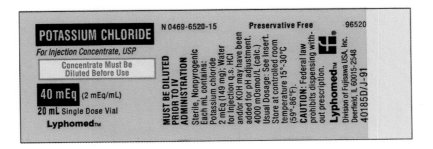

89. Atropine gr ¹⁄₁₂₀ I.M. stat. Atropine is available in an ampule containing gr ¹⁄₁₅₀ per ml. Give _____ ℳ.

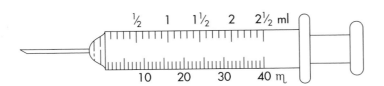

90. Your patient has Thorazine 15 mg I.M. q.6 h. ordered for severe agitation. Give _____ .

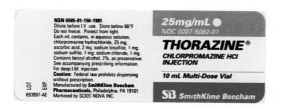

91. Vancocin 500 mg I.V.S.S. q.12 h. Vancocin 250 mg per 5 ml is available after reconstitution. Give _____ .

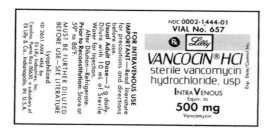

92. Mr. Ray receives tobramycin 90 mg I.V.P.B. q.8 h. for his abdominal wound infection. You have tobramycin 80 mg per 2 ml. Give _____ .

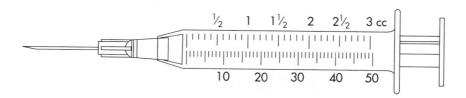

93. Your patient with delerium tremens receives Valium 2 mg. I.M. q.6 h. Valium is available in a vial containing 5 mg per ml. Give _____ .

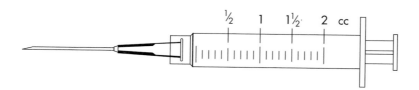

94. The physician orders Flagyl 500 mg I.V. q.6 h. to treat Ms. King's yeast infection. After reconstitution you have Flagyl 100 mg per ml. Give _____ .

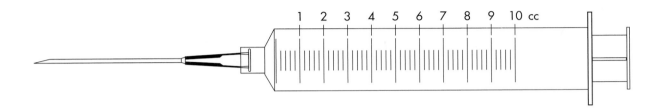

95. Streptomycin 0.64 g I.M. q.d. After reconstitution you have streptomycin 400 mg per ml. Give _____ .

96. Your patient receives nafcillin 500 mg I.M. q.6 h. for treatment of *S. aureas*. You have nafcillin 250 mg per ml. Give _____ .

97. Isuprel 0.2 mg stat I.M. The drug is available in 5 ml ampules containing 1 mg of Isuprel. Give _____ .

98. The physician orders Imferon 100 mg I.M. q.o.d. for your patient with pernicious anemia. The drug is supplied in ampules containing 25 mg per 0.5 ml. Give _____ .

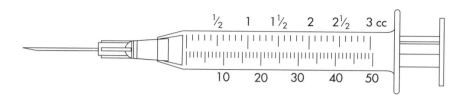

99. Your arthritic patient receives Solganal 10 mg I.M. Solganal is supplied 50 mg per ml. Give _____ .

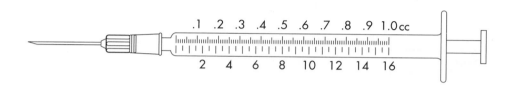

100. Aramine 4 mg I.M. stat. Give _____ .

MSD   NDC 0006-3222-10
10 ml INJECTION
ARAMINE®
(METARAMINOL BITARTRATE, MSD)
1% Metaraminol Equivalent
10 mg per ml
MERCK SHARP & DOHME
DIVISION OF MERCK & CO., INC.
WEST POINT, PA 19486, USA

MULTIPLE DOSE VIAL

Protect from light. Store contents in carton until contents have been used.

USUAL ADULT DOSAGE: See accompanying circular.

CAUTION: Federal (USA) law prohibits dispensing without prescription.

10 ml | No. 3222X   7217609

Answers on pp. 454-471.

Chapter 12 Parenteral Dosages

POSTTEST 1

Name _____

Date _____

ACCEPTABLE SCORE __**18**__

YOUR SCORE _____

Directions: The medication order is listed at the beginning of each problem. Calculate the parenteral dosages. Show your work. Shade the syringe when provided to indicate the correct dosage.

1. The physician orders Vistaril 25 mg I.M. t.i.d. q.4-6 h. p.r.n. to enhance the effects of pain medication for your thyroidectomy patient. Give _____ .

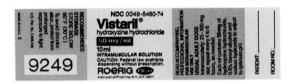

2. Your septoplasty patient complains of nausea and has Phenergan 5.5 mg I.M. q.i.d. Phenergan 25 mg per ml is available. Give _____ ℳ.

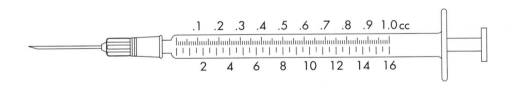

3. Your status post–tympano-mastoidectomy patient complains of pain and has codeine 30 mg I.M. q.2 h. p.r.n. ordered. Codeine is supplied in a 1 ml ampule containing gr ¼. Give _____ .

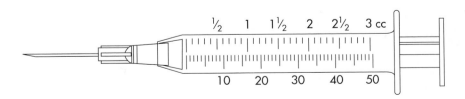

4. The physician orders Keflin 500 mg I.M. q.6 h. for your patient with *Klebsiella*. Keflin 1 g per 10 ml is available. Give _____ .

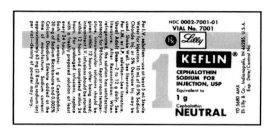

5. Your patient, status post–medullary carcinoma excision, has hydrocortisone 50 mg I.M. b.i.d. ordered. You have hydrocortisone 100 mg per 2 ml available. Give _____ .

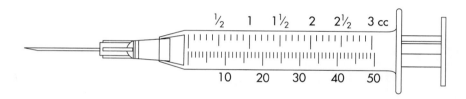

6. Dilaudid 0.5 mg I.M. q.4 h. p.r.n. Give _____ .

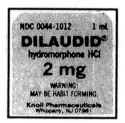

7. Your patient with epilepsy has phenobarbital gr iv I.M. b.i.d. ordered. Phenobarbital is supplied in a 1 ml ampule containing 120 mg per ml. Give _____ .

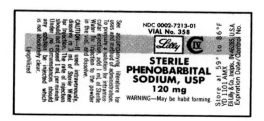

8. The physician orders scopolamine gr ⅟₃₀₀ I.M. at 6 A.M. before surgery. Give _____ .

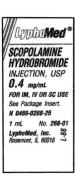

9. Thorazine 100 mg I.M. stat. Thorazine is supplied in a 10 ml vial containing 25 mg per ml. Give _____ .

10. Your severely agitated patient has Valium 2 mg I.M. q.6 h. p.r.n. ordered. You have a 10 ml vial of the drug containing 5 mg per ml. Give _____ .

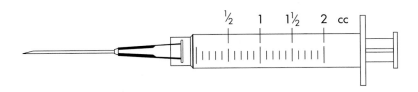

11. Atropine is ordered for your patient 0.7 mg I.M. stat before surgery. You have atropine gr ⅟₁₂₀ per ml. Give _____ .

12. Your patient with a medication reaction complains of pruritis and has Benadryl 25 mg I.M. p.r.n. ordered. You have Benadryl 50 mg per ml available. Give _____ .

13. Your status postmastectomy patient has Demerol 42 mg I.M. q.4 h. p.r.n. ordered. You have an ampule containing 25 mg per 0.5 ml. Give _____ .

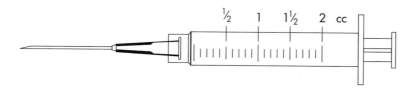

14. The physician orders ampicillin 500 mg I.M. q.4 h. for your lumbar laminectomy patient. You have ampicillin 2.5 g per 10 ml available. Give _____ .

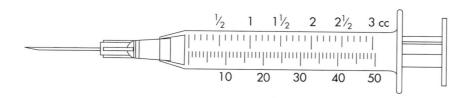

15. Your patient has Librium 0.5 ml I.M. q.i.d. ordered for anxiety. The drug is available in a 5 ml ampule containing 100 mg. Give _____ mg.

16. Morphine 6 mg I.M. q.3 h. p.r.n. Give _____ .

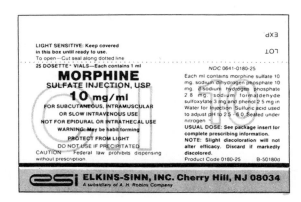

17. Achromycin 300 mg I.V. q.12 h. Achromycin is supplied in a vial containing 500 mg per 10 ml. Give _____ .

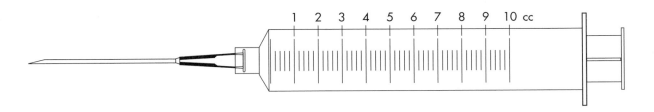

18. Your congestive heart failure patient has furosemide 10 mg I.M. q.6 h. ordered. Give _____ .

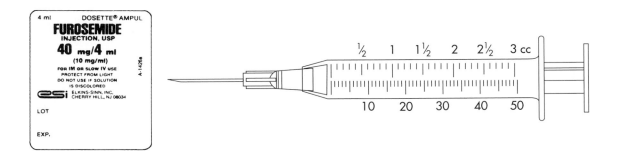

19. The physician orders Lanoxin 20 mcg I.M. q.12 h. for your patient with atrial flutter. You have Lanoxin 0.1 mg per 1 ml. Give _____ m.

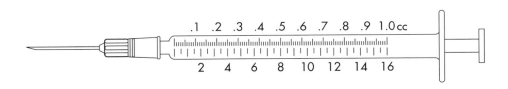

20. D_5W 500 ml plus KCl 5 mEq at 40 ml per h. KCl is supplied in a 10 ml ampule containing 20 mEq per ml. How many ml of KCl will be added to the 500 ml of D_5W? _____ .

Answers on pp. 472-475.

POSTTEST 2

Name _____

Date _____

ACCEPTABLE SCORE __**18**__

YOUR SCORE _____

Directions: The medication order is listed at the beginning of each problem. Calculate the parenteral dosages. Show your work. Shade the syringe when provided to indicate the correct dosage.

1. Your motor vehicle accident patient complains of pain and has Dilaudid 2 mg I.M. q.3 h. p.r.n. ordered. Give _____ .

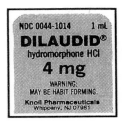

2. Your preop patient complains of anxiety and has Ativan 2 mg I.M. q.6 h. ordered. Ativan is supplied 4 mg per ml. Give _____ .

3. Erythromycin 0.4 g I.V. today. The drug is supplied in vials containing 500 mg per 10 ml. Prepare _____ .

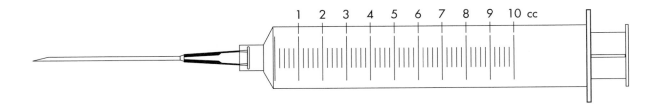

4. The physician orders Seconal 75 mg I.M. h.s. p.r.n. for your septoplasty patient.
Give _____ .

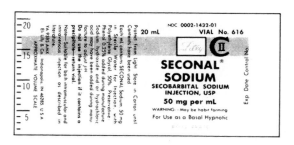

5. Your status postlumpectomy patient has codeine 60 mg I.M. q.3 h. ordered. Give _____ .

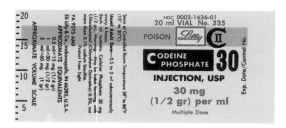

6. Demerol 15 mg I.M. q.4 h. p.r.n. Demerol is available in an ampule containing 25 mg per
0.5 ml. Give _____ .

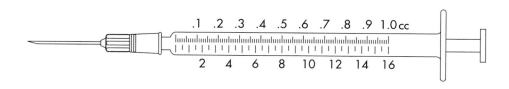

7. Atropine gr ¹⁄₂₀₀ I.M. at 6 A.M. Give _____ .

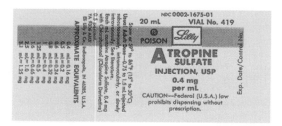

8. The physician orders Benadryl 25 mg I.V.P.B. now for your patient with a mild medication reaction. Benadryl 10 mg per ml is available. Give _____ .

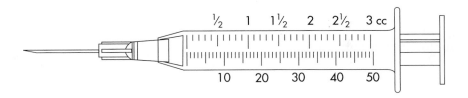

9. Your status postethmoidectomy patient receives tobramycin sulfate 55 mg I.V. q.8 h. Tobramycin 40 mg per ml is available. Give _____ .

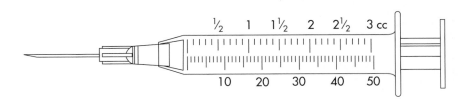

10. The physician orders Thorazine 30 mg I.M. p.r.n. for your obsessive-compulsive patient. Thorazine is supplied in 10 ml vial containing 25 mg per ml. Give _____ .

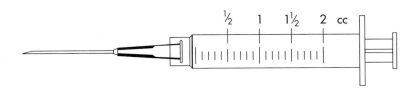

11. Your status postparathyroidectomy patient receives ampicillin 200 mg I.V. q.6 h. Ampicillin 100 mg per ml is available. Give _____ .

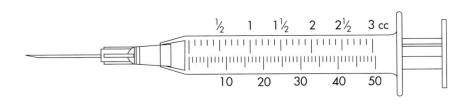

12. Scopolamine gr ⅟₁₅₀ I.M. at 7 A.M. Scopolamine gr ⅟₂₀₀ per ml is available. Give _____ ℳ.

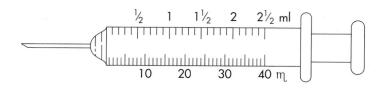

13. The physician orders piperacillin 2 g I.V. q.8 h. for your septic patient. Piperacillin 1 g per 2.5 ml is available. Give _____ .

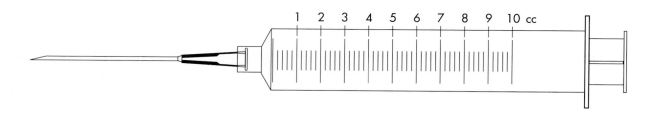

14. Gentamicin 26 mg I.V. q.8 h. Prepare _____ ℳ.

Usual Adult Dose See package insert
Each ml of aqueous solution contains:
gentamicin sulfate, USP equivalent to
40 mg gentamicin, 1.8 mg methylparaben
and 0.2 mg propylparaben as preserva
tives, 3.2 mg sodium bisulfite, and
0.1 mg edetate disodium.
Store between 2° and 30°C (36° and 86°F).
GARAMYCIN Injectable should not be
physically premixed with other drugs.

SCHERING

20 ml Multiple Dose Vial   Sterile
For use in preparation of large volume parenterals

Garamycin₍₎ **Injectable**
brand of gentamicin sulfate injection, USP

40 mg/ml
20 ml = 800 mg

For Parenteral Administration
Caution: Federal law prohibits dispensing without prescription.
Schering Pharmaceutical Corporation (PRI), Manati, Puerto Rico 00701
An Affiliate of Schering Corporation, Kenilworth, N.J. 07033
11788815 Rev.1/81

Read accompanying directions carefully

Control No
Exp. Date

15. Meperidine 6 ℳ I.M. q.3 h. p.r.n. The drug is available in an ampule containing 50 mg per ml. How many mg of the drug will you give? _____ .

16. Your patient, status post–tricuspid valve repair, has Lanoxin 80 mcg I.M. b.i.d. ordered. Give _____ ℳ.

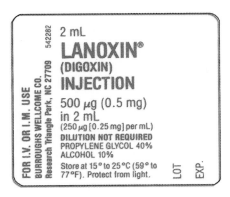

17. Morphine 4 mg subq. q.4 h. p.r.n. Morphine is supplied in a 1 ml ampule containing gr ⅛. Give _____ ℳ.

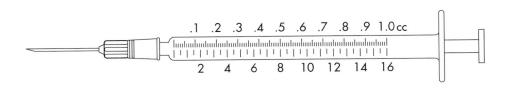

18. Your patient with a history of seizures has Dilantin 100 mg I.V. q.8 h. ordered. Dilantin 50 mg per 2 ml is available. Give _____ .

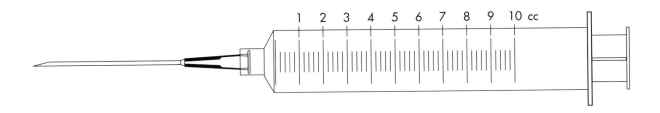

19. The physician orders phenobarbital 0.2 g I.M. q.4 h. for your epileptic patient. Phenobarbital is supplied in a 1 ml ampule containing 120 mg. Give _____ .

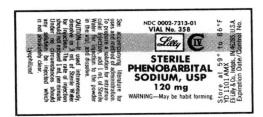

20. D_5W 500 ml plus $CaCl_2$ 10 mEq at 10 ml per h. $CaCl_2$ is supplied in a 10 ml ampule
containing 13.6 mEq. How many ml of $CaCl_2$ will be added to the 500 ml of
D_5W? _____ .

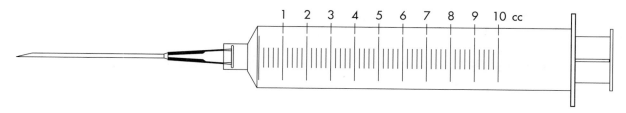

Answers on pp. 475-478.

13 | Dosages Measured in Units

Learning Objectives

On completion of the materials provided in this chapter, you will be able to perform computations accurately by mastering the following mathematical concepts:

1. Use a proportion to solve problems involving drugs measured in unit dosages
2. Draw a line through an illustration of an insulin syringe to indicate the dosage of units desired

A unit (U) is the amount of a drug needed to produce a given result. Various drugs are measured in units; the examples used in this chapter are among the more common drugs used in hospitals and health care centers daily.

Drugs used in this chapter include the following:

Penicillin—antibiotic. Reduces organisms within the body that cause infection.

Heparin—anticoagulant. Inhibits clotting of the blood.

Insulin—hormone secreted by the pancreas, which lowers blood sugar.

Penicillin can be administered orally or parenterally, but heparin and insulin must be given subcutaneously or intravenously.

Before administering penicillin, the nurse must confer with the patient regarding previous allergies to the drug. After administration of the drug, the nurse must still observe the patient for signs of an allergic reaction.

Because heparin prolongs the time blood takes to clot, the dosage must be accurate. A larger dose may cause hemorrhage, and an insufficient dose may not have the desired result. After the administration of the drug, the nurse should observe the patient for signs of hemorrhage.

Insulin is used in the treatment of diabetes mellitus. Accuracy is important in the preparation of insulin. A higher dosage than needed may cause insulin shock. An insufficient amount of insulin may result in diabetic coma. Both conditions are extremely serious, and the nurse must be able to recognize the symptoms of each condition so that immediate treatment may be initiated to stabilize the patient. In many institutions, both insulin and heparin dosages are observed for accuracy by another nurse before the drug is administered to the patient.

A U-100 insulin syringe and U-100 insulin are necessary to ensure an accurate insulin dosage. U-100 insulin means that 100 U of insulin are contained in 1 ml of liquid. U-100 insulin is a universal insulin preparation that all persons requiring insulin can use. Another type of U-100 syringe is the

U-100 Lo-Dose syringe, which measures 50 U; however, for accuracy, no more than 40 U should be measured in the U-100 Lo-Dose syringe. Because the doses are minute, the U-100 syringe provides the most accurate measurement of insulin dosages. The 30 unit, U-100 syringe is used for insulin doses that equal less than 30 units.

Powder Reconstitution

A drug of a powdered form is necessary when a medication is unstable as a liquid form for a long period. This powdered drug must be reconstituted—dissolved with a sterile diluent—before administration. The diluents commonly used include sterile water, sterile normal saline, and 5% dextrose.

Before reconstituting the medication, several principles must be followed.

1. Carefully read the information and directions on the vial or package insert for reconstitution of the medication.
2. If no directions are available with the medication, consult the P.D.R., hospital drug formulary, pharmacology text, or hospital pharmacy.
3. Identify the type and amount of diluent as well as the route of administration.
4. Note the drug strength or concentration after reconstitution and circle or place on the label, if not already written.
5. Note the length of time for which the medication is good once reconstituted as well as the directions for storage.
6. Be aware that the total reconstitution amount will be greater than the amount of diluent.
7. After reconstitution, place your initials, date of preparation, time of preparation, date of expiration, and time of expiration on the label.

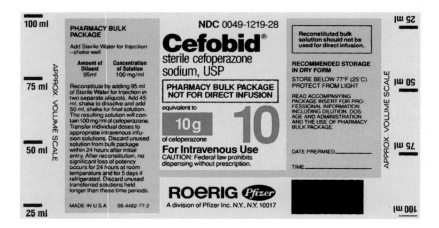

Example:

    a. What is the route of administration?   I.V.
    b. What type of diluent can be used?   sterile water
    c. How much diluent must be added?   95 ml
    d. What is the medication concentration?   100 mg/ml
    e. How long will the medication maintain
       its potency at room temperature?   24 hours
    f. The physician orders 1 g I.V. q.6 h. How
       many ml will you give? Shade the syringe.   10 ml
           a. 100 mg : 1 ml ::
           b. 100 mg : 1 ml :: _____ mg : _____ ml
           c. 100 mg : 1 ml :: 1000 mg : x ml

d. $100x = 1000$

$$x = \frac{1000}{100}$$

$x = 10$

e. $x = 10$ ml

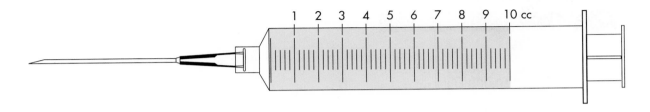

Dosages Measured in Units Involving Oral and Parenteral Medications

Example: Penicillin V 250,000 U p.o. q.i.d. The drug is supplied 200,000 U per 5 ml after reconstitution. Give _____ .

a. On the left side of the proportion, place what you know or have available. In this example, each 5 ml contains 200,000 U. So the left side of the proportion would be

200,000 U : 5 ml ::

b. The right side of the proportion is determined by the physician's order and the abbreviations on the left side of the proportion. Only *two* different abbreviations may be used in a single proportion. The abbreviations must be in the same position on the right side as on the left side.

200,000 U : 5 ml :: 250,000 U : _____ ml

We need to find the number of milliliters to be administered, so we use the symbol x to represent the unknown.

200,000 U : 5 ml :: 250,000 U : x ml

c. Rewrite the proportion without using the abbreviations.

200,000 : 5 :: 250,000 : x

d. Solve for x.

200,000 : 5 :: 250,000 : x

$200,000x = 250,000 \times 5$

$200,000x = 1,250,000$

$$x = \frac{1,250,000}{200,000}$$

$x = 6.25$

e. Label your answer as determined by the abbreviation placed next to x in the original proportion.

$x = 6.25$ ml

6.25 ml would be measured to administer 250,000 U of penicillin V.

Dosages Measured in Units Involving Parenteral Medications

Example: Heparin 12,000 U subq. q.8 h. Give _____ .

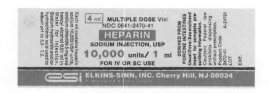

        a. 10,000 U : 1 ml ::
        b. 10,000 U : 1 ml :: _____ U : _____ ml
            10,000 U : 1 ml :: 12,000 U : x ml
        c. 10,000 : 1 :: 12,000 : x
        d. $10,000x = 1 \times 12,000$

$$10,000x = 12,000$$

$$x = \frac{12000}{10000}$$

$$x = 1.2$$

        e. $x = 1.2$ ml

Therefore 1.2 ml of heparin would be the amount of each individual dose of heparin given q.8 h.

Insulin Given with a Lo-Dose Insulin Syringe

Example: Lente insulin 36 U subq. in A.M. Lente insulin U-100 and a U-100 Lo-Dose syringe are available. Draw a vertical line through the syringe to indicate the correct dosage.

Lo-Dose   ┤ 5   15   25   35   45   ½ cc
           ╞ 10   20   30   40   50   units

With a Lo-Dose insulin syringe, 36 U of U-100 insulin would be measured as indicated.

Mixed Insulin Administration

The physician may prescribe two types of insulin to be administered at the same time. These insulins will be drawn up in the same syringe to avoid injecting the patient twice.

Several guidelines apply to this type of administration.

1. Air equal to the amount of insulin being withdrawn should be injected into each vial. Do *not* touch the solution with the tip of the needle.
2. Using the same syringe, draw up the desired amount of insulin from the regular insulin bottle first.
3. Remove the syringe from the regular insulin bottle. Check the syringe for any air bubbles and remove them.

4. Using the same syringe, draw up the amount of cloudy insulin to the desired dosage.
5. Some hospitals require that you check your insulin with another nurse before administration. Consult your hospital policy and procedures.

Example: The physician orders administration of 10 U regular insulin plus 20 U of NPH insulin.

The total amount of insulin is 30 U (10 U + 20 U = 30 U).

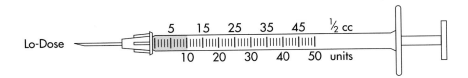

10 U of regular insulin

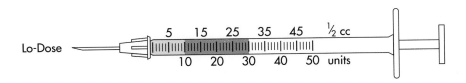

10 U of regular insulin + 20 U of NPH insulin

Regular Insulin Given with Another Type of Insulin in the Same U-100 Syringe

Example: Lente humulin insulin 46 U subq. q.A.M. Regular humulin insulin 20 U. Lente humulin insulin U-100, regular humulin insulin U-100, and a U-100 insulin syringe are available. Draw a vertical line through the syringe to indicate the amount of Lente humulin insulin to be given, and a second line to indicate the total dosage.

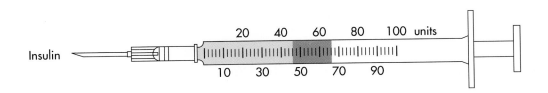

The Lente humulin insulin dosage is indicated at 46 U. Add 20 U of regular humulin insulin for a total dosage of 66 U of insulin.

Complete the following work sheet, which provides for extensive practice in the calculation of dosages measured in units. Check your answers. If you have difficulties, go back and review the necessary material. When you feel ready to evaluate your learning, take the first posttest. Check your answers. An acceptable score as indicated on the posttest signifies that you have successfully completed this chapter. An unacceptable score signifies a need for further study before taking the second posttest.

WORK SHEET

Directions: The medication order is listed at the beginning of each problem. Calculate the dosages. Show your work. Mark the syringe when provided to indicate the correct dosage.

1. Your pneumonia patient receives penicillin V 200,000 U q.i.d. You have penicillin V oral solution 400,000 U per 5 ml available. Give _____ .

2. The physician orders heparin 7500 U subq. q.12 h. for your postop patient. You have heparin 5000 U per ml available. Give _____ .

3. NPH insulin 20 U subq. q.A.M. Draw a vertical line through the syringe to indicate the amount of NPH insulin to be given.

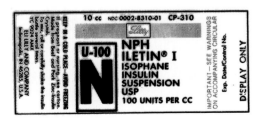

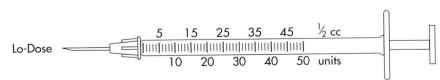

4. A patient with a temporal bone infection receives penicillin G 500,000 U I.M. q.6 h. How much diluent should be added? _____ . What is the medication concentration? _____ . Give _____ .

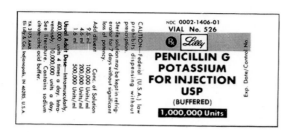

5. The physician orders heparin 2500 U subq. q.12 h. for your jejunostomy patient. You have heparin 5000 U per ml available. Give _____ . Draw a vertical line through the syringe to indicate the dosage.

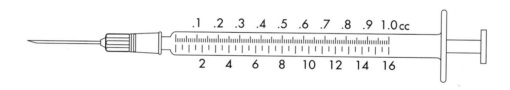

6. Regular humulin insulin 2 U subq. q.P.M. Draw a vertical line through the syringe to indicate the dosage.

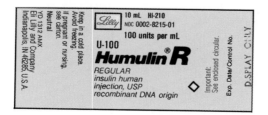

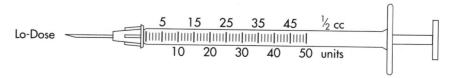

7. Your gastric pull-up patient receives heparin 5000 U subq. q.8 h. Give _____ .

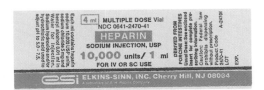

8. V-Cillin K suspension 400,000 U p.o. q.6 h. V-Cillin K suspension is supplied 200,000 U per 5 ml. Give _____ .

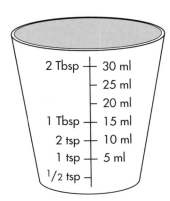

9. Lente insulin 14 U, regular insulin 6 U subq. q.a.m. Lente insulin U-100, regular insulin U-100, and a U-100 Lo-Dose syringe are supplied. Draw a vertical line through the syringe to indicate the amount of Lente insulin to be given and a second line to indicate the total dosage.

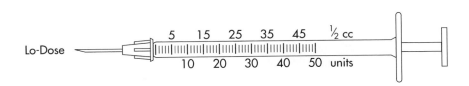

10. Your appendectomy patient has penicillin V 300,000 U p.o. q.i.d. ordered. You have penicillin V oral solution 400,000 U per 5 ml available. Give _____ ml. Draw a vertical line through the syringe to indicate the dosage.

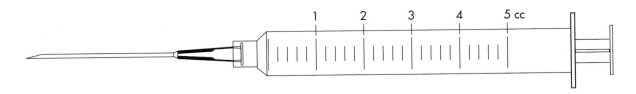

11. The physician orders heparin 6000 U subq. q.d. for your corneal transplant patient. Give _____ .

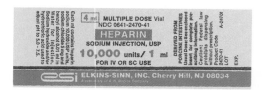

12. Regular insulin 18 U subq. q.A.M. Draw a vertical line through the syringe to indicate the dosage.

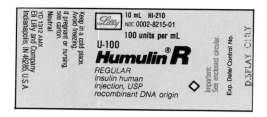

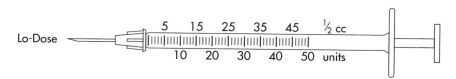

13. NPH insulin 32 U subq. tomorrow at 7:45 A.M. You have NPH insulin U-100 and a U-100 Lo-Dose syringe. Draw a vertical line through the syringe to indicate the dosage.

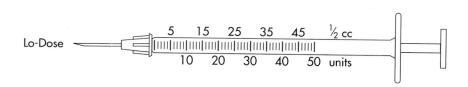

14. Your thoracotomy patient receives penicillin G 600,000 U I.M. b.i.d. How much diluent should be added? _____ . What is the medication concentration? _____ . Give _____ .

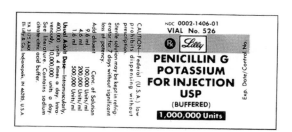

15. The physician orders heparin 10,000 U subq. q.12 h. for your below-the-knee amputation patient. You have heparin 5000 U per ml available. Give _____ . Draw a vertical line through the syringe to indicate the dosage.

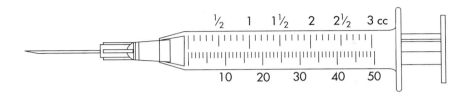

16. Your status post–Nissen procedure patient receives heparin 5000 U q.12 h. Give _____ .

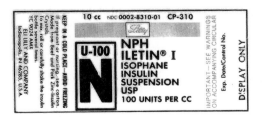

17. Your stapendectomy patient receives penicillin V 300,000 U p.o. q.i.d. The drug is supplied in oral solution 200,000 U per 5 ml. Give _____ .

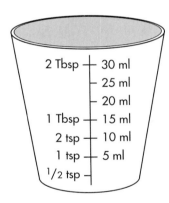

18. Your insulin-dependent patient receives NPH insulin 24 U subq. q.A.M. Draw a vertical line through the syringe to indicate the dosage.

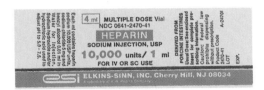

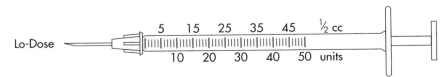

19. Your lumbar laminectomy patient receives heparin 0.5 ml when I.V. is not infusing. Give _____ . Draw a vertical line through the syringe to indicate the dosage.

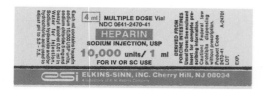

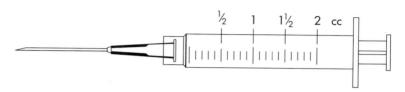

20. Your gastric pull-up patient receives penicillin G 200,000 U I.M. q.6 h. You have penicillin G 250,000 U per ml available. Give _____ . Draw a vertical line through the syringe to indicate the dosage.

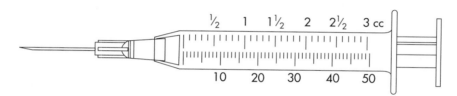

Answers on pp. 479-482.

POSTTEST 1

Name _____

Date _____

ACCEPTABLE SCORE __**13**__

YOUR SCORE _____

Directions: The medication order is listed at the beginning of each problem. Calculate the dosages. Show your work. Mark the syringe when provided to indicate the correct dosage.

1. The physician orders penicillin V 500,000 U p.o. q.i.d. for your hysterectomy patient. Penicillin V pediatric suspension 400,000 U per 5 ml is supplied. Give _____ . Draw a vertical line through the syringe to indicate the dosage.

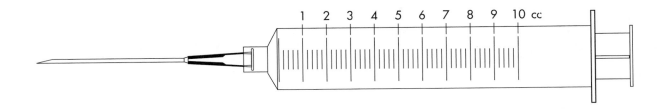

2. Lente insulin 40 U subq. q.A.M. Draw a vertical line through the syringe to indicate the dosage.

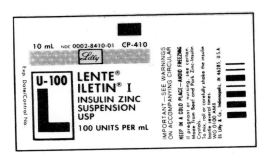

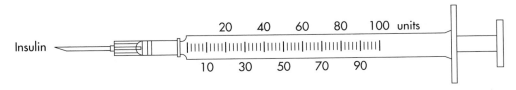

3. Your lumbar laminectomy patient receives heparin 7500 U subq. q.i.d. You have heparin 5000 U per ml available. Give _____ .

4. Regular humulin insulin 6 U subq. Draw a vertical line through the syringe to indicate the dosage.

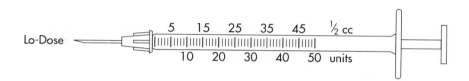

5. The physician orders penicillin G potassium 3,000,000 U I.M. q.6 h. for your ethmoidectomy patient. What is the best amount of diluent to add? _____ . What is the medication concentration? _____ . Give _____ .

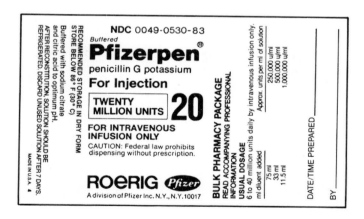

6. Your insulin-dependent patient has NPH insulin 60 U subq. q.A.M. You have NPH insulin U-100 and a U-100 syringe. Draw a vertical line through the syringe to indicate the dosage.

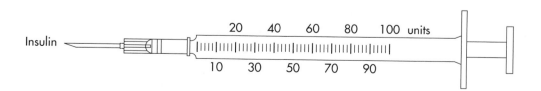

7. Heparin 20,000 U subq. today. Give _____ .

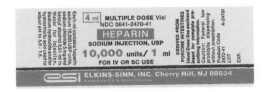

8. Lente insulin 38 U, regular insulin 18 U subq. q.A.M. Lente U-100, regular insulin U-100, and a U-100 syringe are supplied. Draw a vertical line through the syringe to indicate the amount of Lente insulin to be given, and a second line to indicate the total dosage.

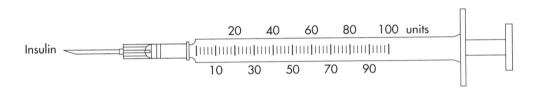

9. The physician orders penicillin V 300,000 U p.o. q.i.d. for your chronic otitis patient. The drug is supplied in oral solution 200,000 U per 5 ml. Give _____ .

10. Streptomycin 0.5 g I.M. b.i.d. How much diluent should be added? _____ . What is the medication concentration? _____ . Give _____ .

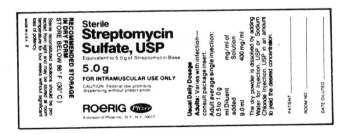

11. Your patient with a sacral decubitus receives penicillin V 200,000 U p.o. q.i.d. You have penicillin V oral solution 400,000 U per 5 ml. Give _____ .

12. Your lumbar laminectomy patient receives heparin 7500 U subq. q.12 h. Heparin 5000 U per ml is available. Give _____ .

13. Your patient with meningitis receives penicillin G 500,000 U I.M. q.6 h. Give _____ .

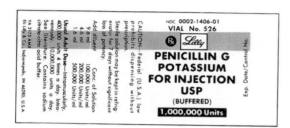

14. Mrs. Daisy receives nafcillin 600 mg I.M. q.6 h. for treatment of *S. aureas*. How much diluent should be added? _____ . What is the medication concentration? _____ . Give _____ .

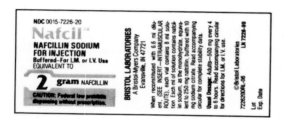

15. Your lumbar discectomy patient requires heparin 5000 U subq. q.8 h. Give _____ .

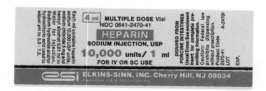

Answers on pp. 482-484.

POSTTEST 2

Name _____

Date _____

ACCEPTABLE SCORE **13**

YOUR SCORE _____

Directions: The medication order is listed at the beginning of each problem. Calculate the dosages. Show your work. Mark the syringe when provided to indicate the correct dosage.

1. Regular insulin 10 U subq. tomorrow A.M. Regular insulin U-100 and a U-100 Lo-Dose syringe are supplied. Draw a vertical line through the syringe to indicate the dosage.

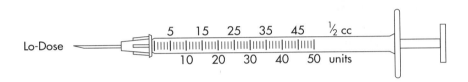

2. Heparin 1000 U per L to be added to I.V. fluids. How many minims would you add to 1 L? _____ .

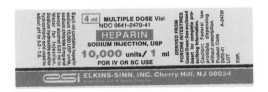

3. Your septoplasty patient receives V-Cillin K 500,000 U p.o. q.6 h. You have 200,000 U per ℥ available. Give _____ ℥.

4. NPH insulin 28 U subq. at 7:45 A.M. Draw a vertical line through the syringe to indicate the NPH insulin to be given.

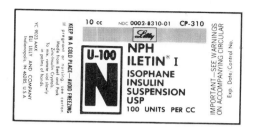

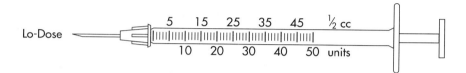

Lo-Dose

5. The physician orders heparin 1500 U subq. today for your total hip replacement patient. Give _____ .

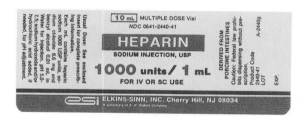

6. The physician orders penicillin G potassium 1.2 million U I.V. q.4 h. for your dental extraction patient. You have a vial containing 1,000,000 U per ml. Give _____ .

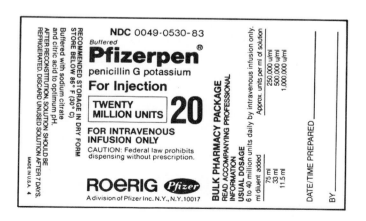

7. Lente insulin 54 U subq. q.A.M. You have Lente insulin U-100 and a U-100 syringe. Draw a vertical line through the syringe to indicate the amount of Lente insulin to be given.

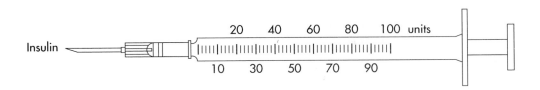

8. NPH insulin 16 U, regular insulin 8 U subq. q.A.M. You have NPH insulin U-100, regular insulin U-100, and a U-100 Lo-Dose syringe. Draw a vertical line through the syringe to indicate the amount of regular insulin to be given and a second line to indicate the total dosage.

9. Your chronic sinusitis patient receives penicillin V 300,000 U p.o. q.i.d. You have penicillin V oral solution 400,000 U per 5 ml. Give _____ .

10. Your jejunostomy patient requires heparin 6000 U subq. q.d. You have heparin 5000 U per ml available. Give _____ . Draw a vertical line through the syringe to indicate the dosage.

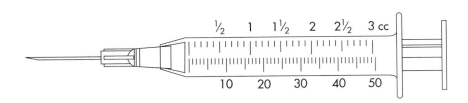

11. Your osteomyelitis patient receives penicillin G 600,000 U I.M. b.i.d. How much diluent should be added? _____ . What is the medication concentration? _____ . Give _____ .

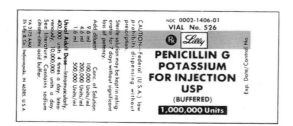

12. Your total hip replacement patient requires heparin 10,000 U subq. q.12 h. You have heparin 5000 U per ml available. Give _____ .

13. Your insulin-dependent patient receives Lente insulin 25 U subq. q.A.M. Draw a vertical line through the syringe to indicate the amount of Lente insulin to be given.

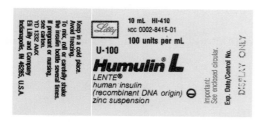

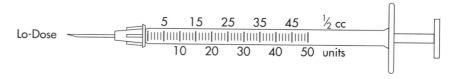

14. Your gastrectomy patient requires heparin 7500 U subq. q.i.d. You have heparin 5000 U per ml. Give _____ .

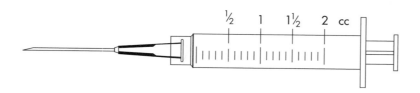

15. Your cholecystectomy patient receives heparin 20,000 U subq. today. Give _____ .

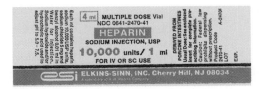

Answers on pp. 485-487.

Chapter *14* | *Intravenous Flow Rates*

Learning Objectives

On completion of the materials provided in this chapter, you will be able to perform computations accurately by mastering the following mathematical concepts:

1 Calculate ml/h. of I.V. flow rates when total volume and length of time over which the I.V. is to infuse is given

2 Calculate ml/min of I.V. flow rates when total volume and length of time over which the I.V. is to infuse is given

3 Calculate gtt/min of I.V. flow rates when total volume and length of time over which the I.V. is to infuse is given

4 Calculate ml/min of I.V. flow rates when ml/h. is given

5 Calculate gtt/min of I.V. flow rates when ml/h. is given

It is sometimes necessary to deliver fluids and medications to a patient intravenously. Intravenous solutions and medications are placed directly into a vein. Infusions are injections of moderate to large quantities of fluids and nutrients into the patient's venous system. An intravenous medication or infusion may be prepared and administered by a physician, nurse, or technician as regulated by state law and the policies of the particular health care agency. Medications and electrolyte milliequivalents are commonly ordered as additives to I.V. fluids. Medications may also be diluted and given in conjunction with I.V. solutions.

I.V. fluids are administered via an intravenous infusion set. This set includes the sealed bottle or bag containing the fluids, a drip chamber connected to the bottle or bag by a small tube or spike, and tubing that leads from the drip chamber down to and connecting with the needle or catheter at the site of insertion into the patient (Figure 14-1). The flow rate is adjusted to the desired drops per minute by a clamp placed around the tubing. The nurse must be knowledgeable about the equipment being used and, in particular, about the flow rate or drops per milliliter that a particular set of tubing will deliver.

Infusion sets come in a variety of sizes. The larger the diameter of the tubing where it enters the drip chamber, the bigger the drop will be. The drop factor of an infusion set is the number of drops contained in 1 ml (1 cc). This equivalent may vary with different manufacturers. The most common drop factors are 10, 12, 15, 20, and 60. Sets that deliver 10, 12, 15, or 20 drops per milliliter are

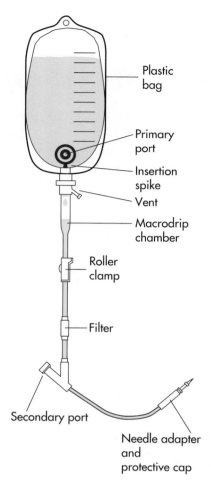

FIGURE 14-1
Intravenous infusion set. *(From Edmunds MW:* Introduction to clinical pharmacology, *ed 2, St Louis, 1995, Mosby.)*

called macrodrip sets. A set that delivers 60 drops per milliliter is called a microdrip set. The macrodrip sets are larger than the microdrips.

If large volumes of fluid must be administered (125 ml/h. or more), a macrodrip set is required. Microdrip sets are unable to deliver large volumes per hour because their drop size is so small. When an I.V. solution is to run at a rate of 50 ml/h. or less, a microdrip set should be used. Some hospitals may even require a microdrip set for rates of 60 to 80 ml/h., for accuracy of flow rate and to help maintain the patency of the line. The number of drops per milliliter for the I.V. administration set is written on the outside of the box. This is essential information in solving problems related to the regulation of I.V. flow rates.

The physician is responsible for writing the order for the type of intravenous or hyperalimentation fluids and amount. The number of hours or rate of infusion is also ordered by the physician. It is usually the nurse's responsibility to regulate and maintain the infusion flow rate. It is the nurse's goal to ensure that the I.V. flow is regular. If the rate is irregular, too much or too little fluid may be infused. This may lead to complications such as fluid overload, dehydration, or medication overdose. Sometimes the rate of flow must be adjusted because of interruptions caused by needle placement, condition of the vein, or infiltration.

Intravenous flow rates often are controlled by an electronic device or pump. The I.V. pumps are programmed to deliver a set amount of fluid per hour. Safety for the patient is an advantage of electronic I.V. pumps. The pumps are used on regular medical-surgical patients and in critical care areas, pediatrics, the operating room, and ambulatory care.

Many electronic pumps are on the market today. These vary from simple one-channel models to those that are four multichannel pumps. Many of the newer models will actually calculate flow rates and automatically start infusions at a later time. Convenience, safety, accuracy, and time-saving options are driving forces in the innovations currently available.

Some examples of equipment are pictured in Figures 14-2, 14-3, and 14-4. Figure 14-2, *A* and *B*, shows a single-channel unit that may be stacked easily to become a multichannel unit. In Figure 14-3, models of one, two, and four channels are shown. In Figure 14-4, two-channel models are being used on a patient in a critical care setting. Each company offers special tubing for use with its pumps.

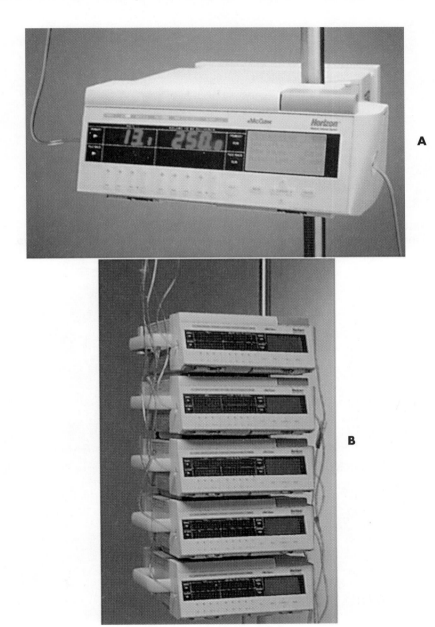

FIGURE 14-2
A, Single-channel unit. **B,** Multichannel unit. *(Courtesy McGaw Inc., Irvine, Calif.)*

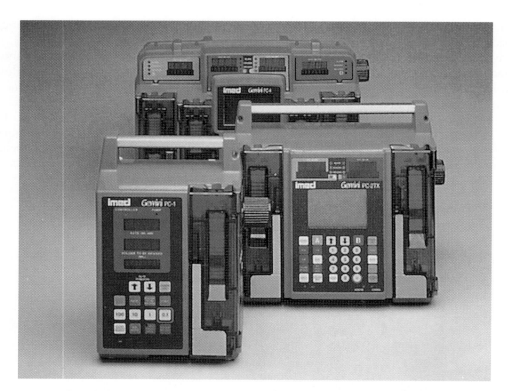

FIGURE 14-3
One-, two-, and four-channel units. *(Courtesy IMED Corporation, San Diego.)*

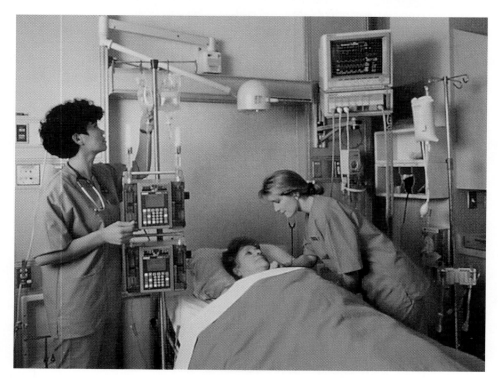

FIGURE 14-4
Two-channel models being used on a patient in a critical care setting. *(Courtesy IMED Corporation, San Diego.)*

The nurse must be able to determine the number of drops per minute that the patient must receive for the infusion to be completed within the specified time. To accomplish this task, the nurse must calculate three different pieces of information in the following manner:

1. milliliters given per hour (ml/h.)
2. milliliters given per minute (ml/min)
3. drops given per minute (gtt/min)

All three of these items may be calculated by the use of a proportion.

Example 1: Amigen 500 ml in 3 h. The drop factor is 15 gtt/ml. How many ml must be given per hour? _____ . How many ml must be given per minute? _____ . How many gtt must be given per minute? _____ .

    1. ml/h.

$$500 \text{ ml} : 3 \text{ h.} :: x \text{ ml} : 1 \text{ h.}$$

$$500 : 3 :: x : 1$$

$$3x = 500$$

$$x = \frac{500}{3}$$

$$x = 166.66 \text{ ml}$$

$$166.66 \text{ ml/h.}$$

    2. ml/min

To determine the drops per minute, the nurse must first calculate the number of milliliters the patient must receive per minute. We have already determined that the patient must receive 166.66 ml per 1 hour, or 60 minutes. Therefore the following proportion may be written:

$$166.66 \text{ ml} : 60 \text{ min} :: x \text{ ml} : 1 \text{ min}$$

$$166.66 : 60 :: x : 1$$

$$60x = 166.66$$

$$x = \frac{166.66}{60}$$

$$x = 2.777 \ldots$$

$$x = 2.78 \text{ ml}$$

$$2.78 \text{ ml/min}$$

3. gtt/min
    This number and calculation depend on the drop factor of the tubing being used. Remember, this information is found on the package. For the problems in this workbook, the drop factor is indicated. The drop factor for this problem is 15. We have just determined that the patient must receive 2.78 ml each minute. Therefore the following proportion may be written:

$$15 \text{ gtt} : 1 \text{ ml} :: x \text{ gtt} : 2.78 \text{ ml}$$

$$15 : 1 :: x : 2.78$$

$$x = 15 \times 2.78$$

$$x = 41.70$$

$$x = 41.70, \text{ or rounded to 42 gtt}$$

The nurse thus knows how to regulate the I.V. to drip at 42 drops per minute, for the full 500 ml to be infused within the 3 hours ordered.

4. Shortcut
    When the volume per hour is known, a different formula may be used by the nurse who has a great deal of mathematical expertise. This formula combines steps 2 and 3.

$$\text{drops per minute} = \frac{\text{volume per hour}}{60 \text{ minutes}} \times \frac{\text{drop factor}}{1}$$

We have determined that the hourly rate is 166.66 or 167 ml per hour or 60 minutes. The problem indicates the drop factor is 15. Therefore the equation would be as follows:

$$x \text{ (gtt/min)} = \frac{167 \text{ (volume per hour)}}{60 \text{ (minutes per hour)}} \times \frac{15 \text{ (drop factor)}}{1}$$

$$x = \frac{167}{\underset{4}{60}} \times \frac{\overset{1}{\cancel{15}}}{1}$$

$$x = \frac{167}{4}$$

$$x = 41.75, \text{ or rounded to 42 gtt/min}$$

Once again the nurse knows to regulate the I.V. to drip at 42 drops per minute for the full 500 ml to be infused within the 3 hours ordered.

Example 2: 250 ml D$_5$W in 24 h. The drop factor is 60. How many ml will be given per hour? _____ . How many ml/min will be given? _____ . How many gtt will be given per minute? _____ .

1. ml/h.

$$250 \text{ ml} : 24 \text{ h.} :: x \text{ ml} : 1 \text{ h.}$$

$$250 : 24 :: x : 1$$

$$24x = 250$$

$$x = \frac{250}{24}$$

$$x = 10.41 \text{ ml}$$

$$x = 10.41 \text{ ml/h.}$$

2. ml/min

$$10.41 \text{ ml} : 60 \text{ min} :: x : 1 \text{ min}$$

$$10.41 : 60 :: x : 1$$

$$60x = 10.41$$

$$x = \frac{10.41}{60}$$

$$x = 0.17$$

$$x = 0.17 \text{ ml/min}$$

3. gtt/min

$$60 \text{ gtt} : 1 \text{ ml} :: x \text{ gtt} : 0.17 \text{ ml}$$

$$60 : 1 :: x : 0.17$$

$$x = 60 \times 0.17$$

$$x = 10.2$$

$$x = 10.2 \text{ or } 10 \text{ gtt/min}$$

4. Shortcut

$$x \text{ (gtt/min)} = \frac{10 \text{ (volume per hour)}}{60 \text{ (minutes per hour)}} \times \frac{60 \text{ (drop factor)}}{1}$$

$$x = \frac{10}{\overset{1}{\underset{1}{\cancel{60}}}} \times \frac{\overset{1}{\cancel{60}}}{1}$$

$$x = 10$$

$$x = 10 \text{ gtt/min}$$

Note: When a microdrip set (drop factor of 60) is used, the drops per minute will be the same as the number of milliliters per hour.

Sometimes the physician writes the order for the type of fluid plus the rate at which it is to infuse. In that case, only the second and third calculations need to be made.

Example 3: $D_5\frac{1}{2}$ N.S. at 120 ml/h. The drop factor is 12. How many ml/min will be given? _____ . How many gtt/min will be given? _____ .

1. 120 ml/h. given in order
2. ml/min

$$120 \text{ ml} : 60 \text{ min} :: x \text{ ml} : 1 \text{ min}$$

$$120 : 60 :: x : 1$$

$$60x = 120$$

$$x = \frac{120}{60}$$

$$x = 2$$

$$x = 2 \text{ ml/min}$$

3. gtt/min

$$12 \text{ gtt} : 1 \text{ ml} :: x \text{ gtt} : 2 \text{ ml}$$

$$12 : 1 :: x : 2$$

$$x = 24$$

$$x = 24 \text{ gtt/min}$$

4. Shortcut

$$x \text{ (gtt/min)} = \frac{120 \text{ (volume per hour)}}{60 \text{ (minutes per hour)}} \times \frac{12 \text{ (drop factor)}}{1}$$

$$x = \frac{120}{\underset{5}{\cancel{60}}} \times \frac{\overset{1}{\cancel{12}}}{1}$$

$$x = \frac{120}{5}$$

$$x = 24$$

$$x = 24 \text{ gtt/min}$$

Critical Care I.V. Medications and Flow Rates

Critically ill patients in a hospital often receive special medications that are very potent and therefore need to be monitored closely. Some of these medications may be ordered at a set amount of the drug measured in units to be infused over a given period; for example, regular insulin or heparin. Other drugs used in the critical care setting may be ordered to be infused by amount of drug per kilogram of body weight per minute. These are called titrations. They are based on the manufacturer's provided recommended dosage and the patient's body weight measured in kilograms. In most health care institutions, these situations will occur in the emergency room, an intensive care unit, or a step-down unit. It is extremely important to accurately monitor the flow of these medications; therefore most are delivered through an I.V. machine. Because of the nature of these drugs, route of administration, and state of the patient, it cannot be overemphasized how important the accuracy of the calculation of the drug dosage and I.V. flow rates is. It is truly a matter of life and death.

This chapter provides a sampling of these types of calculations. However, to become competent and develop expertise in this area, we recommend further in-depth study in a clinical setting with experienced supervision.

I.V. Administration of Regular Insulin and Heparin

Example 1: 0.9% N.S. 500 ml with 200 U regular insulin. Infuse 10 U/h. The drop factor is 60. Amount of drug/ml _____ . How many ml/h.? _____ . How many ml/min? _____ . How many gtt/min? _____ .

1. First determine the amount of drug in each milliliter. This may be done by using a proportion.

$$500 \text{ ml N.S.} : 200 \text{ U insulin} :: 1 \text{ ml N.S.} : x \text{ U insulin}$$

$$500 : 200 :: 1 : x$$

$$500x = 200$$

$$x = \frac{200}{500}$$

$$x = 0.4$$

$$x = 0.4 \text{ U insulin/ml}$$

2. ml/h.

$$0.4 \text{ U insulin} : 1 \text{ ml} :: 10 \text{ U insulin} : x \text{ ml}$$

$$0.4 : 1 :: 10 : x$$

$$0.4x = 10$$

$$x = \frac{10}{0.4}$$

$$x = 25$$

$$x = 25 \text{ ml/h.}$$

3. ml/min

$$25 \text{ ml} : 60 \text{ min} :: x : 1 \text{ min}$$

$$25 : 60 :: x : 1$$

$$60x = 25$$

$$x = \frac{25}{60}$$

$$x = 0.416$$

$$0.42 \text{ ml/min}$$

4. gtt/min

$$60 \text{ gtt} : 1 \text{ ml} :: x \text{ gtt} : 0.42 \text{ ml}$$

$$60 : 1 :: x : 0.42$$

$$x = 25.2$$

$$x = 25.2 \text{ gtt/min}$$

5. Shortcut

$$x \text{ (gtt/min)} = \frac{25 \text{ (volume per hour)}}{60 \text{ (minutes per hour)}} \times \frac{60 \text{ (drop factor)}}{1}$$

$$x = \frac{25}{\cancel{60}} \times \frac{\cancel{60}}{1}$$

$$x = 25 \text{ gtt/min}$$

Example 2: D_5W 1000 ml with 40,000 U heparin. Infuse at 2000 U/h. The drop factor is 60. Amount of drug/ml _____ . How many ml/h.? _____ . How many ml/min? _____ . How many gtt/min? _____ .

1. Amount of drug/ml

1000 ml D_5W : 40,000 U heparin :: 1 ml D_5W : x U heparin

1000 : 40,000 :: 1 : x

$1000x = 40,000$

$x = 40$

40 U heparin/ml

2. ml/h.

40 U heparin : 1 ml D_5W :: 2000 U heparin : x ml D_5W

40 : 1 :: 2000 : x

$40x = 2000$

$x = 50$

50 ml/h.

3. ml/min

50 ml : 60 min :: x ml : 1 min

50 : 60 :: x : 1

$60x = 50$

$x = 0.833$

0.83 ml/min

4. gtt/min

60 gtt : 1 ml :: x : 0.83 ml

60 : 1 :: x : 0.83

$x = 49.8$

$x = 49.8$ gtt/min

5. Shortcut

$$x \text{ (gtt/min)} = \frac{50 \text{ (volume per hour)}}{60 \text{ (minutes per hour)}} \times \frac{60 \text{ (drop factor)}}{1}$$

$$x = \frac{\overset{1}{\cancel{50}}}{\underset{1}{\cancel{60}}} \times \frac{\cancel{60}}{1}$$

$$x = 50 \text{ gtt/min}$$

I.V. Administration of Medication per Kilogram per Minute

Example: Dopamine 1 g in 250 ml D$_5$½ N.S. Infuse at 3 mcg/kg/min for a patient weighing 65 kg. The drop factor is 60. Amount of drug/min for 65 kg patient _____ . Amount of drug/ml _____ . How many ml/min? _____ . How many gtt/min? _____ .

1. Amount of drug per minute for 65 kg patient

$$3 \text{ mcg} : 1 \text{ kg} :: x \text{ mcg} : 65 \text{ kg}$$

$$3 : 1 :: x : 65$$

$$x = 195$$

195 mcg/min for this 65 kg patient

2. Amount of drug/ml
   Because the order is in micrograms, change 1 g to micrograms (see Chapter 6). You should know that 1 g equals 1,000,000 mcg. To find the amount of drug in each milliliter, use the following proportion:

$$1,000,000 \text{ mcg} : 250 \text{ ml} :: x \text{ mcg} : 1 \text{ ml}$$

$$1,000,000 : 250 :: x : 1$$

$$250x = 1,000,000$$

$$x = \frac{1,000,000}{250}$$

$$x = 4000$$

4000 mcg/ml

3. ml/min

$$4000 \text{ mcg} : 1 \text{ ml} :: 195 \text{ mcg} : x \text{ ml}$$

$$4000 : 1 :: 195 : x$$

$$4000x = 195$$

$$x = \frac{195}{4000}$$

$$x = 0.048 \text{ ml}$$

0.048 ml/min must be infused for this 65 kg patient

4. gtt/min

$$60 \text{ gtt} : 1 \text{ ml} :: x \text{ gtt} : 0.048 \text{ ml}$$

$$60 : 1 :: x : 0.048$$

$$x = 2.88$$

$$x = 2.88 \text{ or } 3 \text{ gtt/min}$$

I.V. Piggybacks

Sometimes the physician will order medications to be administered in a small amount of I.V. fluid. This medication will need to infuse in addition to the regular I.V. fluids; it is called an I.V. piggyback (Figure 14-5). The medication for the piggyback (I.V.P.B.) may be received premixed by the pharmacy or may need to be prepared by the nurse. The time frame for the I.V. piggyback infusion is usually 60 minutes or less.

If the physician does not include an infusion time or rate, it is the responsibility of the nurse to follow the manufacturer's guidelines. The hospital pharmacy and drug books such as the *Hospital Formulary* and *A Handbook for Intravenous Medication* published by Mosby are known resources for fluid rates. The nurse should always refer to any standing fluid limits and rates before I.V. piggyback administration.

Example 1: The physician orders cefuroxime 1.0 g in 50 ml of N.S. to run over 30 minutes. Drop factor is 60 gtt/ml. What is the flow rate *(R)* in gtt/min?

$$\frac{V}{T} \times C = R$$

$$\frac{50}{\overset{}{\underset{1}{30}}} \times \frac{\overset{2}{60}}{1} = 100 \text{ gtt/min}$$

Example 2: The physician orders gentamicin 1.5 g in 100 ml D$_5$W to run over 60 minutes. Drop factor is 60 gtt/ml.

$$\frac{V}{T} \times C = R$$

$$\frac{100}{\overset{}{\underset{1}{60}}} \times \frac{\overset{1}{60}}{1} = 100 \text{ gtt/min}$$

Heparin Locks

Heparin locks commonly are used in a variety of health care settings. A heparin lock is an I.V. catheter that is inserted into a peripheral vein. It may be used for medications or fluids, usually on an intermittent basis. The use of a heparin lock prevents the patient from having to endure numerous venipunctures. Also, when fluid is not infusing, the patient enjoys greater mobility and freedom of movement. Each institution will have its own policy concerning the use and care of heparin locks—whether the locks are flushed with only 2 to 3 cc of normal saline, or also with heparin flush solution of 10 units of heparin per 1 cc. This practice is called heparinization and prevents clotting of the heparin lock.

Central Venous Catheter

Occasionally, a patient will have to have a central venous catheter. Central venous catheters are indwelling, semipermanent central lines that are inserted into the right atrium of the heart via the cephalic, subclavian, or jugular veins (Figures 14-6 and 14-7).

This type of catheter may be required for clients who need frequent venipuncture, long-term I.V. infusions, hyperalimentation, chemotherapy, intermittent blood transfusions, or antibiotics. These catheters may be referred to as triple lumen catheters or Hickman lines.

Central venous catheter management involves flushing the catheter with 2.5 cc of 10 U per cc of heparin when the catheter access is routinely capped or clamped after blood draws. Please consult your institution's procedure/policy about central venous line flushes. If continuous fluids are

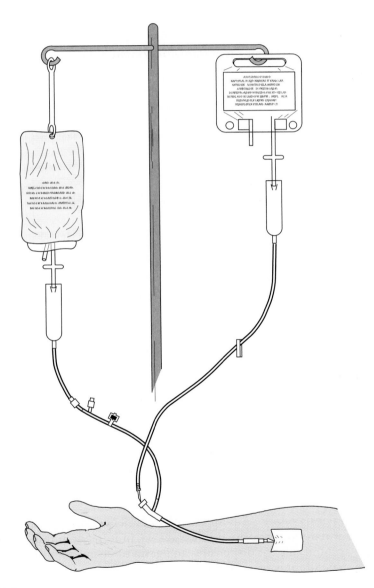

FIGURE 14-5
Intravenous piggyback (I.V.P.B.) administration setup. Note that the smaller bottle is hung higher than the primary bottle. *(From Dison N:* Simplified drugs and solutions for nurses, *St Louis, 1997, Mosby.)*

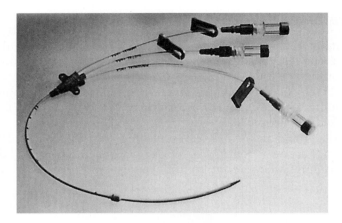

FIGURE 14-6
Multilumen subclavian catheter. *(Courtesy Arrow International, Inc., Reading, Pa.)*

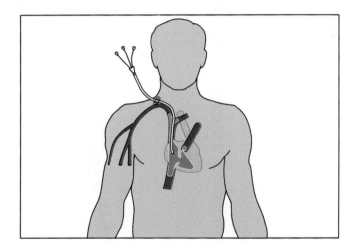

FIGURE 14-7
Multilumen subclavian catheter. *(From LaRocca JC, Otto S: Pocket guide to intravenous therapy, ed 2, St Louis, 1993, Mosby.)*

ordered, these fluids must be regulated via an infusion pump. All central venous catheter management must be under the supervision of a registered nurse.

The central venous catheter site must be assessed regularly. The catheter site should always remain sterile under an occlusive dressing that is changed according to the institution's procedure regarding the central venous catheter.

Patient-Controlled Analgesia

Patient-controlled analgesia or a PCA pump involves patients giving themselves an intravenous narcotic. This intravenous narcotic is given at intervals via an infusion pump (Figure 14-8). Only a registered nurse can be accountable for dispensing analgesia to be given in this manner. In addition, only a registered nurse may administer a PCA loading dose.

Several considerations are crucial in the administration of a PCA. I.V. narcotics may cause depressed respirations, hypotension, sedation, dizziness, and nausea or vomiting in the patient. The patient must have absence of allergy to the narcotic, capability to understand instructions, and compliance as well as a desire to use the PCA. The materials needed for infusion include a PCA

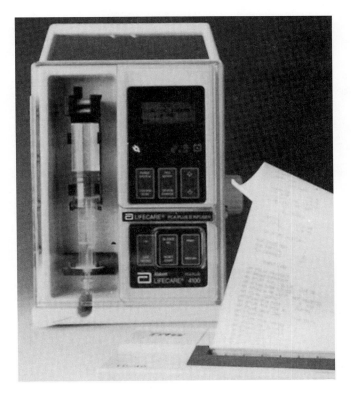

FIGURE 14-8
Patient-controlled analgesia. Life Care PCA Plus II infusor. *(Courtesy Abbott Laboratories, Abbott Park, Ill.)*

pump, PCA tubing, a PCA pump key, a narcotic injector vial, and maintenance I.V. fluids through which the intravenous narcotic will infuse.

Example 1:   The physician orders morphine sulfate 1 mg every 10 minutes to a maximum of 30 mg in 4 hours. Morphine concentration is 1 mg/ml per 30 cc injector vial. What is the pump setting?

1 ml per 10 min, 4-hour limit is 30 ml

Example 2:   The physician orders Demerol 10 mg every 10 minutes to a maximum of 300 mg in 4 hours. Demerol concentration is 10 mg/ml per 30 cc injector vial. What is the pump setting?

1 ml per 10 min, 4-hour limit is 30 ml

Complete the following work sheet, which provides for extensive practice in the calculation of I.V. flow rates. Check your answers. If you have difficulties, go back and review the necessary material. When you feel ready to evaluate your learning, take the first posttest. Check your answers. An acceptable score as indicated on the posttest signifies that you have successfully completed this chapter. An unacceptable score signifies a need for further study before taking the second posttest.

WORK SHEET

Directions: The I.V. fluid order is listed in each problem. Calculate the I.V. flow rates by the use of proportions or the shortcut method, using the indicated drop factors. Show your work.

1. The physician orders dextran 12% 1000 ml within 8 hours for a posttrauma victim. Drop factor is 12 gtt/ml. _____ ml/h. _____ ml/min. _____ gtt/min.

2. Your malnourished patient has an order for Amigen 800 ml to infuse within 8 hours. Drop factor is 10 gtt/ml. _____ ml/h. _____ ml/min. _____ gtt/min.

3. Your patient begins chemotherapy today. The physician orders Cytoxan 475 mg in 250 ml of D_5W over 2 hours. Drop factor is 15 gtt/ml. _____ ml/h. _____ ml/min. _____ gtt/min.

4. Your cardiac catheterization patient is to receive 1.5 L of 5% glucose in DW within 10 hours. Drop factor is 15 gtt/ml. _____ ml/h. _____ ml/min. _____ gtt/min.

5. The physician has ordered N.S. 3000 ml within 48 hours for your dehydrated patient. Drop factor is 10 gtt/ml. _____ ml/h. _____ ml/min. _____ gtt/min.

6. You have a new order for 1000 ml D_5W with 100 mEq KCl to infuse at 100 ml/h. for your hypokalemic patient. Drop factor is 12 gtt/ml. _____ ml/h. _____ ml/min. _____ gtt/min.

7. The burn victim you receive has an order for blood plasma 500 ml within 4 hours. Drop factor is 15 gtt/ml. _____ ml/h. _____ ml/min. _____ gtt/min.

8. A postpartum patient is to receive Ringer's lactate 1500 ml within 16 hours. Drop factor is 10 gtt/ml. _____ ml/h. _____ ml/min. _____ gtt/min.

9. You receive a status post–aortic valve repair patient with orders for $D_{10}\frac{1}{4}$ N.S. with 20 mEq KCl + 1000 U heparin/L at 10 ml/h. Drop factor is 60 gtt/ml. _____ ml/h. _____ ml/min. _____ gtt/min.

10. Your patient is admitted with pernicious anemia. The physician orders packed red blood cells 1 U (0.5 L) within 4 hours. Drop factor is 12 gtt/ml. _____ ml/h. _____ ml/min. _____ gtt/min.

11. An electrolyte-deficient patient is to receive multiple electrolytes 0.8 L within 6 hours. Drop factor is 15 gtt/ml. _____ ml/h. _____ ml/min. _____ gtt/min.

12. The physician has ordered your patient who has had a total hip replacement to receive $D_{10}W$ 250 ml + 7.5 mEq KCl at 2 ml/h. Drop factor is 60 gtt/ml. _____ ml/h. _____ ml/min. _____ gtt/min.

13. You have an order for your diabetic patient to receive 0.9% N.S. 250 ml with 100 U regular insulin. Infuse at 12 U/h. Drop factor is 60 gtt/ml. _____ ml/h. _____ ml/min. _____ gtt/min.

14. The physician's order in problem 13 is reduced to 0.9% N.S. 500 ml with 100 U regular insulin to infuse at 8 U/h. Drop factor is 60 gtt/ml. _____ ml/h. _____ ml/min. _____ gtt/min.

15. A mitral valve patient has D_5W 500 ml with 10,000 U heparin ordered to infuse at 100 U/h. Drop factor is 60 gtt/ml. _____ ml/h. _____ ml/min. _____ gtt/min.

16. A patient admitted with thrombosis is to receive 0.9% N.S. 1000 ml with 30,000 U heparin. Infuse at 1000 U/h. Drop factor is 60 gtt/ml. _____ ml/h. _____ ml/min. _____ gtt/min.

17. The physician orders dobutamine 1 g in 250 ml $D_5\frac{1}{2}$ N.S. for your patient who suffered a myocardial infarction. Infuse at 12 mcg/kg/min for a patient weighing 75 kg. Drop factor is 60 gtt/ml. _____ amt. drug/min for 75 kg patient. _____ amt. drug/ml. _____ ml/min. _____ gtt/min.

18. Your asthma patient has an order for aminophylline 2 g in 1000 ml D_5W. Infuse at 0.4 mg/kg/h. for a patient weighing 55 kg. Drop factor is 60 gtt/ml. _____ amt. drug/min for 55 kg patient. _____ amt. drug/ml. _____ ml/min. _____ gtt/min.

19. Mr. Baxter is having chest pain and has an order for nitroglycerin 100 mg in 500 ml D_5W to infuse at 3 mcg/kg/min for a patient weighing 66 kg. Drop factor is 60 gtt/ml. _____ amt. drug/min for 66 kg patient. _____ amt. drug/ml. _____ ml/min. _____ gtt/min.

20. The physician orders dobutamine 250 mg in 250 ml D$_5$W for your cardiogenic shock patient. Infuse at 500 mcg/kg/min for an 80 kg patient. Drop factor is 60 gtt/ml. _____ amt. drug/min for 80 kg patient. _____ amt. drug/ml. _____ ml/min. _____ gtt/min.

21. Your hyperglycemic patient is admitted with a blood glucose level of 562. The physician orders 0.9% N.S. 500 ml with 200 U regular insulin I.V. Infuse at 10 U/h. Drop factor is 60 gtt/ml. _____ ml/h. _____ ml/min. _____ gtt/min.

22. Your patient is admitted with severe anemia. The physician orders packed red blood cells 1 U (0.5 L) within 4 hours. Drop factor is 12 gtt/ml. _____ ml/h. _____ ml/min. _____ gtt/min.

23. Your patient returns from aortic valve repair. The physician orders D$_5$W 1000 ml with 40,000 U heparin to infuse at 200 U/h. Drop factor is 60 gtt/ml. _____ ml/h. _____ ml/min. _____ gtt/min.

24. The physician orders blood plasma 0.5 L in 4 hours for your trauma patient. Drop factor is 12 gtt/ml. _____ ml/h. _____ ml/min. _____ gtt/min.

25. The physician orders Ringer's lactate 1000 ml within 12 hours for your patient after vaginal delivery. Drop factor is 15 gtt/ml. _____ ml/h. _____ ml/min. _____ gtt/min.

Answers on pp. 487-491.

POSTTEST 1

Name _____

Date _____

ACCEPTABLE SCORE __**13**__

YOUR SCORE _____

Directions: The I.V. fluid order is listed in each problem. Calculate the I.V. flow rates by the use of proportions or the shortcut method, using the indicated drop factor. Show your work.

1. Ringer's lactate 1000 ml is ordered to be given within 12 hours for your hyperthermic patient. Drop factor is 15 gtt/ml. _____ ml/h. _____ ml/min. _____ gtt/min.

2. The physician has ordered blood plasma 0.5 L to be given within 4 hours to your trauma patient. Drop factor is 12 gtt/ml. _____ ml/h. _____ ml/min. _____ gtt/min.

3. Mr. Simpson has a new order for N.S. to infuse at 150 ml/h. after a transesophageal echocardiogram. Drop factor is 15 gtt/ml. _____ ml/h. _____ ml/min. _____ gtt/min.

4. Mrs. Britton requires a bolus of $D_{10}W$ 750 ml to infuse in 10 hours after cardiac catheterization. Drop factor is 10 gtt/ml. _____ ml/h. _____ ml/min. _____ gtt/min.

5. The physician orders Otic 150 mg in 50 ml D$_5$W over 30 minutes for your postop patient. Drop factor is 12 gtt/ml. _____ ml/min. _____ gtt/min.

6. Your diabetic patient has an order for 0.9% N.S. 1000 ml with 500 U regular insulin. Infuse at 9 U/h. Drop factor is 60 gtt/ml. _____ ml/h. _____ ml/min. _____ gtt/min.

7. The tricuspid valve repair patient has orders for D$_5$W 1000 ml with 30,000 U heparin. Infuse at 500 U/h. Drop factor is 60 gtt/ml. _____ ml/h. _____ ml/min. _____ gtt/min.

8. Your hypertensive patient has orders for Nipride 50 mg in 250 ml D$_5$W. Infuse at 3 mcg/kg/min for a patient weighing 82 kg. Drop factor is 60 gtt/ml. _____ amt. drug/min for 82 kg patient. _____ amt. drug/ml. _____ ml/min. _____ gtt/min.

9. Your mitral valve patient has orders for D$_5$W 500 ml with 10,000 U heparin to infuse at 100 U/h. Drop factor is 60 gtt/ml. _____ ml/h. _____ ml/min. _____ gtt/min.

10. The physician orders D$_5$½ N.S. with 20 mEq KCl/L at 30 ml/h. for your septoplasty patient. Drop factor is 20 gtt/ml. _____ ml/h. _____ ml/min. _____ gtt/min.

11. Your hyperglycemic patient receives 0.9% N.S. 250 ml with 250 U regular insulin to infuse at 7 U/h. Drop factor is 60 gtt/ml. _____ ml/h. _____ ml/min. _____ gtt/min.

12. Your patient arrives after a thrombectomy of the left leg. The doctor orders N.S. 1000 ml with 30,000 U heparin to infuse at 1500 U/h. Drop factor is 60 gtt/ml. _____ ml/h. _____ ml/min. _____ gtt/min.

13. The physician orders ½ N.S. 1000 ml within 18 hours for your tympanomastoidectomy patient. Drop factor is 10 gtt/ml. _____ ml/h. _____ ml/min. _____ gtt/min.

14. The physician orders 250 ml N.S. in 24 hours for your lumbar laminectomy patient. Drop factor is 60 gtt/ml. _____ ml/h. _____ ml/min. _____ gtt/min.

15. The physician orders Ringer's lactate 1500 ml within 16 hours for your patient after vaginal delivery. Drop factor is 10 gtt/ml. _____ ml/h. _____ ml/min. _____ gtt/min.

Answers on pp. 491-493.

POSTTEST 2

Name _____

Date _____

ACCEPTABLE SCORE __13__

YOUR SCORE _____

Directions: The I.V. fluid order is listed in each problem. Calculate the I.V. flow rates by the use of proportions or the shortcut method, using the indicated drop factor. Show your work.

1. Your anemic patient needs to be transfused with whole blood 500 ml within 6 hours. Drop factor is 15 gtt/ml. _____ ml/h. _____ ml/min. _____ gtt/min.

2. Mr. Boone has a new order for $D_5\frac{1}{2}$ N.S. with 20 mEq KCl/L at 30 ml/h. after left-leg debridement. Drop factor is 20 gtt/ml. _____ ml/h. _____ ml/min. _____ gtt/min.

3. The physician orders boluses for your dehydrated patient of 5% glucose in N.S. 1000 ml, followed by 1000 ml D_5W, followed by N.S. 1000 ml within 24 hours. Drop factor is 12 gtt/ml. _____ ml/h. _____ ml/min. _____ gtt/min.

4. Your pulmonary edema patient has continuous fluids reduced to D_5W 250 ml at 3 ml/h. ordered. Drop factor is 60 gtt/ml. _____ ml/h. _____ ml/min. _____ gtt/min.

5. Mr. Connick has orders for ½ N.S. 1000 ml within 18 hours after a lumbar laminectomy.
   Drop factor is 10 gtt/ml. _____ ml/h. _____ ml/min. _____ gtt/min.

6. The physician orders 0.9% N.S. 250 ml with 250 U regular insulin to infuse at 7 U/h. for
   your diabetic patient. Drop factor is 60 gtt/ml. _____ ml/h. _____ ml/min.
   _____ gtt/min.

7. Your patient has a blood clot in the left leg. The physician orders D_5W 1000 ml with 30,000 U
   heparin. Infuse at 1500 U/h. Drop factor is 60 gtt/ml. _____ ml/h. _____ ml/min.
   _____ gtt/min.

8. The physician orders Nipride 50 mg in 500 ml D_5W for your patient with hypertension.
   Infuse at 0.5 mcg/kg/min for a patient weighing 75 kg. Drop factor is 60 gtt/ml. _____ amt.
   drug/min for 75 kg patient. _____ amt. drug/ml. _____ ml/min. _____ gtt/min.

9. Your patient returns from cardiac catheterization. The physician orders 250 ml N.S. within
   12 hours. Drop factor is 60 gtt/ml. _____ ml/h. _____ ml/min. _____ gtt/min.

10. Your malnourished patient receives Intralipid 20% 500 ml I.V. today over 12 hours. Drop factor is 12 gtt/ml. _____ ml/h. _____ ml/min. _____ gtt/min.

11. The physician orders 0.9% N.S. 500 ml with 100 U regular insulin to infuse at 2 U/h. for your hyperglycemic patient. Drop factor is 60 gtt/ml. _____ ml/h. _____ ml/min. _____ gtt/min.

12. The physician orders N.S. at 250 ml/h. today for your dehydrated patient. Drop factor is 10 gtt/ml. _____ ml/h. _____ ml/min. _____ gtt/min.

13. The physician orders N.S. 250 ml with 50,000 U heparin to infuse at 1200 U/h. for your mitral valve repair patient. Drop factor is 60 gtt/ml. _____ ml/h. _____ ml/min. _____ gtt/min.

14. The physician orders ½ N.S. at 120 ml/h. for your patient after septoplasty. Drop factor is 12 gtt/ml. _____ ml/h. _____ ml/min. _____ gtt/min.

15. Your patient receives packed red blood cells 1 U (0.5 L) for trauma and blood loss to infuse over 6 hours. Drop factor is 12 gtt/ml. _____ ml/h. _____ ml/min. _____ gtt/min.

Answers on pp. 494-496.

15 Dimensional Analysis and the Calculation of Drug Dosages

Learning Objectives

On completion of the materials provided in this chapter, you will be able to perform computations accurately by mastering the following mathematical concepts:

1 Use the dimensional analysis format to solve oral dosage problems

2 Use the dimensional analysis format to solve parenteral dosage problems

---

Dimensional analysis is another format for setting up problems to calculate drug dosages. The advantage of dimensional analysis is that only one equation is needed. This is true even if the information supplied indicates a need to convert to like units before setting up the proportion to perform the actual calculation of the amount of medication to be given to the patient.

Example: Ampicillin 500 mg q.i.d. The drug is supplied in 250 mg capsules. Give _____ .

    a. On the left side of the equation, place the name or abbreviation of the drug form of x, or what you are solving for.

$$x \text{ capsule} =$$

    b. On the right side of the equation, place the available information related to the measurement or abbreviation that was placed on the left side. In this example, that is *capsule*. This information is placed in the equation as a common fraction; match the appropriate abbreviation or measurement. Thus, the abbreviation that matches the x quantity must be placed in the numerator. We also know from the problem that each capsule contains 250 mg of ampicillin. This information is the denominator of our fraction.

$$x \text{ capsule} = \frac{1 \text{ capsule}}{250 \text{ mg}}$$

357

c. Next, find the information that matches the measurement or abbreviation used in the denominator of the fraction you created. In this example, mg is in the denominator and our order is for 500 mg. Therefore the full proportion is

$$x \text{ capsule} = \frac{1 \text{ capsule}}{250 \ mg} \times \frac{500 \ mg}{1}$$

d. Then cancel out the like abbreviations on the right side of the equation. If you have set up the problem correctly, the remaining measurement or abbreviation should match that used on the left side of the equation. Now solve for x.

$$x \text{ capsule} = \frac{1 \text{ capsule}}{250 \ \cancel{mg}} \times \frac{500 \ \cancel{mg}}{1}$$

$$x = \frac{1 \times 500}{250}$$

$$x = 2$$

The answer to the problem is 2 capsules.

As stated earlier, the advantage of this method is not having to convert into like systems of measurement as would be required if the usual proportion method were used. With dimensional analysis, remember that only one equation is necessary. Let's take a look at an example of this type.

Example: Kantrex 400 mg. I.M. q.12 h. The drug is supplied 0.5 g per 2 ml. Give _____ .

a. On the left side of the equation, place the name or abbreviation of the drug form for which you are solving, or x.

$$x \text{ ml} =$$

b. On the right side of the equation, place the available information related to the measurement or abbreviation that was placed on the left side. In this example, that is *ml*. This information is placed in the equation as part of a fraction; match the appropriate abbreviation. Remember that the abbreviation that matches the x quantity must be placed in the numerator. We know from the problem that each 2 ml contains 0.5 g of Kantrex.

$$x \text{ ml} = \frac{2 \text{ ml}}{0.5 \text{ g}}$$

c. Because the order is for 400 mg and the medication is supplied to us as 0.5 g, a conversion would normally be required. However, with the dimensional analysis method, an additional fraction is added on the right side of the equation. From information supplied in earlier chapters, we know that 1 g equals 1000 mg. This information is then placed in the equation next in the form of the fraction $\frac{1 \text{ g}}{1000 \text{ mg}}$. Note that the abbreviation or measurement in the *numerator* of this fraction must match the abbreviation or measurement in the *denominator* of the immediate previous fraction. The equation now looks like

$$x \text{ ml} = \frac{2 \text{ ml}}{0.5 \text{ g}} \times \frac{1 \text{ g}}{1000 \text{ mg}}$$

d. Next, place the amount of drug ordered in the equation. Note that this will once again match the measurement or abbreviation of the denominator of the fraction immediately before. In this example, that is 400 mg. Therefore the full equation is

$$x \text{ ml} = \frac{2 \text{ ml}}{0.5 \text{ g}} \times \frac{1 \text{ g}}{1000 \text{ mg}} \times \frac{400 \text{ mg}}{1}$$

e. For the final step, cancel out the like abbreviations on the right side of the equation. If the equation has been set up correctly, the remaining abbreviation should match that located on the left side. Now solve for *x*.

$$x \text{ ml} = \frac{2 \text{ ml}}{0.5 \text{ g}} \times \frac{1 \text{ g}}{1000 \text{ mg}} \times \frac{400 \text{ mg}}{1}$$

$$x = \frac{2 \times 400}{0.5 \times 1000}$$

$$x = \frac{800}{500}$$

$$x = 1.6$$

The answer to the problem is 1.6 ml.

WORK SHEET

Directions: Calculate the following drug dosages by using the dimensional analysis method. Show your work and check your answers.

1. Your diabetic patient receives Glipizide 10 mg p.o. q.a.m. The drug is supplied in 5 mg scored tablets. Give _____ .

2. Mr. Theson receives Vistaril 60 mg p.o. q.6 h. for nausea after his acoustic neuroma revision. Vistaril oral suspension 25 mg per 5 ml is supplied. Give _____ .

3. Your status post–lumbar laminectomy patient receives Demerol 0.025 g p.o. q.4 h. p.r.n. for pain. Demerol 50 mg tablets are available. Give _____ .

4. Mrs. Fare receives codeine 30 mg q.3 h. p.r.n. for pain after knee replacement surgery. You have codeine tablets gr ¼ available. Give _____ .

5. Your patient receives Keflex 0.5 g p.o. q.i.d. You have Keflex 250 mg capsules available. Give _____ .

6. Your patient may receive Dilaudid 3 mg I.M. q.3 h. for pain caused by a total hip replacement. Dilaudid is supplied in 1 ml ampules containing 4 mg. Give _____ .

7. Mr. Grey receives Lanoxin 40 mcg I.M. q.12 h. for cardiac arrhythmias. Lanoxin 0.1 mg per ml is available. Give _____ .

8. The physician prescribes Stadol 1 mg I.V. q.4 h. for your patient with a below-the-knee amputation. Stadol 2 mg per ml is available. Give _____ .

9. The physician orders heparin 2500 U subq. q.12 h. for your jejunostomy patient. You have heparin 5000 U per ml available. Give _____ .

10. Gantrisin 2 g p.o. stat. Gantrisin is supplied in 500 mg tablets. Give _____ .

Answers on pp. 496-497.

Chapter 16

Automated Medication Dispensing Systems

Learning Objectives

On completion of the materials provided in this chapter, you will be able to:

1. Recognize an automated medication dispensing system
2. Identify the advantages of using an automated medication dispensing system

Health care delivery systems continue to strive to improve the efficiency and accuracy of the delivery of medications to patients. In recent years, more and more hospitals and other care center areas have moved to the use of automated medication dispensing systems.

Each patient care unit is provided a special cabinet that houses the medications that will be dispensed from that unit. These cabinets are connected to the central pharmacy for order verifications and accuracy, as well as for automation of usage reports that are provided for many facets of the medication process. Depending on the vendor chosen by the institution, a variety of medications may be housed in the cabinet, ranging from only controlled substances to inclusion of first doses, p.r.n.s, and regularly scheduled medications. Having a wide range of medications within the patient care area allows a quick response to changes in a patient's condition or acuity. For example, a new medication order does not require a special trip to the central pharmacy to obtain the needed medication, allowing the new drug regimen to be initiated quickly. With a computerized system, the patient has the added benefit of more time being available to the nurse for all aspects of patient care, and the pharmacist has more time to confer with physicians and resource nurses and to analyze drug studies and usage.

An automatic drug dispensing system also leads to a reduction in medication errors. This is especially true as vendors market new options that allow only the designated drawer housing the medication that is being given at that time to open. The automated medication dispensing system also enhances patient satisfaction. This is especially evident in postsurgical patients or oncology patients who require the administration of pain medications in a timely manner. Pain medications are usually

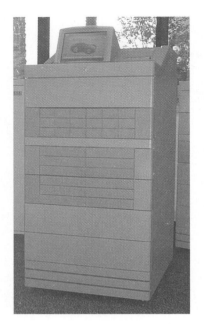

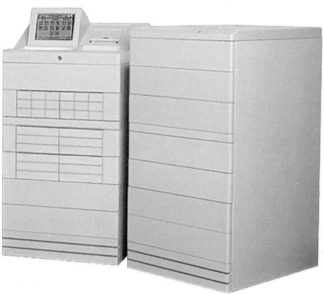

FIGURE 16-1
Automated drug dispensing systems. *(Courtesy MedStation.)*

controlled substances that necessitate the nurse to first locate the narcotic keys from a peer, then open the narcotic supply, find and remove the right medication, relock the supply area, sign out the controlled substance, and then take the medication to the patient for administration. With an automated system, the nurse is able to access the medication from the cabinet through her authorization code. The machine then allows the nurse to confirm the accuracy of the controlled substance count immediately. The medication may then be given quickly to the patient with the least amount of time and effort expended (Figure 16-1).

Another advantage of an automated medication dispensing system is reduction in the time that is required for end-of-shift narcotic counts. This count is performed by two nurses, usually one from

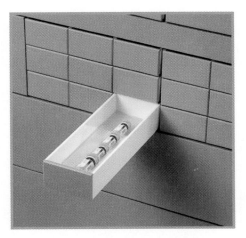

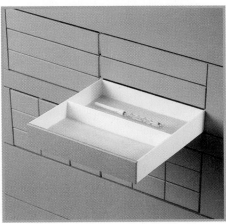

FIGURE 16-2
Cabinet system for housing medications. *(Courtesy MedStation.)*

the ending shift and one from the starting shift. It is also standard practice that until the narcotic count is completed and correct, all staff that are ending their shift may not leave. This results in staff dissatisfaction and unnecessary overtime costs that can be better spent on actual patient care. This scenario is prevented because automated systems require the confirmation of the count of controlled substance medications after each withdrawal.

These medication dispensing systems are also beneficial for patients who are transferred from one unit to another. The medications are already housed in the cabinet if it is one that has been expanded to include most patient medications (Figure 16-2). This allows the patient to continue to progress without delays caused by medications being unavailable.

Some of the systems currently on the market actually interface with the health care system's program for charting of medications. With some dispensing systems, charting is done at the cabinet on the unit, whereas other manufacturers are designing programs to document the administration of medication at the bedside. With the automatic documentation of the administration of the patient's medications, the nurse is not required to return to the paper medication administration record and manually chart that the medicine has been given.

As health care continues to monitor costs and at the same time to improve patient and staff satisfaction, the use of automated medication dispensing systems will become more widespread. This is a new area in which nursing students will need to become knowledgeable and competent because the accurate and efficient delivery of medications is one of the most important skills of patient care that the nurse is required to perform.

Chapter 17 | *Pediatric Dosages*

Learning Objectives

On completion of the materials provided in this chapter, you will be able to perform computations accurately by mastering the following mathematical concepts:

1. Convert the weight of a child from pounds to kilograms
2. Use a formula based on body weight to determine the correct dosage of a medication to be administered to a child
3. Calculate body surface area (BSA) using the West nomogram
4. Estimate body surface area using a formula
5. Calculate pediatric dosages using a formula based on body surface area expressed as square meters (m^2)

Because of their age, weight, height, and physical condition, children are more sensitive to medications than adults. Therefore careful attention must be given when preparing and administering medications to children. The right amount of the right medication must be given to the right child at the right time, in the right way.

Although the physician prescribes the medication, the nurse who administers it is responsible for errors in the calculation of the dosage and in the preparation and administration of the drug. The medication order must be accurate—a dosage that is too high may be unsafe, and a dosage that is too low may not have the desired therapeutic effect.

Pediatric Dosages Calculated by mg/kg/h.

Pediatric dosages are most commonly calculated by the mg/kg/h. method. This is the amount of drug in relation to the child's weight in kilograms, usually for a 24-hour period. Package inserts and reference books such as the current year's *Mosby's Nursing Drug Reference* show the safe amount of the drug that should be given per mg/kg/h. Normally the amount of medication given to children is less than that given to adults. The amount of medication to be given in 24 hours is calculated and then divided into an equal number of doses. The number of doses is determined by the recommended frequency of administration.

Example: Amoxicillin 125 mg p.o. t.i.d. for a child weighing 34.32 lb. You have amoxicillin suspension 125 mg/5 ml. The recommended daily p.o. dose for a child is 20 to 40 mg/kg/day in divided dosages q.8 h. Child's weight is _____ kg. Safe recommended dosage or range for this child is _____ . Is the order safe? _____ . If yes, give _____ .

a.   Change the child's weight to kg (see Chapter 8). Remember, there are 2.2 lb in each kilogram.

$$2.2 \text{ lb} : 1 \text{ kg} :: 34.32 \text{ lb} : x \text{ kg}$$

$$2.2 : 1 :: 34.32 : x$$

$$2.2x = 34.32$$

$$x = \frac{34.32}{2.2}$$

$$x = 15.6 \text{ kg}$$

b.   Write a proportion(s) using the recommended dosage and child's weight as your known values to determine the safe recommended dosage or range for this child.

$$20 \text{ mg} : 1 \text{ kg} :: x \text{ mg} : 15.6 \text{ kg}$$

$$20 : 1 :: x : 15.6$$

$$x = 312 \text{ mg}$$

$$40 \text{ mg} : 1 \text{ kg} :: x \text{ mg} : 15.6 \text{ kg}$$

$$40 : 1 :: x : 15.6$$

$$x = 624 \text{ mg}$$

The safe recommended range for this child, who weighs 15.6 kg, is 312 to 624 mg in a 24-hour period.

c. Determine the total amount of medication ordered per 24-hour period.

$$125 \text{ mg} : 1 \text{ dose} :: x \text{ mg} : 3 \text{ doses}$$

$$125 : 1 :: x : 3$$

$$x = 375 \text{ mg/24 hr period}$$

The order is safe because it falls within the recommended 24-hour range of 312 to 624 mg for this medication and this child.

d. Calculate the actual dosage amount to be given by the use of a proportion (see Chapter 10).

$$125 \text{ mg} : 5 \text{ ml} :: 125 \text{ mg} : x \text{ ml}$$

$$125 : 5 :: 125 : x$$

$$125x = 625$$

$$x = 5 \text{ ml}$$

Therefore 5 ml is the amount of each individual t.i.d. dose.

Body Surface Area Calculations

Body surface area (BSA) is determined by using a child's height and weight along with the West nomogram. If the child has a normal height and weight for his or her age, the BSA may be ascertained by the weight alone. For example, in Figure 17-1 showing the West nomogram, you can see that a child who weighs 70 pounds has a BSA of 1.10 m^2.

When using the West nomogram, take a few minutes to assess the markings of each column. Note that the markings are not at the same intervals throughout each column.

If the child is not of normal height and weight for his or her age, an extended use of the nomogram is required. The far right column is for weight in pounds and kilograms. The far left column is for height measured in centimeters and inches. Place a ruler on the nomogram and draw a line connecting the height and weight points. Where the line crosses the surface area (SA) column, the SA in m^2 will be indicated.

Practice problems—Using the West nomogram, state the BSA in m^2 for each child of normal height and weight listed below:

A. 1. Child weighs 22 lb   BSA = _____
   2. Child weighs 4 lb   BSA = _____
   3. Child weighs 75 lb   BSA = _____
   4. Child weighs 10 lb   BSA = _____
   5. Child weighs 32 lb   BSA = _____

Using the West nomogram, calculate the BSA for each child with the following heights and weights:

B. 1. Child weighs 6 kg, height is 110 cm   BSA = _____
   2. Child weighs 5 lb, height is 19 in   BSA = _____
   3. Child weighs 25 kg, height is 70 cm   BSA = _____
   4. Child weighs 30 lb, height is 90 cm   BSA = _____
   5. Child weighs 160 lb, height is 200 cm   BSA = _____

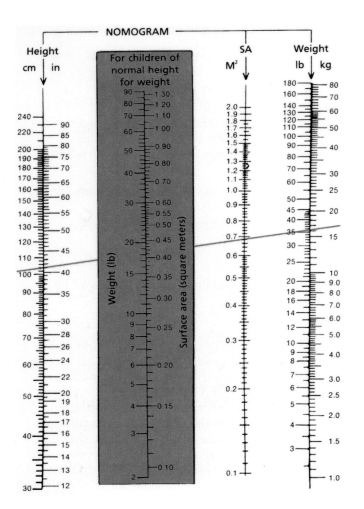

FIGURE 17-1
West nomogram for estimation of body surface areas in children. A straight line is drawn between height and weight. The point where the line crosses the surface area column is the estimated body surface area. *(From Behrman RE, Saunders VC, editors: Nelson textbook of pediatrics, ed 13, Philadelphia, 1987, Saunders; modified from data of E Boyd, by CD West.)*

Calculation of Dosage Based on Body Surface Area

The calculation of dosage may be based on BSA. There are three steps to the calculation using this method.

1. Determine the child's weight in kilograms.
2. Calculate the BSA in square meters (m²). The formula for this calculation is as follows:

$$\frac{4 \text{ W (child's weight in kilograms)} + 7}{\text{W (child's weight in kilograms)} + 90} = \text{BSA in m}^2$$

3. Calculate the pediatric dosage using the following formula. The formula is based on the premise that an adult who weighs 140 pounds has a BSA of 1.7 m².

$$\frac{\text{BSA in m}^2}{1.7} \times \text{adult dose} = \text{child's dose}$$

Example: Child weighs 24 lb and the adult dose is 100 mg.

1. First, convert the child's weight to kilograms.

$$\begin{array}{r} 10.90 \\ 2.2 \wedge \overline{)240.0} \\ \underline{22} \\ 20 \\ \underline{00} \\ 20\ 0 \\ \underline{19\ 8} \\ 20 \end{array}$$

The child weighs approximately 10.9 kg.

2. Next, calculate the child's BSA in m².

$$\frac{4(10.9) + 7}{10.9 + 90} = \frac{43.6 + 7}{10.9 + 90} = \frac{50.6}{100.9} = 0.5$$

Child's BSA = 0.5 m²

3. Finally, calculate the appropriate child dosage.

$$\frac{0.5}{1.7} \times 100 = 29.4 \text{ mg}$$

Practice problems—Calculate the following children's dosages.

C. 1. Child weighs 40 lb, adult dose = 300 mg   child's dose = _____
2. Child weighs 65 lb, adult dose = 30 ml   child's dose = _____
3. Child weighs 20 lb, adult dose = 50 mg   child's dose = _____
4. Child weighs 90 lb, adult dose = 10 ml   child's dose = _____
5. Child weighs 14 lb, adult dose = 2 g   child's dose = _____

Complete the following work sheet, which provides for extensive practice in the calculation of pediatric dosages. Check your answers. If you have difficulties, go back and review the necessary material. When you feel ready to evaluate your learning, take the first posttest. Check your answers. An acceptable score as indicated on the posttest signifies that you have successfully completed this chapter. An unacceptable score signifies a need for further study before taking the second posttest.

Answers to practice problems on p. 372.

Answers to practice problems:

p. 369

A. 1. 0.46 m^2
2. 0.15 m^2
3. 1.15 m^2
4. 0.27 m^2
5. 0.62 m^2

p. 369

B. 1. 0.41 m^2
2. 0.18 m^2
3. 0.74 m^2
4. 0.58 m^2
5. 2.0 m^2

p. 371

C. 1. 132 mg
2. 18.5 ml
3. 13 mg
4. 7.65 ml
5. 0.4 g

WORK SHEET

Directions: The medication order is listed at the beginning of each problem. Calculate the child's weight in kilograms, determine the safe recommended dosage or range, determine the safety of the order, and calculate the drug dosage. Show your work.

1. Keflex 250 mg p.o. q.i.d. for a child weighing 50 lb. You have Keflex 250 mg capsules.
   The recommended daily p.o. dosage for a child is 25 to 50 mg/kg/day in divided doses q.6 h.
   Child's weight is _____ kg. Safe recommended dosage or range for this child is _____ .
   Is the order safe? _____ . If yes, give _____ .

2. Lanoxin 12.5 mg p.o. q.d. for an infant weighing 6½ lb. You have Lanoxin 0.05 mg/ml.
   The recommended daily dosage for an infant is 0.035 to 0.06 mg/kg/day in divided doses
   q.8 h. Child's weight is _____ kg. Safe recommended dosage or range for this child
   is _____ . Is the order safe? _____ . If yes, give _____ .

3. Benadryl 25 mg I.V. q.6 h. for a child weighing 50 lb. You have Benadryl 10 mg/ml. The recommended daily dosage for a child greater than 12 kg is 5 mg/kg/day in four divided doses. Child's weight is _____ kg. Safe recommended dosage or range for this child is _____ . Is the order safe? _____ . If yes, give _____ .

4. Thorazine 10 mg I.V. q.6 h. for a child weighing 44 lb. You have Thorazine 25 mg/ml. The recommended daily dosage is 0.55 mg/kg/q.6 to 8 h. Child's weight is _____ kg. Safe recommended dosage or range for this child is _____ . Is the order safe? _____ . If yes, give _____ .

5. Thioguanine 60 mg p.o. today for a child weighing 78 lb. You have thioguanine 40 mg tablets. The recommended p.o. dosage is 2 mg/kg/day. Child's weight is _____ kg. Safe recommended dosage or range for this child is _____ . Is the order safe? _____ . If yes, give _____ .

6. Initial dose of Furadantin 10 mg p.o. q.d. for a child weighing 30.31 lb. You have Furadantin 5 mg/ml. The recommended p.o. dosage is 2 mg/kg/day. Child's weight is _____ kg. Safe recommended dosage or range for this child is _____ . Is the order safe? _____ . If yes, give _____ .

NDC 0149-0735-15
LIST 73515

5 mg/ml

Furadantin
(nitrofurantoin)
oral suspension

Store below 86°F (30°C).
Protect from freezing.
SHAKE VIGOROUSLY TO
BREAK GEL.

URINARY TRACT
ANTIBACTERIAL
60 ml

CAUTION: Federal law
prohibits dispensing
without prescription.

USUAL ADULT DOSE: 50 to 100
mg q.i.d. with meals and with food
or milk on retiring.
CHILDREN: 2.2 to 3.2 mg per lb of
body weight per 24 hours.
Each teaspoonful (5 ml) contains
25 mg Furadantin, brand of
nitrofurantoin.

Manufactured by
Eaton Laboratories, Inc.
Manati, Puerto Rico 00701
Distributed by
Norwich Eaton Pharmaceuticals, Inc.
Norwich, New York 13815
A Procter & Gamble Company

Norwich Eaton

7. Theophylline 16 mg p.o. q.6 h. for a child weighing 28 lb. You have theophylline elixir 11.25 mg/ml. The recommended p.o. dosage should not exceed 12 mg/kg/24 h. Child's weight is _____ kg. Safe recommended dosage or range for this child is _____ . Is the order safe? _____ . If yes, give _____ .

8. Dilantin 75 mg p.o. q.12 h. for a child weighing 66 lb. You have Dilantin chewable 50 mg tablets. The recommended p.o. dosage for a child is 5 to 7 mg/kg/day in divided doses q.12 h. Child's weight is _____ kg. Safe recommended dosage or range for this child is _____ . Is the order safe? _____ . If yes, give _____ .

Answers on pp. 497-498.

POSTTEST 1

Name _____

Date _____

ACCEPTABLE SCORE __**17**__

YOUR SCORE _____

Directions: The medication order is listed at the beginning of each problem. Calculate the child's weight in kilograms, determine the safe recommended dosage or range, determine the safety of the order, and calculate the drug dosage. Show your work.

1. Phenobarbital 60 mg p.o. q.12 h. for a child weighing 55 lb. Elixir of phenobarbital 20 mg/ 5 ml is available. The recommended daily dosage for a child is 4 to 6 mg/kg/day in divided doses q.12 h. Child's weight is _____ kg. Safe recommended dosage or range for this child is _____ . Is the order safe? _____ . If yes, give _____ .

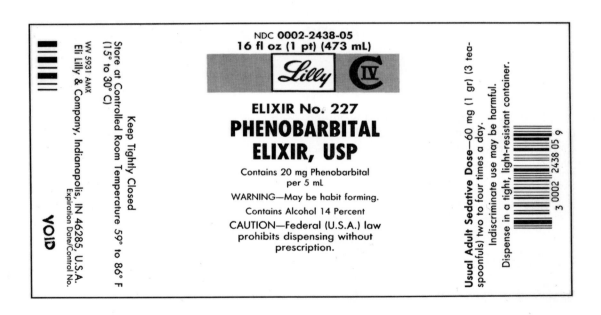

2. Lincocin 500 mg p.o. q.6 h. for a child weighing 44 lb. Lincocin is supplied in 250 mg capsules. The recommended daily p.o. dosage for a child is 30 to 60 mg/kg/day in divided doses q.6 h. Child's weight is _____ kg. Safe recommended dosage or range for this child is _____ . Is the order safe? _____ . If yes, give _____ .

3. Procaine penicillin G 150,000 U I.M. q.12 h. for a child weighing 6¾ lb. You have procaine
penicillin G 300,000 U/ml. The recommended daily I.M. dosage for a child is 50,000 U/kg
I.M. q.d. Child's weight is _____ kg. Safe recommended dosage or range for this child
is _____ . Is the order safe? _____ . If yes, give _____ .

4. Keflex 250 mg p.o. t.i.d. for a child weighing 44 lb. Keflex is supplied in 125 mg/5 ml.
The recommended daily p.o. dosage for a child is 20 to 40 mg/kg/day in divided doses q.8 h.
Child's weight is _____ kg. Safe recommended dosage or range for this child is _____ .
Is the order safe? _____ . If so, give _____ .

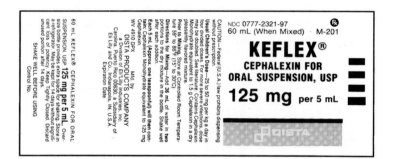

5. Morphine 4 mg I.M. stat for a child weighing 78 lb. You have morphine sulfate 15 mg/ml. The
recommended I.M. dosage for a child is 0.1 to 0.2 mg/kg/day. Child's weight is _____ kg.
Safe recommended dosage or range for this child is _____ . Is the order safe? _____ . If yes,
give _____ .

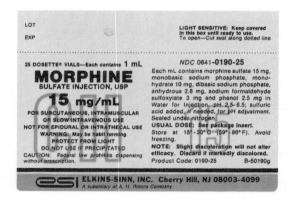

Answers on p. 499.

POSTTEST 2

Name _____

Date _____

ACCEPTABLE SCORE __**17**__

YOUR SCORE _____

Directions: The medication order is listed at the beginning of each problem. Calculate the child's weight in kilograms, determine the safe recommended dosage or range, determine the safety of the order, and calculate the drug dosage. Show your work.

1. Cleocin 225 mg I.V. q.6 h. for a child weighing 58 lb. You have Cleocin 150 mg/ml. The recommended daily dosage for a child is 15 to 40 mg/kg/day in divided doses q.6-8 h. Child's weight is _____ kg. Safe recommended dosage or range for this child is _____ . Is the order safe? _____ . If yes, give _____ .

2. Dilantin 50 mg p.o. q.12 h. for a child weighing 70 lb. You have Dilantin 125 mg/5 ml. The recommended daily p.o. dosage for a child is 5 to 7 mg/kg in divided doses q.12 h. Child's weight is _____ kg. Safe recommended dosage or range for this child is _____ . Is the order safe? _____ . If yes, give _____ .

N 0071-2214-20   **Shake Well**

Dilantin-125®
(Phenytoin Oral Suspension, USP)

125 mg per 5 mL potency

Important—Another strength available; verify unspecified prescriptions.

Caution—Federal law prohibits dispensing without prescription.

8 fl oz (237 mL)

PARKE-DAVIS
Div of Warner-Lambert Co/ Morris Plains, NJ 07950 USA   2214G013

Shake well before using.

Each 5 mL contains phenytoin, 125 mg with a maximum alcohol content not greater than 0.6 percent.

Usual Dose—Adults, 1 teaspoonful three times daily; Children, see package insert.

See package insert for complete prescribing information.

Store below 30° C (86° F). Protect from freezing.

Keep this and all drugs out of the reach of children.

Exp date and lot

6505-00-890-1110

3. Amoxil 250 mg p.o. q.8 h. for a child weighing 58 lb. You have Amoxil 125 mg/5 ml. The recommended daily p.o. dosage for the child is 20 to 40 mg/kg/day in divided doses q.8 h. Child's weight is _____ kg. Safe recommended dosage or range for this child is _____ . Is the order safe? _____ . If yes, give _____ .

NDC 0029–6008–23

AMOXIL® for oral suspension
125 mg/5 mL

AMOXIL®

amoxicillin
for oral suspension

Equivalent to
2.5 g Amoxicillin

When reconstituted
each 5 mL will contain

125 mg
Amoxicillin
as the trihydrate

100 mL

Beecham
laboratories

Tear along perforation

C89

BEECHAM LABORATORIES
DIV. OF BEECHAM INC. BRISTOL, TENN. 37620

**STORE DRY POWDER AT
ROOM TEMPERATURE**

CAUTION: Federal law prohibits dispensing without prescription.

U.S. PATENT 3,192,198
& RE. 28,744

**READ ACCOMPANYING INSERT
BEFORE USE**

DIRECTIONS FOR MIXING:
Tap bottle until all powder flows freely. Add approximately ⅔ of the total amount of water for reconstitution (total~78 mL) and shake vigorously to wet powder. Add the remainder of the water and again shake vigorously. Each 5 mL (1 teaspoonful) will then contain Amoxicillin Trihydrate equivalent to 125 mg Amoxicillin.

USUAL DOSAGE:
Adults: 250 mg–500 mg every 8 hours—
Children: 20–40 mg/kg/day in divided doses every 8 hours—
depending on age, weight and severity of infection.

Tear along perforation

**KEEP TIGHTLY CLOSED
SHAKE WELL BEFORE USING**
Refrigeration preferable, but not required.

Any unused portion of the reconstituted suspension must be discarded after 14 days.

Exp. Date:

Control No.:

9405791

4. Keflex 500 mg p.o. q.6 h. for a child weighing 99 lb. You have Keflex 250 mg capsules available. The recommended daily p.o. dosage for a child is 25 to 50 mg/kg/day in four equal doses q.6 h. Child's weight is _____ kg. Safe recommended dosage or range for this child is _____ . Is the order safe? _____ . If yes, give _____ .

5. Cloxacillin 500 mg p.o. q.6 h. for a child weighing 66 lb. You have cloxacillin 125 mg/ml available. The recommended daily p.o. dosage for a child is 50 to 100 mg/kg in divided doses q.6 h. Child's weight is _____ kg. Safe recommended dosage or range for this child is _____ . Is the order safe? _____ . If yes, give _____ .

Answers on p. 500.

18 Special Considerations for the Elderly

Learning Objectives

On completion of the materials provided in this chapter, you will be able to:

1 Understand the implications of the physiological changes of aging on medication administration for the elderly

2 Understand the special problems and issues related to medication administration for the elderly

People are living longer than at any period in history, and we are continuing to increase our knowledge of how to protect our health and prevent illness. By practicing good health habits, such as proper diet, an exercise program, and a positive attitude, people are enjoying better health. As research continues, cures and maintenance regimens are being found for major health problems. Life expectancy continues to increase. "Old-old" persons over the age of 85 are the most rapidly increasing portion of the population in the United States. This group is also using more of the nation's health care resources.

Aging is a normal process, beginning at infancy and continuing throughout the life cycle. Aging is not the cause of specific diseases, but certain chronic illnesses are more prevalent in the elderly and may lead to additional health problems. Chronic illnesses usually require an increase in drug use to control the symptoms or progression of the condition.

Changes Experienced by the Elderly

Biological and physiological changes occur that affect all body systems and conflict with the action of some medications. Medication problems are more likely to occur in the older age group. These problems can be drug interactions, adverse reactions, drug and food interactions, or medication errors. Reflexes slow and there is an inability to adapt quickly to changes in temperature. A decrease in the sense of touch may be a safety issue. There is a decrease in saliva, which may slow the absorption of buccal medications. Some elderly persons may have difficulty in swallowing, especially large tablets. An advantage of aging is a diminished sense of taste—elderly people may have no difficulty with some of the bitter-tasting medications.

Biological and physiological changes also affect the metabolism and excretion of drugs. Chronic conditions, such as hypertension, diabetes, heart conditions, and arthritis, interfere with homeostasis and may cause medications to be less effective. Absorption is affected by changes in the motility of the gastrointestinal tract. A decrease in motility may cause an increase in drug actions. Many elderly persons resort to the regular use of laxatives. Laxatives increase the motility of the gastrointestinal tract and therefore allow less time for the prescribed medication to be absorbed.

Changes in cardiac output may also decrease the flow of blood to the liver and kidneys. Another major change with aging is the decrease in renal function. This may lead to medications being removed from the body more slowly and perhaps less completely.

A decrease in body weight of many elderly persons is reason to reassess the dosages of medications ordered. The actual weight of the patient should be used to validate the correct dosage of each drug. At times it may be difficult to select a proper site for an injection. This is because of a decrease in muscle mass. However, an advantage to aging may be a decrease in the perception of pain from injections because of a decrease in some sensory perceptions.

These changes in concert with a person's genetic programming add to the severity of health problems in the elderly. It is difficult for a person who has had an active life to deal with these changes. The nurse must be understanding in order to assist an elderly person to adapt to a limited lifestyle.

Physical illness affects the mental posture of a person, which adds to anxiety and further deterioration. Occasionally, an elderly person feels unable to make the most basic decisions. The nurse, in collaboration with other members of the health team, can assist the patient, the family, and the person(s) responsible for giving care to understand the process of change or aging.

Problems of the Elderly

Some older persons are in the habit of visiting an internist for an annual physical examination. Because the elderly have more aches and pains than other age groups, they may also visit a physician in family practice to deal with minor problems that occur. If these aches and pains do not resolve, they may visit a third physician. If each physician writes a prescription(s), the patient may end up with several medications that duplicate their actions or cause drug interaction or overdosage.

The patient should be encouraged to visit only one physician unless referred to a specialist. Should the patient visit another physician, he or she should prepare a list of all medications taken routinely or as needed and give it to the new physician. The physician can then prescribe medication and instruct the patient to delete duplicated medications or those that cause drug interactions.

Inadequate income is a major problem confronted by many older people. To lower medical costs, they may take less than the prescribed amount of a prescription drug so that it will last longer. They may also stop taking the medication if they perceive it to be ineffective. They may go to the drug store and buy nonprescription drugs. Such drugs will save a physician's fee and are less expensive than prescription drugs, but they may be ineffective. However, the patient may perceive them to be a cure. Another method used to lower costs of drugs is to use a medication of a family member or friend. Misuse of drugs is widespread among the elderly and may cause various problems, such as fluid imbalance, nutritional disturbances, or psychological and neurological problems.

As older persons become forgetful, they may not take their medications or may not take them at the prescribed time. Often family members find medications on the floor, and they do not know whether the medication was taken.

When it becomes unsafe for an elderly person to stay at home alone, a day-care center can relieve the pressure on family members who are employed. People enjoy being with others of their age to discuss memories and similar experiences. They can join in crafts and activities as they wish. There are opportunities to discuss thoughts and concerns with personnel at the center. Then the medication regimen can be continued during the day, meals served, and activities planned. Activities at the center stimulate the elderly and give them something interesting to discuss at home in the evening.

More elderly persons are electing to live in their own home rather than in a retirement home or a nursing home. Sometimes they share their home with someone near their age. If an elderly person or a couple cannot care for themselves, they may choose to share their home with an individual or a couple who will not only be homemakers but also give care as needed. Apart from providing a home for the one(s) giving care, a monetary compensation may be provided.

Medical Alert System

A medical alert system is a valuable tool for a homebound person living alone or if the caregiver must be away for a few minutes. It is also used in retirement homes. In an emergency a button is pushed on the monitoring system or on a chain worn by the patient. The system alerts medical personnel to the emergency situation. Such a system gives a feeling of security to homebound persons and their families.

Medications for the Elderly in the Home

When purchasing medications from a pharmacy, elderly persons should request that childproof containers *not* be used. Containers that are available to prepare medications for a day or a week at a time should be purchased and used (Figure 18-1). Such containers have a special compartment for each hour the medications are to be given. The time can be written on the lid of the individual compartment and easily removed if the time changes. These containers are especially helpful if someone outside the home assists the patient in preparing medications.

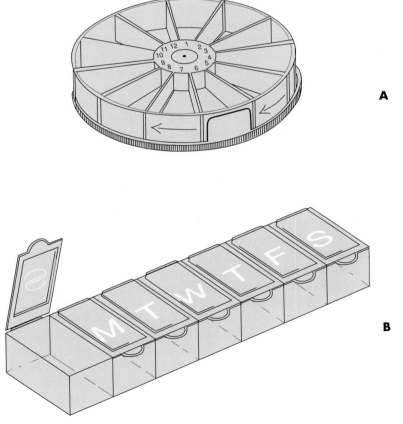

FIGURE 18-1
Examples of containers that hold medications for a day **(A)** or a week **(B)** at a time.

An appointment book with the day and date, a spiral notebook, or a writing tablet with the day and date added can be an efficient and safe way to plan medications taken in the home. The medications and the times they are to be taken each day are listed. The entry is crossed off after the medication has been taken.

Thursday, March 25, 1999
Motrin 300 mg after each meal
   8:00 A.M. 1:00 P.M. 6:00 P.M.
Naprosyn 250 mg two times a day
   8:00 A.M. 4:00 P.M.
Persantin 25 mg two times a day
   10:00 A.M. 6:00 P.M.
Lanoxin 40 mg daily
   10:00 A.M.
Mylanta 2 tablespoons after meals

The used medication sheet is discarded and a new one completed each day.

The Visiting Nurse

At such time that the patient, the family, or the person giving care believes that an assessment of the patient's health status is needed, a request can be made to the physician for assistance from a visiting nurse. The visiting nurse provides skilled care and consultation in the home under the supervision of the patient's physician.

The nurse assesses the patient's condition, gives nursing care as needed, and assists the family and the person giving care to better understand the patient. The nurse should review the patient's medication regimen with the person giving care. If some time has elapsed since the medication was ordered, the nurse should review the medication orders with the physician. The service provided by the visiting nurse will help the patient and family feel secure that the patient is receiving optimum health care in the home.

Medication Errors with the Elderly

The elderly at home are more prone to medication errors than those in health care facilities. The most common error is that of omission. This may be because of the cost of medication or the person's forgetfulness. An incorrect dosage, wrong time, or lack of understanding of directions may be the cause of other medication errors.

The decrease in gross and fine motor skills may affect how well the packaging of medications can be handled. For example, arthritis may make it difficult for an insulin-dependent diabetic to draw up and self-administer the correct dose of insulin.

It is important that the nurse makes sure that the elderly understand the directions for taking their medications safely. Many elderly persons are hearing impaired to some degree. The nurse should ask the patient to verbally repeat the instructions. Older people, beginning with middle age, often are also visually impaired. It is necessary to make certain they can read the labels of their drugs, and any written directions should be printed in a large, easy-to-read format.

Medication errors with the elderly can be reduced if time is taken to explain the reason for medication, its importance, and how it works. This is especially important if timing is critical in maintaining a therapeutic blood level of the medication. Some elderly patients fear becoming addicted to their medication because they do not understand its purpose.

A careful and complete drug history should be taken from all patients, but especially older ones. This history should include over-the-counter drugs. Many people think that over-the-counter drugs are completely safe. However, they may be unaware of the negative interactions that may occur if these products are taken with other medicines that have been prescribed by their physician.

Alcohol is one of the most abused drugs in the elderly population. The combination of alcohol and certain medicines may be a problem for the chronic drinker and the occasional drinker. The nurse's assessment should include the patient's use of alcohol. This information should be validated with other family members.

Medication for the Elderly in the Hospital

Professional nurses will plan nursing care for older patients in the hospital. As our older population continues to increase in numbers, nurses will be employed not only in hospitals and nursing homes but also in day-care centers and retirement communities. The nurse will work with the patient and the family, as well as other health care practitioners, including the physician, dietitian, pharmacist, occupational therapist, social worker, and clinical nurse specialist or nurse practitioner.

Although the physician orders the medications and the pharmacist prepares them, the nurse is responsible for administering the medication to the patient. It is important that the right amount of the right medicine be given to the right patient at the right time in the right way. The patient must also be observed for reactions. The physician must be notified if drug reactions occur. The nurse must record the date, time, medication, dosage, and route of administration.

Before administering the medication to the patient, the nurse should tell the patient the name of the drug and why it was prescribed. The nurse must also be sure that the medication was taken. Sometimes an older patient may hold the medication in the mouth and then remove it after the nurse leaves the bedside. The patient may save the medication in case he or she needs it later. This could cause an overdose. The nurse should observe the patient after administering the medication for any unusual symptoms and record these observations on the patient's chart. The patient's physician must be notified if serious symptoms occur.

Administration of medications is one of the most important responsibilities of the nurse. However, without good skin care, oral hygiene, body alignment and exercise, and a well-balanced diet, the patient will not maintain the potential for health and a satisfying life. Care of the whole person is essential for health and well-being.

Remember, the elderly should be viewed as experienced and mature adults no matter what the functional state of the body. Older adults are capable of learning, but their learning is most successful when there is no time constraint. Allow for plenty of time for their learning to take place and relate the new material to something familiar, if possible. For these reasons discharge planning needs to be done *before the day of discharge*. When teaching the elderly, use visual material, simple language, large print, and involve their support persons. The elderly especially should be encouraged to administer their own medications in the hospital if possible. This allows the nurse to answer questions and assess the level of learning that has occurred.

Chapter 19 | *Home Care Considerations*

Learning Objectives

On completion of the materials provided in this chapter, you will be able to:

1. Understand the unique issues of nursing practice in a home care setting
2. Understand the administration of I.V. therapy in a home care setting

HOME HEALTH NURSING

Home health nursing is one of the fastest growing sectors in the health care industry. To promote cost-effective health care, quality nursing care is being delivered to patients in their homes. These services may be provided on a scheduled or intermittent basis. Home health care is often more conducive to restoring or maintaining a patient's quality of life. Patient satisfaction may also be increased by being at home rather than separated from family while in an acute-care setting.

Nurses working in the field of home care enjoy an increase in autonomy of practice. They must have a medical-surgical background (usually 1 year of clinical experience) and be able to demonstrate expert critical thinking skills. These skills include assessment, communication, judgment, and problem solving. Home care nurses need to be self-directed. Their patient's acuity has likely increased because of the shortened length of stays in hospitals, resulting in an increase in the technology used in the home. These nurses need to be independent and innovative in their practice. The technical skills required of them often will be the same as for nurses working in intensive care units. Many states require home care agencies to be available 24 hours a day.

Home care nursing may involve dressing changes, tracheostomy and/or ventilator care, patient/family teaching, bathing, rehabilitation services, and hospice care. However, the home infusion market is the area of greatest growth in home care. This involves the administration and management of medications in the home. Administration of I.V. medications at home costs substantially less than if the patient must stay in a hospital. The design of portable infusion pumps has improved the safety, accuracy, and ease of home infusion therapy (Figure 19-1).

The principles of medication administration are the same in the home setting as in a hospital. The physician writes the order for the medication. Medication calculations are done in exactly the same way as has been discussed earlier in this book. The guiding principles include the five rights of medication administration. The nurse must follow the rights as discussed in Chapter 9, "Interpretation of the Physician's Orders."

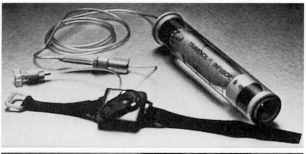

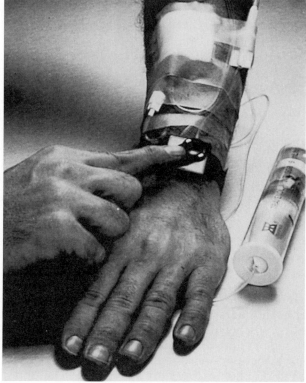

FIGURE 19-1
Portable wrist-model continuous-infusion pump. *(Courtesy Baxter Healthcare Corporation, Deerfield, Ill.)*

Five Rights of Medication Administration

1. Drug
2. Dose
3. Patient
4. Route
5. Time

The sixth right of *documentation* is also required in home administration of medications. This is not only for a legal record; it also plays a significant role in cost reimbursement and payments. The nurse needs to be very knowledgeable about home health care policies. This information is then used to provide the clinical documentation that results in the greatest amount of reimbursement for the patient.

I.V. THERAPY IN THE HOME

Central Venous Catheter

A central venous catheter (CVC) is often used in home care. The CVC may be used for antibiotic therapy, fluid replacement, chemotherapy, hyperalimentation, narcotic pain control, and blood components. These devices prevent repeated venipunctures in the management of patients with cancer, malnutrition, and long-term antibiotic needs. Central lines may also be used for drawing blood from a patient without another needlestick.

Depending on the brand name, the CVC may be called a Hickman, Broviac, or Groshong. The line is placed by a physician using sterile technique, and the patient is put under local or general anesthesia. The line is threaded into a subclavian, jugular, or superior vena cava. The catheter is sutured on the outside of the body to secure placement. Before using the line for administration of fluids or medications, a radiograph is done to confirm appropriate placement. A subclavian catheter is for short-term use of less than 60 days (Figure 19-2). Tunneled catheters such as a Hickman are for long-term use of 1 to 2 years (Figure 19-3).

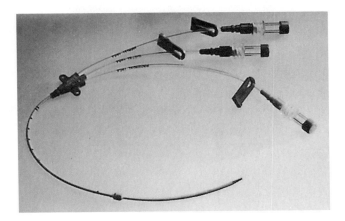

FIGURE 19-2
Multilumen subclavian catheter. *(Courtesy Arrow International, Inc., Reading, Pa.)*

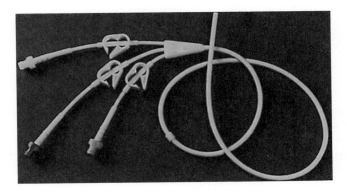

FIGURE 19-3
Hickman tunneled catheter. *(Courtesy CR Bard, Inc., Cranston, RI.)*

Peripherally Inserted Central Catheter

A current trend in home care is to favor the use of a peripherally inserted central catheter (PICC) line. The line is inserted peripherally by a physician or specially certified nurse at the bedside, using strict aseptic technique (Figures 19-4 and 19-5). This catheter is used for 1 to 8 weeks of therapy. Placement should be confirmed by radiography.

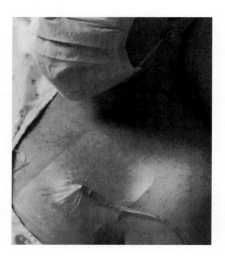

FIGURE 19-4
Continuous infusion with a peripherally inserted central catheter (PICC). *(From Perry A, Potter P:* Clinical nursing skills and techniques, *ed 4, St Louis, 1998, Mosby.)*

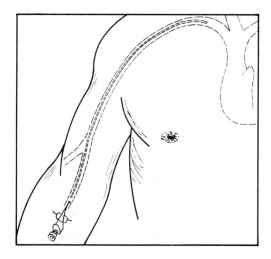

FIGURE 19-5
Insertion of a peripherally inserted central catheter (PICC). *(From LaRocca JC, Otto S:* Pocket guide to intravenous therapy, *ed 3, St Louis, 1997, Mosby.)*

Implantable Venous Access Devices, or Ports

An implantable or subcutaneous port is placed in the subcutaneous layer beneath the skin of the patient. The port is seen as a raised area of 0.2 inch beneath the skin (Figure 19-6). The dome of the port is made of a self-sealing silicone septum. This access may be used for long-term therapy of 1 to 2 years.

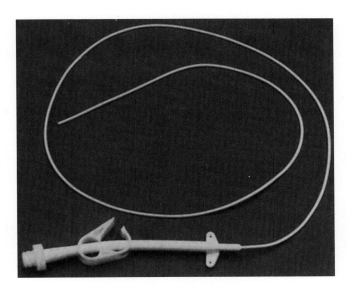

FIGURE 19-6
Peripherally inserted central venous catheter. *(Courtesy Cook Critical Care, Blooming-ton, Ind.)*

Landmark Midline Venous Access Device

The midline catheter follows the same principle of other peripherally inserted central catheters with one exception. This catheter is inserted into the antecubital area and is advanced into the upper veins of the arm. It does not advance into the chest area. Therefore placement does not require an x ray.

The Landmark catheter is constructed of a new material called Aquavane. This catheter is introduced by an over-the-needle method. After placement, the Aquavane material absorbs fluid from the blood and softens. At the same time, the gauge expands and provides an increased flow rate. This catheter also should be placed following strict aseptic technique.

Implications for Home Care Nursing

With home I.V. therapy, it is important that the nurse managing the patient be aware of the care and precautions required by an I.V. line. Routine dressing changes and assessment of the insertion site and area are mandatory. Assessment for infiltration and signs and symptoms of infection are necessary also. Education of the patient and the family is vital for the successful use of home I.V. therapies. Routine line care must be followed accurately to prevent clotting and infection. The patient also needs to be assessed for systemic complications such as circulatory overload and an air embolus. The routine care will be delineated by the physician and per agency policies.

For home infusion therapy to be successful, the patient and family need to be informed and educated. The areas to include are medication information, how to administer and manage the I.V. fluids, what complications may occur and how to handle them, principles of infection control, operation of equipment, and clear guidelines as to when to notify the physician. With physicians, nurses, patients, and families working together, true continuity of care may be attained in the home.

COMPREHENSIVE POSTTEST

Name _____

Date _____

ACCEPTABLE SCORE __**68**__

YOUR SCORE _____

Directions: This test contains 39 questions with a total of 76 points possible. Each of the five separate case sections depicts a variety of patient diagnoses. Test items focus on medication dosages, medication calculations, and medication transcription. Use the forms provided and mark syringes where indicated.

CASE 1
(20 PTS.)

Mr. Jones is transferred to your floor from ICU. You receive Mr. Jones and look over his orders. It is 1700 on 2/3/99. Refer to the physician's order sheet and medication profile sheet for the following questions. Show your work where applicable.

1. Mr. Jones complains of pain to his incision. Percocet tablets are ordered on the physician's order sheet. Percocet is supplied in single tablets issued from the pharmacy. Give _____ .

(1 pt.)

2. What regularly scheduled medications would Mr. Jones receive at 0900 each day? Include the amount of medication.   Give _____ .

_____ .

_____ .

_____ .

(4 pts.)

3. How much I.V. fluid will Mr. Jones receive every 8 hours? _____ ml.

(1 pt.)

PHYSICIAN'S ORDERS

Mr. Jones

1. ADDRESSOGRAPH BEFORE PLACING IN PATIENT'S CHART ▶
2. INITIAL AND DETACH COPY EACH TIME PHYSICIAN WRITES ORDERS
3. TRANSMIT COPY TO PHARMACY
4. ORDERS MUST BE DATED AND TIMED

DATE	ORDERS	TRANS BY
	Diagnosis: *S/P Coronary Art. Bypass Graff* Weight: *184.5#* Height: *5'11"*	
	Sensitivities/Drug Allergies: NKDA	
2/3/99	1. Transfer to step-down unit from ICU	
	2. VS q.4 h. × 24 hours then q.shift	
	3. Up in chair 3×day, asst. to walk in hall 2×day	
	4. I+O q.shift	
	5. Daily WT.	
	6. TED Hose	
	7. Incentive Spirometer q.2 h. while awake	
	8. Diet: 3 gm Na^+, low cholesterol	
	9. Percocet $\frac{..}{ii}$ tabs p.o. q.4 h. p.r.n. pain	
	10. Tylenol GrX p.o. q.4 h. p.r.n. pain or Temp. >38.°	
	11. MOM 30cc p.o. q.day p.r.n. constipation	
	12. Mylanta 30cc p.o. q.4 h. p.r.n. indigestion	
	13. Restoril 15mg p.o. q.h.s. p.r.n. insomnia	
	14. $O_2$3L per nasal cannula	
	15. IVF: Ds $1/2$ NS @ $50^{cc}/_{hr}$, maximum 1200 cc IVF/day	
	16. Digoxin 0.25mg p.o. q.day	
	17. E.C. ASA Gr. V p.o. q.day	
	18. Cimetidine 300mg p.o. t.i.d.	
	19. Lasix 20mg I.V. q.8 h.	
	20. Slow-K 10meq p.o. b.i.d.	
	21. Labs A_7, CBC, CXR q. a.m.	
	M. Doctor, M.D.	

Do Not Write Orders If No Copies Remain; Begin New Form   Copies Remaining

MEDICAL RECORDS COPY	**PHYSICIAN'S ORDERS**							**T-5**
B-CLIN. NOTES	E-LAB	G-X-RAY	K-DIAGNOSTIC	M-SURGERY	Q-THERAPY	T-ORDERS	W-NURSING	Y-MISC.

(Forms courtesy Indiana University Medical Center.)

Transcription of Med Sheet by: _____

Reviewed by: _____ Page _____ of _____

Mr. Jones

Initials	Signature
_____	_____
_____	_____
_____	_____
_____	_____
_____	_____
_____	_____
AN	A. Nurse R. N.

Allergies: ☑ NKDA

Injection Sites:
A = RUE
B = LUE   E = Abdomen
C = RLE   F = R Glut
D = LLE   G = L Glut

Special Notes:

See Legend on Back

☐ Inpatient   ☐ Outpatient

DATE	DRUG	dose	route	interval	08 09 10 11	12 13 14 15	16 17 18 19	20 21 22 23	24 01 02 03	04 05 06 07	2/3	2/4	2/5	2/6	2/7
1 2/3	Digoxin	0.25 mg	p.o.	qday	09										
2 2/3	E.C. ASA	Gr V	p.o.	qday	09										
3 2/3	Cimetidine	300 mg	p.o.	TID	09	13	17								
4 2/3	Lasix	20 mg	IV	q8°	08		16		24						
5 2/3	Slow-K	10 meq	p.o.	BID	09		17								
6		dose	route	interval											
7		dose	route	interval											
8		dose	route	interval											
9		dose	route	interval											
10 2/3	Percocet	·· ̄1̄1̄ dose	p.o.	q.4 h. p.r.n. pain											
11 2/3	Tylenol	Gr. X dose	p.o.	q.4 h. p.r.n. pain or temp >38°											
12 2/3	MOM	30cc dose	p.o.	q.day p.r.n. constipation											
13 2/3	Mylanta	30cc dose	p.o.	q.4 h. p.r.n. indigestion											
14 2/3	Restoril	15 mg dose	p.o.	q.h.s p.r.n. insomnia											

MEDICATION PROFILE | **W-32**

B-CLIN. NOTES	E-LAB	G-X-RAY	K-DIAGNOSTIC	M-SURGERY	Q-THERAPY	T-ORDERS	W-NURSING	Y-MISC.

4. Transcribe each p.r.n. medication from the physician's orders. Include date, medication, dose, route, interval, and time schedule.

(5 pts.)

1														
	dose	route	interval											
2														
	dose	route	interval											
3														
	dose	route	interval											
4														
	dose	route	interval											
5														
	dose	route	interval											

5. Transcribe each regularly scheduled medication from the physician's order sheet. Include date, medication, dose, route, interval, and time schedule.

(5 pts.)

1														
	dose	route	interval											
2														
	dose	route	interval											
3														
	dose	route	interval											
4														
	dose	route	interval											
5														
	dose	route	interval											

6. Mr. Jones complains of insomnia at 2300. What p.r.n. medication is available for him? Give _____ .

(1 pt.)

7. It is time to give Mr. Jones his Lasix. You have a premixed I.V.P.B. of Lasix 20 mg in 50 cc of N.S. Infusion time is 30 minutes. Drop factor is 60 gtt/ml. Give _____ gtt/min.

(1 pt.)

8. Mr. Jones complains of constipation. What is the medication and amount you will give? Give _____ .

(1 pt.)

9. What regularly scheduled medications would Mr. Jones receive at 0800 each day? Include the amount of medication. Give _____ .

(1 pt.)

CASE 2
(12 PTS.)

Mrs. Smith is received by you from the recovery room. You review her orders. It is 1700 on 2/3/99. Refer to the physician's order sheet for the following questions. Show your work where applicable.

1. What regularly scheduled medication(s) would Mrs. Smith receive at 0900 each day? Include the amount of medication. a. _____ . b. _____ .

(2 pts.)

2. Mrs. Smith complains of nausea. You have Phenergan 25 mg per 2 ml available. Give _____ ml.

(1 pt.)

3. How much I.V. fluid will Mrs. Smith receive per shift? per day? _____ ml/shift. _____ ml/day.

(2 pts.)

PHYSICIAN'S ORDERS

Mrs. Smith

1. ADDRESSOGRAPH BEFORE PLACING IN PATIENT'S CHART
2. INITIAL AND DETACH COPY EACH TIME PHYSICIAN WRITES ORDERS
3. TRANSMIT COPY TO PHARMACY
4. ORDERS MUST BE DATED AND TIMED

☐ Inpatient   ☐ Outpatient

DATE	TIME	ORDERS	TRANS BY
2/3/99	1650	**Diagnosis:** S/P Thyroidectomy **Weight:** 146.0# **Height:** 5'10"	
		Sensitivities/Drug Allergies: PCN	
		STATUS: ASSIGN TO OBSERVATION [ ] ; ADMIT AS INPATIENT [ ]	
	1.	Transfer to ward from recovery room.	
	2.	VS q.1 hour ×2 hours, then q.4 hours	
	3.	HOB ↑45 degrees	
	4.	Up in chair 3× day	
	5.	I+O q. shift	
	6.	Incentive Spirometer q.2 hours while awake	
	7.	Diet: Full liquid.	
	8.	Demerol 25mg I.M. q.4 hours p.r.n. pain	
	9.	Phenergan 12.5mg. I.M. q.4-6 hours p.r.n. nausea	
	10.	Tylenol Gr. X p.o. q.4 hours p.r.n. pain or Temp >38°C	
	11.	Restoril 15mg p.o. q.h.s. p.r.n. insomnia	
	12.	O_2 4L per nasal cannula	
	13.	IVF: NS @ 75^{cc}/$_{hr}$	
	14.	Synthroid 0.15mg. p.o. q.day	
	15.	Tagamet 300mg. p.o. q.day	
	16.	Labs: Ca^+ q. 8 hours × 3 days	
		A_7, CBC q. a.m.	
	17.	JP drains × 2 to bulb suction, record output q. shift	
		M. Doctor, M.D.	

Do Not Write Orders If No Copies Remain; Begin New Form   Copies Remaining

MEDICAL RECORDS COPY		**PHYSICIAN'S ORDERS**						**T-5**
B-CLIN. NOTES	E-LAB	G-X-RAY	K-DIAGNOSTIC	M-SURGERY	Q-THERAPY	T-ORDERS	W-NURSING	Y-MISC.

4. Mrs. Smith complains of insomnia at 2200. Restoril is supplied in 30 mg tablets. Give _____ tablet(s).

(1 pt.)

5. What p.r.n. medications are available for complaints of pain? a. _____ . b. _____ .

(2 pts.)

6. Your patient complains of pain shortly after she is received on the ward from the recovery room. Demerol is available 100 mg in 2 ml for injection. Give _____ ml.

(1 pt.)

7. Your patient has a fever of 38.1° C. You have Tylenol 325 mg tablets available. Give _____ tablets.

(1 pt.)

8. Transcribe all regularly scheduled medications from the physician's orders.

(2 pts.)

1												
	dose	route	interval									
2												
	dose	route	interval									

CASE 3
(12 PTS.)

Mrs. Hutsen is received by you after vaginal delivery childbirth without complications. Refer to the physician's order sheet for the following questions. Show your work where applicable.

PHYSICIAN'S ORDERS

1. ADDRESSOGRAPH BEFORE PLACING IN PATIENT'S CHART ▶
2. INITIAL AND DETACH COPY EACH TIME PHYSICIAN WRITES ORDERS
3. TRANSMIT COPY TO PHARMACY
4. ORDERS MUST BE DATED AND TIMED

Mrs. Hutsen

☐ Inpatient   ☐ Outpatient

DATE	TIME	ORDERS	TRANS BY
4/27/99	0815	**Diagnosis:** S/P Childbirth **Weight:** 146.0# **Height:** 5'8"	
		Sensitivities/Drug Allergies: PCN	
		STATUS: ASSIGN TO OBSERVATION ☐ ; ADMIT AS INPATIENT ☐	
		Diet: Regular	
		Activity: Up ad lib c̄ assistance as needed	
		Vital signs: Routine	
		Breast care: per protocol manual breast pump if desired.	
		Incentive spirometer ×10 breaths q.2 h. while awake	
		May shower as desired	
		If pt. unable to void within 6-8 h. or fundus boggy, bladder	
		distended, or uterus displaced, may I+0 cath.	
		Notify M.D. if unable to void 6 h. after catheterization.	
		Call H.O. for Temp >38.5° C, u/o <240 cc/shift.	
		DSLR @ 50cc/hr, may D/C I.V. when tolerating p.o. well.	
		Parlodel 2.5mg p.o. b.i.d. if pt. not breast-feeding.	
		FESO4 0.3gm p.o. b.i.d.	
		Ibuprofen 600mg p.o. q.6 h. p.r.n. pain	
		Tucks to peri-area p.r.n. at bedside.	
		Senokot ī p.o. q.d. p.r.n.	
		Seconal 100 mg I.M. q.h.s. p.r.n. insomnia	
		Tylenol 650mg p.o. q.4 h. p.r.n. pain	
		M. Doctor, M.D.	

Do Not Write Orders If No Copies Remain; Begin New Form

Copies
Remaining

1. What regularly scheduled medication would your patient receive each day? Include the amount. Med. _____ . amt. _____ .

    (2 pts.)

2. Your patient is tolerating p.o. well. Her I.V. fluid was stopped 2 hours before the evening shift ended. How many cc did the patient receive on the evening shift? _____ cc.

    (1 pt.)

3. Your patient complains of insomnia and requests Seconal. Seconal is supplied as 200 mg per ml in a vial. Give _____ ml.

    Mark the syringe at the appropriate amount.

    (2 pts.)

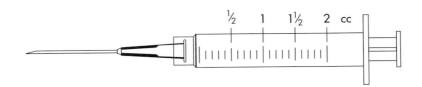

4. Your patient complains of pain and has Ibuprofen ordered. Ibuprofen is supplied as 1200 mg tablets. Give _____ tablet(s).

    (1 pt.)

5. Transcribe all p.r.n. medications from the physician's orders.

    (5 pts.)

10												
	dose	route	interval									
11												
	dose	route	interval									
12												
	dose	route	interval									
13												
	dose	route	interval									
14												
	dose	route	interval									

6. Your patient decides not to breast-feed her baby. You need to start Parlodel. Parlodel is supplied in 1 mg tablets. Give _____ tablet(s).

    (1 pt.)

CASE 4
(15 PTS.)

J. Todd is received on your floor with a diagnosis of acute lymphocytic leukemia. Refer to the physician's order sheet for the following questions. Show your work where applicable.

PHYSICIAN'S ORDERS

Jason Todd

1. ADDRESSOGRAPH BEFORE PLACING IN PATIENT'S CHART ▶
2. INITIAL AND DETACH COPY EACH TIME PHYSICIAN WRITES ORDERS
3. TRANSMIT COPY TO PHARMACY
4. ORDERS MUST BE DATED AND TIMED

☐ Inpatient ☐ Outpatient

DATE	TIME	ORDERS	TRANS BY
10/13/99	0800	**Diagnosis:** Acute Lymphocytic Leukemia **Weight:** 28# **Height:** 3'0"	
		Sensitivities/Drug Allergies: Codeine	
		STATUS: ASSIGN TO OBSERVATION ☐ ; ADMIT AS INPATIENT ☐	
	1.	Diet: Regular	
	2.	Activity: ↑chair t.i.d., Ø rigorous play activity	
	3.	O_2–Biox to keep sats >93%	
	4.	Vital signs: q.4 h.	
	5.	I+O q. shift	
	6.	Daily WT.	
	7.	IVF: D5$\frac{1}{2}$ NS @ 25$^{cc}/_{hr}$.	
	8.	Allopurinol 50mg. p.o. t.i.d.	
	9.	Theophylline 16mg. p.o. q.6 h.	
	10.	Prednisone 2mg./kg/day	
	11.	Vincristine 5.0mg./m^2 in 50ml. of NaCl × $\frac{-}{i}$ now	
	12.	MVI $\frac{-}{i}$ q.day p.o.	
	13.	Compazine 0.07 mg./kg. I.M. q.day p.r.n. nausea	
	14.	Tylenol 120 mg. p.o. t.i.d. p.r.n. pain	
	15.	Call H.O. SBP >140<90, DBP >90<40, Temp. >38.5°C, SOB,	
		$^u/o$ <200 ^{cc}/shift, any problems	
	16.	Labs: CBC c̄ diff., A$_7$, plts., CXR q.day	
		M. Doctor, M.D.	

Do Not Write Orders If No Copies Remain; Begin New Form Copies Remaining

MEDICAL RECORDS COPY		**PHYSICIAN'S ORDERS**						**T-5**
B-CLIN. NOTES	E-LAB	G-X-RAY	K-DIAGNOSTIC	M-SURGERY	Q-THERAPY	T-ORDERS	W-NURSING	Y-MISC.

1. Transcribe all regularly scheduled medications.

(4 pts.)

2. Transcribe all p.r.n. medications.

(2 pts.)

3. Your patient requires theophylline 16 mg p.o. q.6 h. You have theophylline elixir 11.25 mg per ml available. Give _____ ml.

(1 pt.)

4. Your patient requires the allopurinol dose now. You have allopurinol elixir 100 mg per 1 ml available. Give _____ ml.

(1 pt.)

5. Your patient receives prednisone 2 mg/kg/day. You have 10 mg/ml available. Calculate the patient's weight in kg and the correct dose. _____ kg. Give _____ ml.

(2 pts.)

6. Your patient requires a vincristine dosage now. The vincristine is supplied in 50 ml of NaCl and infused over 60 minutes. Drop factor is 60 gtt/ml. _____ gtt/ml.

(1 pt.)

7. Your patient complains of nausea. You have Compazine 1 mg per ml available. Give _____ ml. Mark the syringe at the appropriate amount.

(2 pts.)

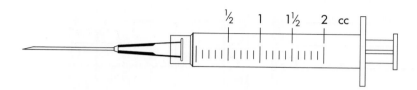

8. Your patient receives D$_5$ ½ N.S. at 25 cc/h. How much fluid will your patient receive each shift? _____ cc.

(1 pt.)

9. Your patient complains of pain. You have Tylenol elixir 360 mg per 2 ml available. Give _____ ml.

(1 pt.)

CASE 5
(18 PTS.)

Mr. Miller is received on your floor from the recovery room. Refer to the physician's order sheet for the following questions. Show your work where applicable.

		PHYSICIAN'S ORDERS	Mr. Miller

1. ADDRESSOGRAPH BEFORE PLACING IN PATIENT'S CHART ▶
2. INITIAL AND DETACH COPY EACH TIME PHYSICIAN WRITES ORDERS
3. TRANSMIT COPY TO PHARMACY
4. ORDERS MUST BE DATED AND TIMED

☐ Inpatient   ☐ Outpatient

DATE	TIME	ORDERS	TRANS BY
6/15/99	1600	**Diagnosis:** S/P Ⓡ total hip replacement **Weight:** 197.0# **Height:** 6'2"	
		Sensitivities/Drug Allergies: NKDA	
		STATUS: ASSIGN TO OBSERVATION ☐ ; ADMIT AS INPATIENT ☐	
		Diet: NPO til fully awake, then clear liquids	
		Activity: Bedrest, log roll side-back-side q.2 h.	
		Vital signs: Every 4 hours	
		Overhead frame trapeze	
		Abductor pillow is necessary whenever pt. is supine.	
		Incentive spirometer q.1 h. while awake.	
		I+O q.8 h.	
		Hemovacs to own reservoirs, record output q.1 h. × 6 h., then q.6 h.	
		I+O catheterization q.shift p.r.n. inability to void.	
		Heparin 5,000 U. S.C. b.i.d.	
		Torecan 10mg. I.M. q.4 h. p.r.n. nausea	
		Mylanta 30cc p.o. p.r.n. indigestion	
		Restoril 15mg. p.o. q. h.s. p.r.n. insomnia	
		Tylenol c̄ codeine p.o. $\frac{\cdot}{i} - \frac{\cdot\cdot}{ii}$ tabs q.4 h. p.r.n. pain	
		Demerol PCA 10mg. I.V. q.10 minutes to maximum 250mg./4 h.	
		Dulcolax supp. $\frac{\cdot}{i}$ p.r. q.shift p.r.n. constipation	
		Labs: CBC q.day × 3	
		Call Orders: Hemovac output >500^{cc}/shift,	
		^{u}/o<250^{cc}/shift, Temp. >38.5°C, Hgb <10.0,	
		SBP >160<80, DBP >90<50.	
		IVF: D$_5$NS @ 50^{cc}/hr.	
		Cefuroxime 1.0 gm. IVPB q.8 h.	
		M. Doctor, M.D.	

Do Not Write Orders If No Copies Remain; Begin New Form   Copies Remaining

MEDICAL RECORDS COPY			**PHYSICIAN'S ORDERS**					**T-5**
B-CLIN. NOTES	E-LAB	G-X-RAY	K-DIAGNOSTIC	M-SURGERY	Q-THERAPY	T-ORDERS	W-NURSING	Y-MISC.

1. Transcribe the regularly scheduled medication below.

(2 pts.)

1										
	dose	route	interval							
2										
	dose	route	interval							

2. Transcribe all p.r.n. medications ordered below.

(7 pts.)

3										
	dose	route	interval							
4										
	dose	route	interval							
5										
	dose	route	interval							
6										
	dose	route	interval							
7										
	dose	route	interval							
8										
	dose	route	interval							
9										
	dose	route	interval							

3. Your patient requires 5000 U heparin subq. You have a vial containing 10,000 U per ml. Give _____ ml. Mark the syringe at the appropriate amount.

(2 pts.)

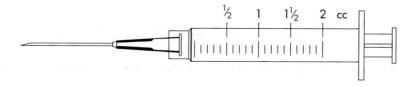

4. Your patient requires a Demerol PCA 10 mg every 10 minutes. You have a Demerol syringe with 300 mg/30 ml available. How many ml will the patient receive every 10 minutes? _____ ml/10 min.

(1 pt.)

5. Your patient complains of nausea and requires Torecan as ordered. You have Torecan 20 mg per 2 ml available per vial. Give _____ ml.

(1 pt.)

6. Your patient receives D_5 N.S. at 50 cc/h. How much I.V. fluid will your patient receive per shift? per day? _____ /shift. _____ /day.

(2 pts.)

7. Your patient receives cefuroxime 1.0 g in 100 cc N.S. I.V.P.B. 30 minutes q.8 h. Drop factor is 60 gtt/ml. _____ ml/h. _____ ml/min. _____ gtt/min.

(3 pts.)

Answers on pp. 501-504.

Glossary

Addends   the numbers to be added

Ampule   a sealed glass container; usually contains one dose of a drug

Buccal   between teeth and cheek

Canceling   dividing numerator and denominator by a common number

Capsule   a small soluble container for enclosing a single dose of medicine

Complex Fraction   a fraction whose numerator, denominator, or both contain fractions

Decimal Fraction   a fraction consisting of a numerator that is expressed in numerals, a decimal point that designates the value of the denominator, and the denominator, which is understood to be 10 or some power of 10

Decimal Numbers   include an integer, a decimal point, and a decimal fraction

Denominator   the number of parts into which a whole has been divided

Difference   the result of subtracting

Dividend   the number being divided

Divisor   the number by which another number is divided

Dosage   the determination and regulation of the size, frequency, and number of doses

Dose   the exact amount of medicine to be administered at one time

Drug   a chemical substance used in therapy, diagnosis, and prevention of a disease or condition

Elixir   a clear, sweet, hydroalcoholic liquid in which a drug is suspended

Equivalent   equal

Extremes   the first and fourth terms of a proportion

Fraction   indicates the number of equal parts of a whole

Improper Fraction   a fraction whose numerator is larger than or equal to the denominator

Infusion   the therapeutic introduction of a fluid into a vein by the flow of gravity

Injection   the therapeutic introduction of a fluid into a part of the body by force

Integer   a whole number

Intramuscular   within the muscle

Intravenous   within the vein

Invert   turn upside down

Lowest Common Denominator   the smallest whole number that can be divided evenly by all denominators within the problem

Means   the second and third terms of a proportion

Medicine   any drug

Milliequivalent   the number of grams of a solute contained in one milliliter of a normal solution

Minuend   the number from which another number is subtracted

Mixed Number   a combination of a whole number and a proper fraction

Multiplicand   the number that is to be multiplied

Multiplier   the number that another number is to be multiplied by

Numerator   the number of parts of a divided whole

Oral Dosage   a medication taken by mouth

Parenteral Dosage   a dosage administered by routes that bypass the gastrointestinal tract and that are generally given by injection

Percent   indicates the number of hundredths

Product   the result of multiplying

Proper Fraction   a fraction whose numerator is smaller than the denominator

Proportion   two ratios that are of equal value and are connected by a double colon

Quotient   the answer to a division problem

Ratio   the relationship between two numbers that are connected by a colon

Reconstitution   the return of a medication to its previous state by the addition of water or other designated liquid

Subcutaneous   beneath the skin

Sublingual   under the tongue

Subtrahend   the number being subtracted

Sum   the result of adding

Suspension   a liquid in which a drug is distributed

Syrup   a sweet, thick, aqueous liquid in which a drug is suspended

Tablet   a drug compressed into a small disk

Topical   on top of the skin or mucous membrane

Unit   the amount of a drug needed to produce a given result

Vial   a glass container with a rubber stopper; usually contains a number of doses of a drug

Answer Key

PART I

Mathematics Pretest, pp. 3-8

1. $^{17}/_{24}$
2. $4^2/_{21}$
3. $1^{16}/_{45}$
4. $4^9/_{40}$
5. 4.364
6. 33.832
7. 13.058
8. 34.659
9. $1^1/_{12}$
10. $^{23}/_{30}$
11. $^5/_8$
12. $1^5/_6$
13. 1.053
14. 0.754
15. 0.585
16. 1.417
17. $1^5/_7$
18. $^5/_9$
19. 9

20. $8^9/_{40}$
21. 27.413
22. 1.827
23. 31.79484
24. 1579.2
25. $^{18}/_{25}$
26. $^5/_{12}$
27. $^2/_{15}$
28. $^{33}/_{80}$
29. 25.9924
30. 0.22625
31. 21.373
32. 6.4771
33. 0.003
34. 0.45
35. 0.0072
36. 0.058
37. 0.155
38. 0.8

39. 0.249
40. 2.99
41. 0.625
42. 0.75
43. 0.55
44. 0.68
45. $^7/_8$
46. $^3/_8$
47. $^1/_{20}$
48. $^1/_8$
49. 43.2%
50. $^{13}/_{20}$
51. 3 : 1000
52. $12^1/_2\%$ or 12.5%
53. 20%
54. 50%
55. $7^1/_2\%$ or 7.5%
56. 0.15
57. 42.3

58. 292.5
59. 3 : 14
60. 9 : 16
61. 329 : 400
62. 5 : 11
63. 17 : 50
64. 400
65. 5
66. 24
67. $7^1/_5$ or 7.2
68. 20
69. 2000
70. 100
71. 500
72. 51
73. $2^1/_2$ or 2.5
74. 68
75. 36,288

Chapter 1 Fractions—Pretest, pp. 9-11

1. $^{19}/_{24}$
2. $1^{10}/_{63}$
3. $9^7/_{20}$
4. $10^2/_3$
5. $9^3/_4$
6. $5^9/_{16}$
7. $9^1/_{22}$
8. $7^8/_9$
9. $3^5/_6$
10. $5^{23}/_{24}$

11. $^3/_{10}$
12. $^7/_8$
13. $^{13}/_{15}$
14. $2^5/_8$
15. $6^3/_{26}$
16. $2^{17}/_{24}$
17. $1^5/_6$
18. $1^4/_5$
19. $1^5/_{16}$
20. $1^5/_6$

21. $^1/_{15}$
22. $^{21}/_{80}$
23. 5
24. $7^{19}/_{63}$
25. $1^1/_{14}$
26. $^1/_{10,000}$
27. $4^5/_{18}$
28. $5^{41}/_{75}$
29. $12^1/_{12}$
30. $2^{25}/_{28}$

31. $^5/_{16}$
32. $^{49}/_{81}$
33. $1^1/_3$
34. $33^1/_3$
35. $^7/_8$
36. $1^1/_3$
37. $^1/_{12}$
38. $^5/_9$
39. $1^7/_{10}$
40. 2

Chapter 1 Fractions—Work Sheet, pp. 25-32

Improper fractions to mixed numbers, pp. 25-26

1. $1\frac{1}{3}$	**7.** $1\frac{3}{7}$	**13.** $1\frac{2}{3}$	**19.** $4\frac{2}{3}$
2. 3	**8.** $3\frac{1}{4}$	**14.** $2\frac{1}{6}$	**20.** $1\frac{3}{8}$
3. $2\frac{1}{4}$	**9.** $3\frac{1}{3}$	**15.** $6\frac{1}{3}$	**21.** $3\frac{1}{2}$
4. $3\frac{1}{5}$	**10.** $2\frac{1}{9}$	**16.** $3\frac{1}{7}$	**22.** $1\frac{3}{25}$
5. $1\frac{7}{10}$	**11.** $1\frac{1}{2}$	**17.** $2\frac{9}{13}$	**23.** $2\frac{7}{15}$
6. $1\frac{1}{2}$	**12.** $1\frac{1}{8}$	**18.** $3\frac{1}{2}$	**24.** $1\frac{1}{2}$

Mixed numbers to improper fractions, pp. 26-27

1. $\frac{3}{2}$	**7.** $\frac{17}{6}$	**13.** $\frac{29}{3}$	**19.** $\frac{53}{8}$
2. $\frac{15}{4}$	**8.** $\frac{8}{5}$	**14.** $\frac{70}{11}$	**20.** $\frac{29}{13}$
3. $\frac{8}{3}$	**9.** $\frac{25}{7}$	**15.** $\frac{307}{100}$	**21.** $\frac{28}{25}$
4. $\frac{33}{8}$	**10.** $\frac{22}{3}$	**16.** $\frac{31}{7}$	**22.** $\frac{17}{4}$
5. $\frac{65}{9}$	**11.** $\frac{39}{8}$	**17.** $\frac{4}{3}$	**23.** $\frac{43}{8}$
6. $\frac{53}{10}$	**12.** $\frac{11}{2}$	**18.** $\frac{27}{10}$	**24.** $\frac{22}{9}$

Addition, pp. 27-28

1. $1\frac{1}{2}$	**7.** $5\frac{13}{20}$	**13.** $7\frac{5}{8}$	**19.** $6\frac{19}{30}$
2. $\frac{29}{35}$	**8.** $3\frac{5}{39}$	**14.** $6\frac{17}{22}$	**20.** $1\frac{7}{12}$
3. $3\frac{19}{24}$	**9.** $3\frac{7}{16}$	**15.** $6\frac{4}{9}$	**21.** $4\frac{3}{20}$
4. $1\frac{8}{9}$	**10.** $10\frac{4}{5}$	**16.** $6\frac{11}{30}$	**22.** 9
5. $3\frac{1}{4}$	**11.** $6\frac{1}{2}$	**17.** $4\frac{17}{24}$	**23.** $6\frac{10}{63}$
6. $\frac{65}{77}$	**12.** $6\frac{14}{15}$	**18.** $6\frac{19}{40}$	**24.** $8\frac{7}{30}$

Subtraction, pp. 28-29

1. $\frac{5}{21}$	**7.** $1\frac{1}{10}$	**13.** $1\frac{15}{16}$	**19.** $1\frac{5}{12}$
2. $\frac{9}{16}$	**8.** $1\frac{1}{6}$	**14.** $\frac{5}{8}$	**20.** $1\frac{7}{24}$
3. $\frac{7}{48}$	**9.** $2\frac{31}{40}$	**15.** $1\frac{1}{3}$	**21.** $1\frac{1}{12}$
4. $\frac{1}{2}$	**10.** $1\frac{1}{24}$	**16.** $2\frac{5}{8}$	**22.** $1\frac{19}{24}$
5. $\frac{1}{5}$	**11.** $\frac{11}{16}$	**17.** $\frac{19}{24}$	**23.** $1\frac{3}{5}$
6. $\frac{3}{16}$	**12.** $1\frac{13}{24}$	**18.** $1\frac{25}{48}$	**24.** $\frac{15}{16}$

Multiplication, pp. 29-31

1. $\frac{4}{15}$	**7.** $8\frac{3}{4}$	**13.** $4\frac{4}{15}$	**19.** $4\frac{1}{10}$
2. $\frac{5}{27}$	**8.** $6\frac{6}{35}$	**14.** $1\frac{25}{32}$	**20.** $4\frac{1}{4}$
3. $\frac{7}{12}$	**9.** $11\frac{7}{8}$	**15.** $5\frac{5}{8}$	**21.** $2\frac{11}{14}$
4. $\frac{4}{7}$	**10.** $5\frac{49}{50}$	**16.** $\frac{1}{5}$	**22.** $6\frac{5}{12}$
5. 4	**11.** $5\frac{2}{15}$	**17.** $4\frac{15}{32}$	**23.** $3\frac{2}{3}$
6. $1\frac{1}{2}$	**12.** $12\frac{11}{16}$	**18.** $\frac{3}{1000}$	**24.** $3\frac{1}{9}$

Division, pp. 31-32

1. $\frac{10}{21}$	**7.** $2\frac{1}{2}$	**13.** $1\frac{29}{40}$	**19.** $1\frac{13}{22}$
2. $1\frac{4}{5}$	**8.** $1\frac{23}{26}$	**14.** $3\frac{47}{51}$	**20.** $2\frac{1}{16}$
3. $2\frac{1}{5}$	**9.** $2\frac{32}{39}$	**15.** $1\frac{29}{176}$	**21.** $2\frac{2}{19}$
4. $2\frac{5}{6}$	**10.** $1\frac{7}{20}$	**16.** $3\frac{1}{2}$	**22.** $1\frac{9}{28}$
5. $1\frac{5}{9}$	**11.** $1\frac{7}{11}$	**17.** $2\frac{5}{17}$	**23.** $1\frac{1}{2}$
6. $2\frac{23}{56}$	**12.** $1\frac{7}{8}$	**18.** $4\frac{23}{24}$	**24.** $1\frac{22}{23}$

Chapter 1 Fractions—Posttest 1, pp. 33-35

1. $1\frac{1}{9}$
2. $\frac{17}{24}$
3. $5\frac{1}{12}$
4. $4\frac{3}{10}$
5. $3\frac{2}{21}$
6. $4\frac{10}{21}$
7. $\frac{39}{50}$
8. $3\frac{19}{24}$
9. $8\frac{3}{20}$
10. $7\frac{7}{12}$

11. $\frac{5}{36}$
12. $\frac{9}{10}$
13. $\frac{5}{6}$
14. $\frac{3}{14}$
15. $1\frac{4}{9}$
16. $1\frac{15}{16}$
17. $1\frac{31}{63}$
18. $1\frac{9}{20}$
19. $5\frac{7}{10}$
20. $1\frac{1}{12}$

21. $\frac{9}{14}$
22. $2\frac{2}{5}$
23. $\frac{2}{5}$
24. 2
25. $3\frac{5}{24}$
26. $3\frac{1}{3}$
27. $14\frac{7}{10}$
28. $3\frac{18}{35}$
29. $\frac{7}{8}$
30. $42\frac{1}{2}$

31. $1\frac{1}{15}$
32. 10
33. $\frac{2}{3}$
34. $1\frac{1}{4}$
35. $\frac{3}{20}$
36. $\frac{9}{14}$
37. $\frac{3}{5}$
38. $1\frac{7}{20}$
39. $4\frac{1}{2}$
40. $1\frac{3}{22}$

Chapter 1 Fractions—Posttest 2, pp. 37-39

1. $1\frac{1}{12}$
2. $4\frac{1}{10}$
3. $3\frac{2}{21}$
4. $7\frac{1}{15}$
5. $5\frac{11}{40}$
6. $4\frac{19}{24}$
7. $11\frac{4}{5}$
8. $6\frac{25}{36}$
9. $3\frac{1}{2}$
10. $3\frac{19}{40}$

11. $\frac{1}{9}$
12. $1\frac{7}{8}$
13. $1\frac{5}{6}$
14. $\frac{32}{35}$
15. $2\frac{5}{16}$
16. $\frac{5}{8}$
17. $1\frac{1}{2}$
18. $3\frac{9}{10}$
19. $\frac{3}{5}$
20. $4\frac{13}{14}$

21. $\frac{4}{21}$
22. $6\frac{1}{5}$
23. $1\frac{1}{3}$
24. $7\frac{21}{22}$
25. $1\frac{17}{18}$
26. $\frac{1}{1000}$
27. $6\frac{6}{11}$
28. 36
29. $3\frac{1}{2}$
30. $11\frac{1}{4}$

31. $\frac{27}{32}$
32. $\frac{21}{26}$
33. $6\frac{2}{9}$
34. $\frac{1}{49}$
35. $\frac{5}{8}$
36. $\frac{21}{32}$
37. $1\frac{23}{32}$
38. $1\frac{11}{16}$
39. $1\frac{19}{26}$
40. $1\frac{1}{8}$

Chapter 2 Decimals—Pretest, pp. 41-44

1. Four hundredths
2. One and six tenths
3. Sixteen and six thousand seven hundred thirty-four hundred thousandths
4. One and fifteen thousandths
5. Nine thousandths
6. 0.02
7. 0.004
8. 1.6
9. 2.082
10. 0.003
11. 1429.421
12. 983.799
13. 25.376
14. 324.3
15. 36.1094
16. 1012.867
17. 150.6736
18. 1003.6135
19. 84.565
20. 552.1326
21. 1.078
22. 863.45

23. 1.008
24. 759.4
25. 1.7
26. 11.69
27. 0.079
28. 10.946
29. 0.48
30. 8.06
31. 0.0567
32. 6.6472
33. 0.0608
34. 0.193272
35. 1.9425
36. 3.2604
37. 29.5336
38. 186.543
39. 0.676

40. 356.546
41. 0.21
42. 17.95
43. 3.94
44. 31,000
45. 0.01
46. 8.98
47. 627
48. 0.70
49. 40.75
50. 0.02
51. $\frac{1}{5}$
52. $\frac{9}{20}$
53. $\frac{1}{125}$
54. $\frac{1}{4}$
55. $16\frac{1}{500}$

56. $\frac{27}{100}$
57. $\frac{3}{10}$
58. $\frac{1}{250}$
59. $\frac{17}{50}$
60. $\frac{19}{20}$
61. 0.6
62. 0.67
63. 0.01
64. 0.35
65. 0.08
66. 0.625, 0.63
67. 0.03
68. 0.375, 0.38
69. 0.01
70. 0.16

Chapter 2 Decimals—Work Sheet, pp. 51-60

1. Two tenths
2. Nine and sixty-eight hundredths
3. One hundred eighty-six and nine hundred thirty-five thousandths
4. Eight one hundred thousandths
5. Eighty-six thousand nine hundred thirty-one hundred thousandths
6. Six hundred ninety-eight thousand four hundred thirty-seven and fifteen hundredths
7. Three ten thousandths
8. Twelve thousand three hundred seventy-five and seven tenths
9. Six and four thousandths
10. One thousand nine hundred sixty-eight and three hundred forty-two thousandths
11. Two hundredths
12. Thirty-five and four thousand seven hundred twenty-six ten thousandths

13. 0.25	**16.** 0.68	**19.** 0.6	**22.** 0.08
14. 0.45	**17.** 1.8	**20.** 0.0003	**23.** 0.007
15. 0.98	**18.** 7.44	**21.** 1.0022	**24.** 3.006

Addition, pp. 52-53

1. 41.755	**7.** 21.919	**13.** 22.833	**19.** 526.173
2. 372.675	**8.** 16.908	**14.** 111.5919	**20.** 55.117
3. 40.9787	**9.** 54.033	**15.** 26.62	**21.** 216.28
4. 888.5997	**10.** 894.842	**16.** 23.391	**22.** 51.555
5. 39.073	**11.** 67.137	**17.** 41.4281	**23.** 142.218
6. 27.851	**12.** 37.394	**18.** 37.9	**24.** 218.05

Subtraction, pp. 53-54

1. 1257.87	**7.** 1.079	**13.** 50.675	**19.** 0.88
2. 1.849	**8.** 4.144	**14.** 62.022	**20.** 0.009
3. 0.71	**9.** 0.461	**15.** 287.371	**21.** 919.57
4. 32.746	**10.** 0.988	**16.** 0.187	**22.** 659.74
5. 174.804	**11.** 3.332	**17.** 9.949	**23.** 0.447
6. 7.418	**12.** 6.893	**18.** 2.939	**24.** 17.67

Multiplication, pp. 54-55

1. 115.3674	**9.** 56.1144	**17.** 13282.75
2. 16.25	**10.** 41.92	**18.** 409.0318
3. 159.84	**11.** 11.696	**19.** 0.512
4. 6.56	**12.** 1.156	**20.** 43.472
5. 609.6	**13.** 33.6813	**21.** 643211.7
6. 52.052	**14.** 35.7	**22.** 0.15113
7. 26.25	**15.** 33.6	**23.** 7147.5
8. 696	**16.** 103.983	**24.** 23.5971

Multiply by 10, p. 56

1. 0.9		**4.** 3.0	
2. 2.0		**5.** 6.25	
3. 1.8		**6.** 23.3	

Multiply by 100, p. 56

1. 2.3		**4.** 12.5	
2. 150		**5.** 865	
3. 0.4		**6.** 7640	

Multiply by 1000, p. 56

1. 200		**4.** 9650	
2. 5		**5.** 460	
3. 187		**6.** 489	

Multiply by 0.1, p. 56

1. 3.0   **4.** 0.095
2. 0.069   **5.** 0.0138
3. 0.17   **6.** 0.567

Multiply by 0.01, p. 56

1. 0.0026   **4.** 0.112
2. 0.908   **5.** 0.00875
3. 0.055   **6.** 0.633

Multiply by 0.001, p. 56

1. 0.056   **4.** 0.0333
2. 0.01255   **5.** 0.009684
3. 0.1265   **6.** 0.241

Round to the nearest tenth, p. 56

1. 0.3   **4.** 0.7
2. 0.9   **5.** 58.4
3. 2.4   **6.** 8.1

Round to the nearest hundredth, p. 56

1. 2.56   **4.** 3.92
2. 4.28   **5.** 6.53
3. 0.28   **6.** 2.99

Round to the nearest thousandth, p. 56

1. 27.863   **4.** 0.849
2. 5.925   **5.** 321.087
3. 2.157   **6.** 455.768

Division, pp. 56-58

1. 1.17   **7.** 1.7   **13.** 740   **19.** 0.48
2. 4140   **8.** 0.13   **14.** 0.05   **20.** 0.8
3. 7.8   **9.** 185   **15.** 0.5   **21.** 2.52
4. 0.03   **10.** 0.02   **16.** 4.53   **22.** 2.63
5. 400   **11.** 0.13   **17.** 1.45   **23.** 47
6. 8.4   **12.** 82.6   **18.** 17.39   **24.** 17.48

Divide by 10, p. 58

1. 0.6   **4.** 0.005
2. 0.02   **5.** 0.0375
3. 0.98   **6.** 0.099

Divide by 100, p. 58

1. 0.007   **4.** 0.0019
2. 0.0811   **5.** 0.12
3. 7   **6.** 0.302

Divide by 1000, p. 58

1. 0.0018   **4.** 0.0546
2. 0.36   **5.** 0.0075
3. 0.00025   **6.** 7.14

Divide by 0.1, p. 58

1. 28   **4.** 9.87
2. 1   **5.** 150
3. 6.5   **6.** 82.5

Divide by 0.01, p. 58

1. 3600   **4.** 959
2. 16   **5.** 80
3. 48   **6.** 9.7

Divide by 0.001, p. 58

1. 6200   **4.** 860
2. 839,000   **5.** 13,800
3. 5000   **6.** 15.6

Decimal fractions to proper fractions, pp. 58-59

1. $3/50$ **7.** $1/400$ **13.** $1/250$ **19.** $4/25$
2. $19/200$ **8.** $17/20$ **14.** $3/25$ **20.** $11/50$
3. $4/5$ **9.** $1/2$ **15.** $11/200$ **21.** $1/200$
4. $17/25$ **10.** $5/8$ **16.** $7/8$ **22.** $1/100$
5. $1/8$ **11.** $1/4$ **17.** $16/25$ **23.** $11/250$
6. $37/50$ **12.** $9/10$ **18.** $3/4$ **24.** $1/5$

Proper fractions to decimal fractions, pp. 59-60

1. 0.125, 0.13   **7.** 0.24   **13.** 0.5   **19.** 0.75
2. 0.55   **8.** 0.6   **14.** 0.9   **20.** 0.34
3. 0.67   **9.** 0.04   **15.** 0.8   **21.** 0.01
4. 0.375, 0.38   **10.** 0.33   **16.** 0.15   **22.** 0.09
5. 0.64   **11.** 0.86   **17.** 0.875, 0.88   **23.** 0.83
6. 0.25   **12.** 0.08   **18.** 0.25   **24.** 0.95

Chapter 2 Decimals—Posttest 1, pp. 61-64

1. Forty-two and sixty-eight thousand five hundred ninety-three hundred thousandths
2. Six hundred thirty-four and eighteen hundredths
3. Nine tenths
4. Three thousandths
5. Sixty-four and two hundred thirty-one thousandths

6. 0.25	28. 20.95	50. 500
7. 0.15	29. 43.6077	51. $9/100$
8. 0.6666	30. 0.211	52. $5/8$
9. 0.6	31. 702.4472	53. $4/25$
10. 5.5	32. 0.13904	54. $1/2$
11. 54.66	33. 5.46875	55. $1/400$
12. 8.235	34. 2366.079981	56. $11/20$
13. 926.043	35. 162	57. $3/8$
14. 22.904	36. 0.850304	58. $2/5$
15. 8.89	37. 44.278	59. $3/500$
16. 2054.74	38. 0.585	60. $3/4$
17. 138.44	39. 924448.47552	61. 0.71
18. 6.352	40. 21.892	62. 0.22
19. 6.104	41. 16.8	63. 0.85
20. 2152.626	42. 4662.5	64. 0.01
21. 88.982	43. 1481.67	65. 0.8
22. 7.137	44. 1880	66. 0.31
23. 0.339	45. 51333.33	67. 0.33
24. 5.32	46. 627	68. 0.004
25. 1.4532	47. 1.41	69. 0.125, 0.13
26. 323.08	48. 55.19	70. 0.09
27. 0.628	49. 2	

Chapter 2 Decimals—Posttest 2, pp. 65-68

1. Five tenths
2. Eight and two thousand six hundred fifty-eight ten thousandths
3. Four and two ten thousandths
4. One hundred twenty-three and sixty-nine hundredths
5. Two and four hundred five thousandths

6. 0.8	23. 0.587	40. 161.975
7. 0.9	24. 7.789	41. 820
8. 0.86	25. 2.766	42. 1.11
9. 0.659	26. 2.513	43. 5
10. 1.222	27. 81.79	44. 0.48
11. 456.8191	28. 3.84	45. 4.08
12. 130.5837	29. 1.085	46. 15,500
13. 16.055	30. 223.98	47. 2
14. 33.209	31. 28.57704	48. 12
15. 280.895	32. 167.04	49. 0.30
16. 285.591	33. 104,552	50. 2.47
17. 2011.306	34. 247.975	51. $1/25$
18. 47.725	35. 27.61018	52. $1/200$
19. 507.629	36. 1.01574	53. $7/20$
20. 339	37. 276.35148	54. $1/8$
21. 612.969	38. 83.2	55. $9/10$
22. 27.9	39. 2560	56. $17/20$

57. $^3/_{1000}$
58. $^4/_5$
59. $^{11}/_{50}$
60. $^3/_5$
61. 0.55

62. 0.17
63. 0.003
64. 0.875, 0.88
65. 0.4
66. 0.75

67. 0.007
68. 0.5
69. 0.008
70. 0.19

Chapter 3 Percents—Pretest, pp. 69-71

Fractions to percents, p. 69

1. $1^2/_3$%, 1.6666%
2. $71^3/_7$%, 71.4285%
3. $12^1/_2$%, 12.5%

4. 30%
5. $133^1/_3$%, 133.3333%

Decimals to percents, p. 69

6. 0.6%
7. 35%
8. 42.7%

9. 382.1%
10. 70%

Percents to fractions, p. 70

11. $^1/_{200}$
12. $^3/_4$
13. $^{19}/_{200}$

14. $^{31}/_{125}$
15. $^3/_{800}$

Percents to decimals, p. 70

16. 0.0116
17. 0.075
18. 0.133

19. 0.0088
20. 0.63

What percent of, pp. 70-71

21. 375%
22. $16^2/_3$%, 16.6666%
23. 65%
24. $^1/_5$%, 0.2%
25. $33^1/_3$%, 33.333%

26. $12^{32}/_{189}$%, 12.1693%
27. $43^7/_{26}$%, 43.2692%
28. 10%
29. $7^1/_7$%, 7.1428%
30. $1^{209}/_{291}$%, 1.7182%

What is, p. 71

31. 1.8
32. 0.15
33. 2.565
34. 0.68
35. 3.08

36. 4.278
37. 0.05999
38. 19.36
39. 11.856
40. 15

Chapter 3 Percents—Work Sheet, pp. 77-83

Fractions to percents, pp. 77-78

1. 75%
2. 50%
3. $37^1/_2$%
4. 80%
5. 32%
6. $^3/_{10}$%

7. $3^1/_2$%
8. $66^2/_3$%
9. $41^2/_3$%
10. $23^1/_3$%
11. $2^1/_4$%
12. $84^3/_8$%

13. 15%
14. $70^{10}/_{17}$%
15. $22^8/_{11}$%
16. 6%
17. $68^3/_4$%
18. $21^3/_7$%

19. $38^2/_{21}$%
20. $83^1/_3$%
21. $^3/_4$%
22. $13^1/_3$%
23. $44^4/_9$%
24. $87^1/_2$%

Decimals to percents, pp. 78-79

1. 40.2%
2. 3.67%
3. 431%
4. 16.3%
5. 622%
6. 98%

7. 32.76%
8. 30%
9. 133.97%
10. 14.5%
11. 28.24%
12. 67%

13. 70%
14. 62.24%
15. 42%
16. 63.37%
17. 620%
18. 15.9%

19. 290.14%
20. 67.3%
21. 40.5%
22. 37.12%
23. 723.4%
24. 220%

Percents to fractions, pp. 79-80

1. $^7/_{200}$
2. $^3/_{400}$
3. $^{203}/_{500}$
4. $^1/_{800}$
5. $^1/_{10}$
6. $^1/_{150}$

7. $^1/_{600}$
8. $^7/_{2000}$
9. $^9/_{20}$
10. $^{101}/_{500}$
11. $^1/_{160}$
12. $^9/_{200}$

13. $^3/_{25}$
14. $^1/_{400}$
15. $^{19}/_{800}$
16. $^{29}/_{50}$
17. $^2/_{25}$
18. $^1/_{16}$

19. $^{21}/_{1000}$
20. $^3/_{2000}$
21. $^1/_{200}$
22. $^{81}/_{250}$
23. $^2/_3$
24. $^9/_{500}$

Percents to decimals, pp. 80-81

1. 0.375	**7.** 0.4	**13.** 0.0023	**19.** 0.0875
2. 0.03	**8.** 0.0135	**14.** 0.726	**20.** 0.005
3. 0.017	**9.** 0.025	**15.** 0.16	**21.** 0.0575
4. 0.0675	**10.** 0.00375	**16.** 0.3064	**22.** 0.0098
5. 0.0042	**11.** 0.05	**17.** 0.0293	**23.** 0.069
6. 0.0025	**12.** 0.8	**18.** 0.003125	**24.** 0.0058

What percent of, pp. 81-82

1. 55%	**7.** $24\frac{6}{11}\%$, 24.5454%	**13.** 15%	**19.** $10\frac{15}{19}\%$, 10.7894%
2. $16\frac{2}{3}\%$, 16.6666%	**8.** 200%	**14.** $23\frac{1}{13}\%$, 23.0769%	**20.** 45%
3. $7\frac{7}{8}\%$, 7.875%	**9.** $5\frac{25}{36}\%$, 5.6944%	**15.** $74\frac{38}{163}\%$, 74.2331%	**21.** 1%
4. 50%	**10.** 2%	**16.** 20%	**22.** $2\frac{2}{25}\%$, 2.08%
5. $46\frac{2}{3}\%$, 46.6666%	**11.** 12%	**17.** 10%	**23.** $3\frac{3}{4}\%$, 3.75%
6. 84%	**12.** 5%	**18.** $4\frac{56}{75}\%$, 4.746%	**24.** 20%

What is, pp. 82-83

1. 119.5	**7.** 30.77	**13.** 0.585	**19.** 168.48
2. 3.4	**8.** 999.9 or 1000	**14.** 0.12	**20.** 0.066
3. 14.28	**9.** 1.995	**15.** 131.712	**21.** 10.752
4. 633.75	**10.** 4.0	**16.** 540.02	**22.** 105
5. 0.14	**11.** 11.52	**17.** 0.17	**23.** 0.10125
6. 1.625	**12.** 0.13	**18.** 11.07	**24.** 5.0868

Chapter 3 Percents—Posttest 1, pp. 85-87

Fractions to percents, p. 85

1. $44\frac{4}{9}\%$, 44.4444%	**4.** $266\frac{2}{3}\%$, 266.6666%
2. $87\frac{1}{2}\%$, 87.5%	**5.** $\frac{3}{10}\%$, 0.3%
3. 55%	

Decimals to percents, p. 85

6. 25.6%	**9.** 167.8%
7. 3330%	**10.** 90%
8. 0.4%	

Percents to fractions, p. 86

11. $\frac{3}{5}$	**14.** $\frac{1}{400}$
12. $\frac{17}{20}$	**15.** $\frac{7}{200}$
13. $\frac{3}{1000}$	

Percents to decimals, p. 86

16. 0.863	**19.** 0.0078
17. 0.04625	**20.** 0.0036
18. 0.2945	

What percent of, pp. 86-87

21. 10%	**26.** 20%
22. 5%	**27.** 50%
23. $\frac{1}{3}\%$, 0.33%	**28.** $7\frac{1}{2}\%$, 7.5%
24. 12%	**29.** $8\frac{6}{13}\%$, 8.4615%
25. $42\frac{6}{7}\%$, 42.8571%	**30.** 8%

What is, p. 87

31. 520	**36.** 42.3
32. 36	**37.** 292.5
33. 0.09	**38.** 0.15
34. 170	**39.** 2.408
35. 1.6875	**40.** 0.4576

Chapter 3 Percents—Posttest 2, pp. 89-91

Fractions to percents, p. 89

1. $12\frac{1}{2}\%$, 12.5%
2. 40%
3. $16\frac{2}{3}\%$, 16.6666%
4. 95%
5. $122\frac{2}{9}\%$, 122.2222%

Decimals to percents, p. 89

6. 6.5%
7. 0.5%
8. 434.6%
9. 57%
10. 20%

Percents to fractions, p. 90

11. $\frac{3}{1000}$
12. $\frac{33}{200}$
13. $\frac{3}{500}$
14. $\frac{7}{400}$
15. $\frac{1}{400}$

Percents to decimals, p. 90

16. 0.004
17. 0.0375
18. 0.07
19. 0.0555
20. 0.65

What percent of, pp. 90-91

21. $22\frac{2}{9}\%$, 22.2222%
22. 50%
23. $2\frac{2}{5}\%$, 2.4%
24. 80%
25. $7\frac{1}{2}\%$, 7.5%
26. 10%
27. $41\frac{7}{23}\%$, 41.3043%
28. $12\frac{1}{2}\%$, 12.5%
29. $40\frac{20}{87}\%$, 40.2298%
30. $126\frac{62}{63}\%$, 126.9841%

What is, p. 91

31. 227.5
32. 0.29
33. 42.3
34. 9.68
35. 14.4
36. 19.575
37. 10.9215
38. 0.56
39. 0.156
40. 97.232

Chapter 4 Ratios—Pretest, p. 93

1. $\frac{1}{3}$, 0.3333, 33.33%
2. 143 : 200, $\frac{143}{200}$, 71.5%
3. 2 : 5, 0.4, 40%
4. 1 : 8, $\frac{1}{8}$, 0.125
5. $\frac{1}{20}$, 0.05, 5%
6. 5 : 32, 0.15625, 15.625%
7. 143 : 500, $\frac{143}{500}$, 28.6%
8. 5 : 7, $\frac{5}{7}$, 0.714
9. 13 : 80, $\frac{13}{80}$, 0.1625
10. 231 : 500, $\frac{231}{500}$, 46.2%

Chapter 4 Ratios—Work Sheet, pp. 99-107

Fractions to ratios, pp. 99-100

1. 3 : 4
2. 1 : 3
3. 3 : 4
4. 2 : 3
5. 3 : 10
6. 1 : 2
7. 2 : 3
8. 14 : 25
9. 1 : 4
10. 2 : 5
11. 31 : 100
12. 1 : 2
13. 5 : 8
14. 3 : 2
15. 10 : 7
16. 67 : 14
17. 67 : 14
18. 16 : 27
19. 10 : 1
20. 7 : 30
21. 3 : 67
22. 155 : 228
23. 1 : 1
24. 25 : 112

Decimals to ratios, pp. 100-101

1. 112 : 125
2. 24 : 25
3. 3369 : 5000
4. 3 : 50
5. 189 : 250
6. 3 : 5
7. 252 : 625
8. 821 : 1000
9. 37 : 50
10. 83 : 500
11. 547 : 1250
12. 13 : 50
13. 123 : 250
14. 33 : 100
15. 41 : 50
16. 19 : 20
17. 1 : 5
18. 47 : 200
19. 67 : 100
20. 1071 : 2000
21. 423 : 500
22. 43 : 250
23. 9 : 10
24. 297 : 625

Percents to ratios, pp. 101-103

1. 1 : 10
2. 1 : 40
3. 1 : 3
4. 3 : 800
5. 1 : 4
6. 27 : 1000
7. 11 : 25
8. 157 : 1000
9. 6 : 125
10. 2781 : 5000
11. 31 : 400
12. 7 : 20
13. 1 : 40
14. 11 : 2500
15. 1 : 2000
16. 39 : 500
17. 1 : 100
18. 27 : 400
19. 77 : 800
20. 7 : 5000
21. 3 : 500
22. 109 : 900
23. 6 : 175
24. 41 : 500

Ratios to fractions, pp. 103-104

1. ½	**7.** ³/₁₀₀	**13.** 3⅕	**19.** 1⁶/₁₁
2. ¾	**8.** 1½	**14.** ½	**20.** ³⁷/₆₇
3. ¹/₁₆	**9.** ⅓	**15.** ⅕	**21.** 3¹¹/₆₃
4. ⅘	**10.** 1³/₇	**16.** ⁸/₄₅	**22.** ⁷/₄₂₉
5. ¹/₂₀₀	**11.** 1	**17.** ²⁶/₅₁	**23.** ⁸²/₁₂₇
6. ¹/₅₀	**12.** ⅓	**18.** ⅓	**24.** ¹²¹/₈₂₁

Ratios to decimal numbers, pp. 104-105

1. 0.5	**7.** 0.5	**13.** 0.5098	**19.** 0.3888
2. 0.25	**8.** 1.5	**14.** 0.9	**20.** 6240
3. 0.375	**9.** 0.0666	**15.** 0.2666	**21.** 2.9166
4. 0.625	**10.** 0.1	**16.** 0.5235	**22.** 12
5. 0.3333	**11.** 0.4	**17.** 0.027	**23.** 0.7777
6. 6.25	**12.** 0.4525	**18.** 0.4772	**24.** 3.5

Ratios to percents, pp. 105-107

1. 50%	**9.** ¹/₁₀%, 0.1%	**17.** 95%
2. 3¹/₃₃%, 3.0303%	**10.** 25%	**18.** 24⁸/₃₃%, 24.2424%
3. 10%	**11.** 56²/₃%, 56.6666%	**19.** 55⁵/₉%, 55.5555%
4. 20%	**12.** 206¼%, 206.25%	**20.** 31¹¹/₁₉%, 31.5789%
5. 128⁴/₇%, 128.5714%	**13.** 52¹/₁₂%, 52.0833%	**21.** 20%
6. 71³/₇%, 71.4285%	**14.** 225%	**22.** 2133⅓%, 2133.3333%
7. 37¹/₂₇%, 37.037%	**15.** ⅕%, 0.2%	**23.** 226²/₂₃%, 226.0869%
8. 175%	**16.** 66²/₃%, 66.6666%	**24.** 56¹²/₂₃%, 56.5217%

Chapter 4 Ratios—Posttest 1, p. 109

1. ⅞, 0.875, 87.5%	**5.** 7 : 20, ⁷/₂₀, 35%	**9.** 41 : 200, ⁴¹/₂₀₀, 20.5%
2. 1 : 250, ¹/₂₅₀, 0.4%	**6.** 6 : 25, 0.24, 24%	**10.** 4 : 11, 0.3636, 36.36%
3. 13 : 20, 0.65, 65%	**7.** ²⁷/₄₀, 0.675, 67.5%	
4. 9 : 400, ⁹/₄₀₀, 0.0225	**8.** 3 : 1000, ³/₁₀₀₀, 0.003	

Chapter 4 Ratios—Posttest 2, p. 111

1. ⁷/₁₀, 0.7, 70%	**5.** 3 : 800, ³/₈₀₀, 0.00375	**9.** 161 : 500, ¹⁶¹/₅₀₀, 32.2%
2. 5 : 16, 0.3125, 31.25%	**6.** 1 : 150, 0.0066, 0.66%	**10.** 91 : 500, ⁹¹/₅₀₀, 0.182
3. 3 : 40, ³/₄₀, 7.5%	**7.** 7 : 1000, ⁷/₁₀₀₀, 0.7%	
4. 3 : 50, ³/₅₀, 0.06	**8.** ²/₇, 0.2857, 28.57%	

Chapter 5 Proportions—Pretest, pp. 113-114

1. 100	**6.** 4	**11.** 80	**16.** 80
2. 7½ or 7.5	**7.** 400 or 399.9	**12.** ⅙	**17.** 10
3. ¹/₆₀₀	**8.** ½	**13.** 14	**18.** 126
4. 3.2	**9.** ³/₇	**14.** 48	**19.** ¹/₁₅₀
5. 128	**10.** 8	**15.** ³/₁₀	**20.** 16¼ or 16.25

Chapter 5 Proportions—Work Sheet, pp. 119-124

1. 84
2. 600
3. 28.125
4. 1⅕
5. 52½
6. 27
7. 7200
8. 1½ or 1.5
9. ¾
10. 1
11. 4⅘
12. 252
13. 240
14. 1½
15. 2000
16. 1
17. 80
18. 1

19. 2400
20. 5
21. 600
22. 40
23. 0.032
24. 128
25. 0.2
26. 8
27. ½ or 0.5
28. 960
29. 25
30. 20
31. ½ or 0.5
32. 1.2
33. 1.17
34. 3
35. 15
36. 30

37. 48
38. 15
39. 0.9
40. 4
41. 18
42. 16
43. 1350
44. 6
45. 36
46. 1⅓
47. 8
48. 3.6
49. 450
50. 18
51. $^{657}/_{1100}$ or 0.597
52. ⅗ or 0.6
53. 2$^7/_{10}$
54. 2000

55. 171.43
56. 500
57. 10
58. 12½ or 12.5
59. 240
60. 18¾
61. 6
62. 500
63. 62.4375
64. 180
65. 12½
66. 80
67. $^1/_{32}$, 0.03125
68. 100
69. 1620
70. 20

Chapter 5 Proportions—Posttest 1, pp. 125-126

1. 2
2. $^{35}/_{48}$
3. 6
4. 6.25
5. 32

6. ½
7. 2½ or 2.5
8. 2
9. $^5/_9$
10. 36

11. 4
12. 4
13. 8
14. 1500
15. 42

16. $^4/_9$
17. 4
18. 100
19. 1
20. 3.2

Chapter 5 Proportions—Posttest 2, pp. 127-128

1. 225
2. 1$^7/_{25}$, 1.28
3. 120
4. 6.84
5. 13⅓

6. 56
7. 1
8. 3.8
9. $^3/_{20}$
10. 40

11. 3.6
12. 105
13. 2$^7/_{10}$
14. $^{35}/_{72}$
15. 10

16. 360
17. 15
18. 72
19. 1$^2/_{25}$ or 1.08
20. 150

Mathematics Posttest, pp. 129-133

1. mixed
   whole
   $^7/_6$
   $^6/_3$
   $^9/_9$
2. fraction
   ½/4
   $^3/_7$/$^4/_2$
   21/$^2/_3$

3. relationship
   two
   4 : 12
   24 : 100
   3 : 100
   13 : 8
   22 : 1000 or 2.2 : 100
     (same value)
   124 : 100

4. denominator
   2 / ③
   4 ÷ ⑧
   10 : ⑤
   ④)̅1̅2̅
   14 / ⑧
   6 ÷ ㉔
   ㊷)̅7̅
   7 : ⑩

5. numerator
10
10
$436/1000$
$51/1000$
$1^{42}/10{,}000$
$9684/10{,}000$
$19/10{,}000$
$1^{2064}/100{,}000$
6. $1^{28}/45$
7. $7^{1}/12$
8. $5^{5}/6$
9. $5^{1}/2$
10. 8.52
11. 46.29
12. 234.93
13. 459.56
14. $1/6$
15. $1^{13}/21$
16. $41/45$
17. $5^{11}/18$
18. 23.9
19. 0.1
20. 4.1
21. 1.0
22. $5^{5}/8$
23. $2/3$
24. $8^{26}/27$

25. $26^{3}/5$
26. 1.93
27. 1.97
28. 4.48
29. 181.79
30. $1^{31}/32$
31. $18/35$
32. $1/225$
33. $473/576$
34. 5.654
35. 0.001
36. 80,000
37. 17.349
38. 0.014, 0.048, 0.407, 0.45, 1.46, 2.401
39. 0.015, 0.15, 0.155, 1.0015, 1.015, 1.15
40. 0.090, 0.90, 0.99, 9.009, 9.09, 90.90
41. 0.24, 0.4, 0.44, 0.52, 0.6, 0.7
42. 0.021, 0.1091, 0.191, 0.2, 0.201, 0.21
43. 0.83
44. 0.56
45. 0.56
46. 0.01
47. $9/40$

48. $93/200$
49. $3/50$
50. $93/250$
51. 27.5%
52. 37.5%
53. $21/50$
54. 62 : 10,000
55. 12.5%
56. 25%
57. 15%
58. 0.24
59. 54.6
60. 149.5
61. 2 : 9
62. 3 : 8
63. 73 : 125
64. 2 : 3
65. 12 : 25
66. 270
67. 1.68
68. 13.04
69. 1.13
70. 150
71. 484
72. 198.33
73. $533^{1}/3$ or 533.33
74. 27
75. 3.75

PART II

Chapter 6 Metric and Household Measurements—Pretest, pp. 137-139

1. 0.8 g
2. 3000 mcg
3. 0.255 g
4. 45 ml
5. 3 mg
6. 680 mg
7. 0.326 L
8. 72.6 lb
9. 2100 L
10. 3 kg

11. 100 ml
12. 12.5 ml
13. 5 cc
14. 800 g
15. 0.25 kl
16. 300 ml
17. 10,000 g
18. 630 ml
19. 0.733 kg
20. 1,250,000 mcg

21. 4 ml
22. 250 mcg
23. 600 L
24. 20.45 kg
25. 0.01 g
26. 1200 g
27. 300 ml
28. 710 mg
29. 0.48 L
30. $1^{43}/100$ lb

Chapter 6 Metric and Household Measurements—Work Sheet, pp. 145-148

1. 0.00023 g
2. 5000 mcg
3. 2,500,000 mcg
4. 4 mg
5. 330 mg
6. 6000 g
7. 0.725 L

8. 0.002 g
9. 30 mm
10. 0.62 kg
11. 36 ml
12. 0.46 L
13. 660 mcg
14. 500,000 mcg

15. 0.474 kl
16. 0.35 g
17. 0.025 g
18. 1460 ml
19. 2500 g
20. 12,000 mcg
21. 3400 g

22. 0.00092 g	**32.** 10 ml	**42.** 15 ml
23. 2.5 cm	**33.** 2 ml	**43.** 17³/₅ lb
24. 0.3 mg	**34.** 7.62 cm	**44.** 8.415 lb
25. 160 ml	**35.** 405 ml	**45.** 17.78 cm
26. 10 mg	**36.** 21 ml	**46.** 1.36 kg
27. 0.5 mg	**37.** 320 ml	**47.** 26²/₅ lb
28. 0.36 g	**38.** 60 ml	**48.** 3²/₂₅ lb
29. 3250 L	**39.** 160 ml	**49.** 10909.09 g
30. 450 mg	**40.** 5 ml	**50.** 68.18 kg
31. 0.24 L	**41.** 270 ml	

Chapter 6 Metric and Household Measurements—Posttest 1, pp. 149-150

1. 0.005 g	**11.** 12727.27 g	**21.** 4000 mcg
2. 10,000 mcg	**12.** 10 cm	**22.** 5¹⁸/₂₅ lb
3. 810 ml	**13.** 0.5 g	**23.** 360 ml
4. 0.035 g	**14.** 0.037 L	**24.** 200 ml
5. 8.75 ml	**15.** 20 cc	**25.** 0.533 kl
6. 120,000 mcg	**16.** 216 ml	**26.** 1,500,000 mcg
7. 35¹/₅ lb	**17.** 2500 mg	**27.** 0.62 g
8. 0.28 L	**18.** 12 ml	**28.** 2300 g
9. 400 g	**19.** 6.7 kg	**29.** 90 ml
10. 3 ml	**20.** 300 L	**30.** 3.18 kg

Chapter 6 Metric and Household Measurements—Posttest 2, pp. 151-152

1. 4 mg	**11.** 100 L	**21.** 16.25 ml
2. 0.15 kg	**12.** 32,000 mcg	**22.** 1400 L
3. 450 ml	**13.** 0.618 L	**23.** 780 mg
4. 1¹⁹/₂₅ lb	**14.** 0.1 g	**24.** 0.225 mg
5. 96⁴/₅ lb	**15.** 6 ml	**25.** 4.5 kg
6. 0.76 g	**16.** 0.714 L	**26.** 200 ml
7. 550 ml	**17.** 0.35 kl	**27.** 30 ml
8. 3.5 cm	**18.** 0.25 g	**28.** 40 ml
9. 80 ml	**19.** 870 mg	**29.** 2,600,000 mcg
10. 965.909 g	**20.** 7000 mcg	**30.** 33.18 kg

Chapter 7 Apothecaries' and Household Measurements—Pretest, pp. 153-154

1. 6 ℥, ¾ ʒ	**6.** 1¾ gal, 224 fl. ʒ, 14 pt
2. 9 ʒ, 4320 gr	**7.** 24 fl. ʒ
3. 1⁹/₁₆ fl. ʒ, 750 ℳ	**8.** 6 fl. ℥
4. 20 fl. ʒ, 1¼ pt, ⅝ qt, ⁵/₃₂ gal	**9.** 1¾ fl. ℥
5. 80 fl. ℥, 640 fl. ʒ, 2½ qt	**10.** 15 fl. ℥

Chapter 7 Apothecaries' and Household Measurements—Work Sheet, pp. 161-162

Arabic to Roman numerals, p. 161

1. xxii	**3.** iii	**5.** xiv	**7.** xv
2. ix	**4.** xxx	**6.** vi	**8.** xii

Roman to Arabic numerals, p. 161

1. 29
2. 7
3. 20
4. 6
5. 16
6. 4
7. 25
8. 240

Equivalents within the apothecaries' system, pp. 161-162

1. ½ ʒ
2. 3 ʒ, 3/8 ℥
3. 12 gr
4. 2 ℥, 960 gr
5. 1½ fl. ʒ, 3/16 fl. ℥
6. 2½ fl. ℥, 5/32 pt, 1200 ♏
7. 15 fl. ℥, 15/16 pt, 15/32 qt
8. 512 fl. ʒ, 64 fl. ℥, 2 qt
9. 40 fl. ℥, 320 fl. ʒ, 19,200 ♏
10. 4 qt, 1 gal
11. 3840 ♏, 64 fl. ʒ, 8 fl. ℥
12. ¾ gal, 768 fl. ʒ, 6 pt
13. 20 pt, 320 fl. ℥, 2½ gal
14. 6 qt, 12 pt, 192 fl. ℥

Household measures to equivalents in the apothecaries' system, p. 162

15. 12 fl. ʒ, 1½ fl. ℥
16. 16 fl. ℥
17. 24 fl. ʒ, 3 fl. ℥
18. 26 fl. ℥, 208 fl. ʒ

Chapter 7 Apothecaries' and Household Measurements—Posttest 1, pp. 163-164

1. 4 ʒ, ½ ℥
2. 1920 gr, 32 ʒ
3. 5 fl. ℥, 2400 ♏, 5/16 pt
4. 80 fl. ʒ, 5/8 pt
5. 1¼ gal, 10 pt, 160 fl. ℥, 1280 fl. ʒ
6. 7 qt, 14 pt, 224 fl. ℥
7. 12 fl. ℥
8. 4½ fl. ℥
9. 12 fl. ʒ
10. 2½ fl. ʒ

Chapter 7 Apothecaries' and Household Measurements—Posttest 2, p. 165

1. 5 ʒ, 5/8 ℥
2. 60 ℥, 28,800 gr
3. 26¼ fl. ℥, 1 41/64 pt, 105/128 qt
4. 576 fl. ʒ, 4½ pt, 2¼ qt
5. 1½ gal, 192 fl. ℥
6. 10 qt, 20 pt, 320 fl. ℥
7. 20 fl. ʒ
8. 13½ fl. ℥, 4/5 pt
9. 4 fl. ℥
10. 1⅓ Tbsp

Chapter 8 Equivalents—Pretest, pp. 167-168

1. 12 ml
2. 28 ml
3. 79 1/5 lb
4. 5250 ml
5. 3 fl. ℥
6. 1.75 L
7. 6 g
8. 67½ ♏
9. 3909.0909 g
10. 1125 ml
11. 210 ml
12. 0.6666 g
13. 5½ qt
14. 0.3333 ml
15. 240 mg
16. 12 fl. ℥
17. 1 1/5 pt
18. 12 1/10 lb
19. 5 fl. ʒ
20. 1/5 gr
21. 0.2 mg
22. 38.6363 kg
23. 1/150 gr
24. 36 ♏
25. 4 1/5 qt
26. 45 ml
27. 12 mg
28. 69 gr
29. 37.1° C
30. 105.8° F
31. 36.4° C
32. 101.3° F
33. 37.7° C
34. 103.3° F
35. 39.2° C
36. 104.4° F

Chapter 8 Equivalents—Work Sheet, pp. 175-178

1. 3⅓ gr
2. 16 ml
3. 96 ml
4. 4 g
5. 75 fl. ℥
6. 10 g
7. 1750 ml
8. 7 fl. ℥
9. 2.6666 ml
10. 22 lb
11. 3½ pt
12. 15 ml
13. 270 mg
14. 9⁶/₂₅ lb
15. 7 gr
16. 75 ℥
17. 3000 ml
18. 3½ qt
19. 300 mg
20. 5 fl. ℥
21. 2 ml
22. 24 ml
23. 49½ gr
24. 3090.909 g
25. 180 ℥
26. 11.25 ml
27. 165 mg
28. 105 gr
29. 2.2727 kg
30. 5²/₅ pt
31. 72 ml
32. 5²/₃ gr
33. 2.5 L
34. 8³/₁₀₀ lb
35. 6 qt
36. 32 ml
37. 120 ℥
38. 3 g
39. 3 ml
40. 120 ml
41. 5454.5454 g
42. 18¾ fl. ℥
43. 45 ℥
44. 34.0909 kg
45. 2125 ml
46. 1²/₃ gr
47. 3½ qt
48. 90 mg
49. 1500 ml
50. 55 lb
51. 37.6° C
52. 38.8° C
53. 40.1° C
54. 36.3° C
55. 104.7° F
56. 95.7° F
57. 98.2° F
58. 102.6° F
59. 91.4° F
60. 36.9° C
61. 106.2° F
62. 39.8° C
63. 105.1° F
64. 39° C
65. 99.3° F
66. 38° C

Chapter 8 Equivalents—Posttest 1, pp. 179-180

1. 180 mg
2. 0.8 ml
3. 20 ml
4. 5 g
5. 90 ml
6. 750 ml
7. ¼ gr
8. 1½ qt
9. 3409.0909 g
10. 17.3333 ml
11. 1⁷/₁₀ qt
12. 0.3333 g
13. 2 fl. ℥
14. 9.0909 kg
15. 10 mg
16. 2 pt
17. 30 ℥
18. ¹/₂₀₀ gr
19. 45 gr
20. 2 fl. ℥
21. 5⁴⁷/₅₀ lb
22. 150 ml
23. 70²/₅ lb
24. ¹/₁₂ gr
25. 22½ ℥
26. 5.33 g
27. 2.75 L
28. 18 fl. ℥
29. 35.2° C
30. 96.1° F
31. 39.6° C
32. 105.4° F
33. 40.1° C
34. 99° F
35. 37.4° C
36. 92.8° F

Chapter 8 Equivalents—Posttest 2, pp. 181-182

1. 64½ ℥
2. 27.2727 kg
3. 2½ qt
4. 0.2666 g
5. 625 ml
6. 15 mg
7. 1¼ qt
8. ⅓ gr
9. 1.5 ml
10. 9090.909 g
11. 375 ml
12. 2375 ml
13. 45 gr
14. 0.5 mg
15. 40 ml
16. 0.4666 g
17. 3.5 L
18. 3 pt
19. 2¹⁶/₂₅ lb
20. 0.6666 ml
21. ¹/₇₅ gr
22. 92²/₅ lb
23. 48 ml
24. 3 mg
25. 21 ℥
26. 19½ gr
27. 1590.909 g
28. 2½ fl. ℥
29. 35.7° C
30. 100.8° F
31. 98.2° F
32. 36.6° C
33. 104.7° F
34. 38.2° C
35. 106.5° F
36. 39.6° C

PART III

Chapter 9 Interpretation of the Physician's Orders—Posttest, p. 191

7 1/12	Cefuroxime																									
	÷ g dose	IV route	q 8 hours interval	08		16		24																		
8 1/12	Lasix																									
	40 mg dose	p.o. route	b.i.d. interval		09		21																			
9 1/12	Slow-K																									
	10 mEq dose	p.o. route	b.i.d. interval		09		21																			

Chapter 10 Reading Medication Labels—Posttest 1, pp. 197-198

1. Lioresal
   baclofen
   10 mg
   tablets
   100 tablets
2. Diabinese
   chlorpropamide
   250 mg
   tablets
   250 tablets

3. Robinul
   glycopyrrolate
   0.4 mg/2 ml or 0.2 mg/ml
   milliliters
   I.M. or I.V.
4. Cefobid
   cefoperazone sodium
   10 g
   milliliters
   intravenous

Chapter 10 Reading Medication Labels—Posttest 2, pp. 199-200

1. Furadantin
   nitrofurantoin
   5 mg/ml
   suspension
   oral
   60 ml
2. Decadron
   dexamethasone
   1.5 mg
   tablets

3. Capoten
   captopril
   25 mg
   tablet
   100 tablets
4. Kefzol
   cefazolin sodium
   225 mg/ml
   milliliters after reconstitution
   injection

Chapter 11 Oral Dosages—Work Sheet, pp. 213-240

Proportion

1. 1 mg : 1 capsule : : 2 mg : x capsule
   1 : 1 : : 2 : x
   x = 2 capsules

Formula

$$\frac{2 \text{ mg}}{1 \text{ mg}} \times 1 \text{ capsule} = 2 \text{ capsules}$$

Proportion

2. 20 mg:5 ml::30 mg:x ml
20:5::30:x
20x = 150
$\quad x$ = 7.5 ml

3. 0.05 mg:1 tab::0.2 mg:x tab
0.05:1::0.2:x
0.05x = 0.2
$\quad\quad x = \dfrac{0.2}{0.05}$
$\quad\quad x$ = 4 tablets

0.05 mg:1 tab::0.15 mg:x tab
0.05:1::0.15:x
0.05x = 0.15
$\quad\quad x = \dfrac{0.15}{0.05}$
$\quad\quad x$ = 3 tablets

4. $\dfrac{1}{6}$ gr = _____ mg

60 mg:1 gr::x mg:⅙ gr
60:1::x:⅙
$x = \dfrac{60}{6}$
x = 10 mg

10 mg:x tablets::10 mg:1 tablet
10:x::10:1
10x = 10
$\quad x$ = 1 tablet

5. 5 mg:5 ml::2.5 mg:x ml
5:5::2.5:x
5x = 12.5
$\quad\quad x = \dfrac{12.5}{5}$
$\quad\quad x$ = 2.5 ml

Formula

$\dfrac{30 \text{ mg}}{20 \text{ mg}} \times 5 \text{ ml} =$

$\dfrac{30}{\overset{4}{\cancel{20}}} \times \dfrac{\overset{1}{\cancel{5}}}{1} = \dfrac{30}{4}$

$\qquad \dfrac{30}{4} = 7.5 \text{ ml}$

$\dfrac{0.2 \text{ mg}}{0.05 \text{ mg}} \times 1 \text{ tab} =$

$\dfrac{0.2}{0.05} = 4 \text{ tablets}$

$\dfrac{0.15 \text{ mg}}{0.05 \text{ mg}} \times \dfrac{1}{1} =$

$\quad \dfrac{0.15}{0.05} = 3 \text{ tablets}$

$\dfrac{10 \text{ mg}}{10 \text{ mg}} \times 1 \text{ tablet} =$

$\quad \dfrac{10}{10} \times 1 = 1 \text{ tablet}$

$\dfrac{2.5 \text{ mg}}{5 \text{ mg}} \times 5 \text{ ml} =$

$\dfrac{2.5}{\underset{1}{\cancel{5}}} \times \dfrac{\overset{1}{\cancel{5}}}{1} = \dfrac{2.5}{1} = 2.5 \text{ ml}$

Proportion   **Formula**

6. 2.5 mg:5 ml::2.5 mg:x ml
2.5:5::2.5:x
2.5x = 12.5
$x = \dfrac{12.5}{2.5}$
x = 5 ml

30 ml:1 ℥::x ml:4 ℥
30:1::x:4
x = 120
x = 120 ml

5 ml:1 dose::120 ml:x doses
5:1::120:x
5x = 120
x = 24 doses

7. 60 mg:1 gr::x mg:$^1/_{12}$ gr
60:1::x:$^1/_{12}$

$x = \dfrac{\overset{5}{\cancel{60}}}{1} \times \dfrac{1}{\underset{1}{\cancel{12}}}$

x = 5 mg
$^1/_{12}$ gr = 5 mg capsules

5 mg:1 capsule::10 mg:x capsule
5:1::10:x
5x = 10
$x = \dfrac{10}{5}$
x = 2 capsules

$\dfrac{10 \text{ mg}}{5 \text{ mg}} \times 1$ capsule =

$\dfrac{10}{5} \times \dfrac{1}{1}$ = 2 capsules

8. 0.5 g:1 tablet::1 g:x tablet
0.5:1::1:x
0.5x = 1
x = 2 tablets

$\dfrac{1 \text{ g}}{0.5 \text{ g}} \times 1$ tablet =

$\dfrac{1}{0.5}$ = 2 tablets

9. 500 mg:5 ml::500 mg:x ml
500:5::500:x
500x = 2500
x = 5 ml

$\dfrac{500 \text{ mg}}{500 \text{ mg}} \times 5$ ml =

$\dfrac{\overset{1}{500}}{\underset{100}{\cancel{500}}} \times \dfrac{\cancel{5}}{1}$ = 5 ml

10. 0.5 mg:1 tab::1 mg: x tab
0.5:1::1:x
0.5x = 1
x = 2 tablets

$\dfrac{1 \text{ mg}}{0.5 \text{ mg}} \times \dfrac{1}{1}$ tab =

$\dfrac{1}{0.5}$ = 2 tablets

Proportion   Formula

11. 60 mg:1 gr::x mg:5 gr
60:1::x:5
$x = 300$ mg

300 mg:1 tablet::300:x tablet $\dfrac{300 \text{ mg}}{300 \text{ mg}} \times 1$ tablet =
300:1::300:x
$300x = 300$ $\dfrac{300}{300} = 1$ tablet
$\quad x = \dfrac{300}{300}$
$\quad x = 1$ tablet

12. 1000 mg:1 gr:x mg:0.6 g
1000:1::x:0.6
$x = 600$

300 mg:1 tablet::600 mg: x tablet $\dfrac{600 \text{ mg}}{300 \text{ mg}} \times 1$ tablet =
300:1::600:x
$300x = 600$ $\dfrac{600}{300} \times 1 = 2$ tablets
$\quad x = \dfrac{600}{300}$
$\quad x = 2$ tablets

600 mg:1 dose::x mg:2 dose
600:1::x:2
$x = 1200$ mg

13. 1000 mg:1 g::x mg:0.25 g
1000:1::x:0.25
$x = 250$ mg

500 mg:1 tablet::250 mg:x tablet $\dfrac{250 \text{ mg}}{500 \text{ mg}} \times 1 = \frac{1}{2}$ tablet
500:1::250:x
$500x = 250$
$\quad x = \dfrac{250}{500}$
$\quad x = \frac{1}{2}$ tablet

14. 50 mg:1 tablet::25 mg:x tablet $\dfrac{25 \text{ mg}}{50 \text{ mg}} \times 1$ tablet =
50:1::25:x
$50x = 25$ $\dfrac{25}{50} = \frac{1}{2}$ tablet
$\quad x = \dfrac{25}{50}$
$\quad x = \frac{1}{2}$ tablet

15. 60 mg:1 gr::x mg:5 gr
60:1::x:5
$x = 300$ mg

300 mg:1 tablet::300 mg:x tablet $\dfrac{300 \text{ mg}}{300 \text{ mg}} \times 1$ tablet =
300:1::300:x
$300x = 300$ $\dfrac{300}{300} = 1$ tablet
$\quad x = \dfrac{300}{300}$
$\quad x = 1$ tablet

Proportion

Formula

16. 0.5 g:1 tab::4 g:x tab
0.5:1::4:x
0.5x = 4
$$x = \frac{4}{0.5}$$
x = 8 tablets

$$\frac{4 \text{ g}}{0.5 \text{ g}} \times 1 \text{ tablet} =$$
$$\frac{4}{0.5} = 8 \text{ tablets}$$

0.5 g:1 tab::2 g:x tab
0.5:1::2:x
0.5x = 2
$$x = \frac{2}{0.5}$$
x = 4 tablets

$$\frac{2 \text{ g}}{0.5 \text{ g}} \times 1 \text{ tablet} =$$
$$\frac{2}{0.5} = 4 \text{ tablets}$$

17. 500 mg:10 ml::90 mg:x ml
500:10::90:x
500x = 900
$$x = \frac{900}{500}$$
x = 1.8 ml

$$\frac{90 \text{ mg}}{500 \text{ mg}} \times 10 \text{ ml} =$$
$$\frac{90}{500} \times \frac{\overset{1}{\cancel{10}}}{1} =$$
$$\underset{50}{}$$
$$\frac{90}{50} = 1.8 \text{ ml}$$

18. 30 ml = 1 ℥ each dose
4 ℥ given each day

19. 12.5 mg:5 ml::30 mg:x ml
12.5:5::30:x
12.5x = 150
$$x = \frac{150}{12.5}$$
x = 12 ml

$$\frac{30 \text{ mg}}{12.5 \text{ mg}} \times \frac{5 \text{ ml}}{1} =$$
$$\frac{30}{12.5} \times \frac{5}{1} =$$
$$\frac{150}{12.5} = 12 \text{ ml}$$

20. 60 mg:1 gr::x mg:¼ gr
$$x = \frac{\overset{15}{\cancel{60}}}{1} \times \frac{1}{\underset{1}{\cancel{4}}}$$
x = 15 mg
15 mg = ¼ gr = 1 tablet

15 mg:1 tab::60 mg:x tab
15:1::60:x
15x = 60
$$x = \frac{60}{15}$$
x = 4 tablets

$$\frac{60 \text{ mg}}{15 \text{ mg}} \times 1 \text{ tablet} =$$
$$\frac{60}{15} = 4 \text{ tablets}$$

Proportion	Formula

21. 125 mg:5 ml::x mg:5.5 ml

125:5::x:5.5

$5x = 125 \times 5.5$

$5x = 687.5$

$x = \dfrac{687.5}{5}$

$x = 137.5$ mg

$\dfrac{x \text{ mg}}{125 \text{ mg}} \times 5 \text{ ml} = 5.5 \text{ ml}$

$\dfrac{x}{\underset{25}{\cancel{125}}} \times \dfrac{\overset{1}{\cancel{5}}}{1} = 5.5$

$\dfrac{x}{25} = 5.5$

$\dfrac{\overset{1}{\cancel{25}}}{1} \times \dfrac{x}{\underset{1}{\cancel{25}}} = 5.5 \times 25$

$x = 137.5$ mg

22. 40 mg:1 tablet::80 mg:x tablet

40:1::80:x

$40x = 80$

$x = \dfrac{80}{40}$

$x = 2$ tablets

$\dfrac{80 \text{ mg}}{40 \text{ mg}} \times \dfrac{1 \text{ tab}}{1} =$

$\dfrac{80}{40} = 2$ tablets

23. 1000 mg:1 g::x mg:0.5 g

1000:1::x:0.5

$x = 500$ mg or 0.5 g

250 mg:1 cap::500 mg:x cap

250:1::500:x

$250x = 500$

$x = \dfrac{500}{250}$

$x = 2$ capsules

2 cap:1 dose::x cap:4 doses

2:1::x:4

$x = 8$ capsules

$\dfrac{500 \text{ mg}}{250 \text{ mg}} \times \dfrac{1}{1}$ tablet $=$

$\dfrac{500}{250} = 2$ capsules

24. 0.5 mg:5 ml::1.5 mg:x ml

0.5:5::1.5:x

$0.5x = 7.5$

$x = \dfrac{7.5}{0.5}$

$x = 15$ ml

30 ml:1 ℥::15 ml:x ℥

30:1::15:x

$30x = 15$

$x = \dfrac{15}{30}$

$x = ½$ ℥

$\dfrac{1.5 \text{ mg}}{0.5 \text{ mg}} \times \dfrac{5 \text{ ml}}{1} =$

$\dfrac{1.5}{0.5} \times \dfrac{5}{1} = \dfrac{7.5}{0.5}$

$\dfrac{7.5}{0.5} = 15$ ml

Proportion

25. $10 \text{ mg} : 5 \text{ ml} :: 15 \text{ mg} : x \text{ ml}$
$10 : 5 :: 15 : x$
$10x = 75$
$x = \dfrac{75}{10}$
$x = 7.5 \text{ ml}$

26. $50 \text{ mg} : 1 \text{ tab} :: 25 \text{ mg} : x \text{ tab}$
$50 : 1 :: 25 : x$
$50x = 25$
$x = \dfrac{25}{50}$
$x = \frac{1}{2} \text{ tablet}$

27. $30 \text{ ml} = 1 \text{ ʒ}$
order is for 1 ʒ
supplied in 12 ʒ bottle
$1 \text{ ʒ} : 1 \text{ dose} :: 12 \text{ ʒ} : x \text{ dose}$
$1 : 1 :: 12 : x$
$x = 12 \text{ doses}$

28. $100 \text{ mg} : 1 \text{ tab} :: 200 \text{ mg} : x \text{ tab}$
$100 : 1 :: 200 : x$
$100x = 200$
$x = \dfrac{200}{100}$
$x = 2 \text{ tablets}$

29. $60 \text{ mg} : 1 \text{ gr} :: x \text{ mg} : \frac{1}{2} \text{ gr}$
$60 : 1 :: x : \frac{1}{2}$

$x = \dfrac{\overset{30}{\cancel{60}}}{1} \times \dfrac{1}{\underset{1}{\cancel{2}}}$

$x = 30 \text{ mg} = \frac{1}{2} \text{ gr}$

$30 \text{ mg} : 1 \text{ tab} :: 15 \text{ mg} : x \text{ tablet}$
$30 : 1 :: 15 : x$
$30x = 15$
$x = \dfrac{15}{30}$
$x = \frac{1}{2} \text{ tablet}$

Formula

$\dfrac{15 \text{ mg}}{10 \text{ mg}} \times 5 \text{ ml} =$

$\dfrac{15}{\overset{}{\underset{2}{\cancel{10}}}} \times \dfrac{\overset{1}{\cancel{5}}}{1} = \dfrac{15}{2}$

$\dfrac{15}{2} = 7.5 \text{ ml}$

$\dfrac{25 \text{ mg}}{50 \text{ mg}} \times \dfrac{1}{1} \text{ tablet} =$

$\dfrac{25}{50} = \frac{1}{2} \text{ tablet}$

$\dfrac{200 \text{ mg}}{100 \text{ mg}} \times \dfrac{1}{1} \text{ tab} =$

$\dfrac{200}{100} = 2 \text{ tablets}$

$\dfrac{15 \text{ mg}}{30 \text{ mg}} \times 1 \text{ tablet} =$

$\dfrac{15}{30} = \frac{1}{2} \text{ tablet}$

Proportion	Formula

30. $250 \text{ mg} : 5 \text{ ml} :: 125 \text{ mg} : x \text{ ml}$
$250 : 5 :: 125 : x$
$250x = 625$
$x = \dfrac{625}{250}$
$x = 2.5 \text{ ml}$

$$\dfrac{125 \text{ mg}}{250 \text{ mg}} \times 5 \text{ ml} =$$

$$\dfrac{125}{\overset{}{\underset{50}{250}}} \times \dfrac{\overset{1}{\cancel{5}}}{1} = \dfrac{125}{50}$$

$$\dfrac{125}{50} = 2.5 \text{ ml}$$

31. $50 \text{ mg} : 1 \text{ tab} :: 25 \text{ mg} : x \text{ tab}$
$50 : 1 :: 25 : x$
$50x = 25$
$x = \dfrac{25}{50}$
$x = \frac{1}{2} \text{ tablet}$

$$\dfrac{25 \text{ mg}}{50 \text{ mg}} \times \dfrac{1}{1} \text{ tablet} =$$

$$\dfrac{25}{50} = \frac{1}{2} \text{ tablet}$$

32. $1000 \text{ mg} : 1 \text{ g} :: x \text{ mg} : 0.6 \text{ g}$
$1000 : 1 :: x : 0.6$
$x = 0.6 \times 1000$
$x = 600 \text{ mg}$

$200 \text{ mg} : 1 \text{ tablet} :: 600 \text{ mg} : x \text{ tablet}$
$200 : 1 :: 600 : x$
$200x = 600$
$x = \dfrac{600}{200}$
$x = 3 \text{ tablets}$

$3 \text{ tablets} : 1 \text{ dose} :: x \text{ tab} : 6 \text{ doses}$
$3 : 1 :: x : 6$
$x = 18 \text{ tablets}$

$$\dfrac{600 \text{ mg}}{200 \text{ mg}} \times 1 \text{ tablet} =$$

$$\dfrac{600}{200} = 3 \text{ tablets}$$

33. $6.25 \text{ mg} : 1 \; \tilde{3} :: 12.5 \text{ mg} : x \; \tilde{3}$
$6.25 : 1 :: 12.5 : x$
$6.25x = 12.5$
$x = \dfrac{12.5}{6.25}$
$x = 2 \; \tilde{3}$

$$\dfrac{12.5 \text{ mg}}{6.25 \text{ mg}} \times 1 \; \tilde{3} =$$

$$\dfrac{12.5}{6.25} = 2 \; \tilde{3}$$

34. $60 \text{ mg} : 1 \text{ gr} :: x \text{ mg} : \frac{1}{4} \text{ gr}$
$60 : 1 :: x : \frac{1}{4}$
$x = \dfrac{60}{4}$
$x = 15 \text{ mg}$

$15 \text{ mg} : 1 \text{ cap} :: 30 \text{ mg} : x \text{ cap}$
$15 : 1 :: 30 : x$
$15x = 30$
$x = \dfrac{30}{15} = 2 \text{ capsules}$

$$\dfrac{30 \text{ mg}}{15 \text{ mg}} \times 1 \text{ cap} =$$

$$\dfrac{30}{15} = 2 \text{ capsules}$$

Proportion	Formula

35. 20 mg : 5 ml : : 100 mg : x ml

20:5::100:x

$20x = 500$

$x = \dfrac{500}{20}$

$x = 25$ ml

$$\dfrac{100 \text{ mg}}{20 \text{ mg}} \times \dfrac{5}{1} \text{ ml} =$$

$$\dfrac{100}{\cancel{20}} \times \dfrac{\cancel{5}}{1} = \qquad \overset{1}{}$$

$$\overset{4}{}$$

$$\dfrac{100}{4} = 25 \text{ ml}$$

36. 40 mEq : 15 ml : : 80 mEq : x ml

40:15::80:x

$40x = 1200$

$x = \dfrac{1200}{40}$

$x = 30$ ml

$$\dfrac{80}{\cancel{40}} \times \dfrac{\overset{3}{\cancel{15}}}{1} = \qquad \overset{8}{}$$

$$\dfrac{240}{8} = 30 \text{ ml}$$

37. 2.5 mg : 1 tab : : 7.5 mg : x tab

2.5:1::7.5:x

$2.5x = 7.5$

$x = \dfrac{7.5}{2.5}$

$x = 3$ tablets

$$\dfrac{7.5 \text{ mg}}{2.5 \text{ mg}} \times \dfrac{1 \text{ tab}}{1} =$$

$$\dfrac{7.5}{2.5} = 3 \text{ tablets}$$

38. 1000 mg : 1 g : : x mg : 0.2 g

1000:1::x:0.2

$x = 200$ mg

100 mg : 1 tab : : 200 mg : x tab

100:1::200:x

$100x = 200$

$x = \dfrac{200}{100}$

$x = 2$ tablets

$$\dfrac{200 \text{ mg}}{100 \text{ mg}} \times 1 \text{ tab} =$$

$$\dfrac{200}{100} = 2 \text{ tablets}$$

39. 60 mg : 1 gr : : x mg : 5 gr

60:1::x:5

$x = 300$ mg

160 mg : 5 ml : : 300 mg : x ml

160:5::300:x

$160x = 1500$

$x = 9.375$ ml or 9.38 ml

$$\dfrac{300 \text{ mg}}{160 \text{ mg}} \times 5 \text{ ml} =$$

$$\dfrac{300}{\underset{32}{\cancel{160}}} \times \dfrac{\overset{1}{\cancel{5}}}{1} = \dfrac{300}{32}$$

$$\dfrac{300}{32} = 9.375 \text{ ml or } 9.38 \text{ ml}$$

Proportion	Formula

40. $0.25 \text{ mg} : 1 \text{ tab} :: 0.5 \text{ mg} : x \text{ tab}$
$0.25 : 1 :: 0.5 : x$
$0.25x = 0.5$
$x = \dfrac{0.5}{0.25}$
$x = 2 \text{ tablets}$

$\dfrac{0.5 \text{ mg}}{0.25 \text{ mg}} \times 1 \text{ tab} =$
$\dfrac{0.5}{0.25} = 2 \text{ tablets}$

41. $5 \text{ mg} : 1 \text{ tab} :: 10 \text{ mg} : x \text{ tab}$
$5 : 1 :: 10 : x$
$5x = 10$
$x = \dfrac{10}{5}$
$x = 2 \text{ tablets}$

$\dfrac{10 \text{ mg}}{5 \text{ mg}} \times 1 \text{ tab} =$
$\dfrac{10}{5} = 2 \text{ tablets}$

42. $50 \text{ mg} : 1 \text{ tab} :: 100 \text{ mg} : x \text{ tab}$
$50 : 1 :: 100 : x$
$50x = 100$
$x = \dfrac{100}{50}$
$x = 2 \text{ tablets}$

$\dfrac{100 \text{ mg}}{50 \text{ mg}} \times 1 \text{ tab} =$
$\dfrac{100}{50} = 2 \text{ tablets}$

43. $\text{grss} = \frac{1}{2} \text{ gr} = 30 \text{ mg}$
$30 \text{ mg} : 1 \text{ tab} :: 30 \text{ mg} : x \text{ tab}$
$30 : 1 :: 30 : x$
$30x = 30$
$x = \dfrac{30}{30}$
$x = 1 \text{ tablet}$

$\dfrac{30 \text{ mg}}{30 \text{ mg}} \times 1 =$
$\dfrac{30}{30} = 1 \text{ tablet}$

44. $0.125 \text{ mg} : 1 \text{ tab} :: 0.25 : x \text{ tab}$
$0.125 : 1 :: 0.25 : x$
$0.125x = 0.25$
$x = \dfrac{0.25}{0.125}$
$x = 2 \text{ tablets}$

$\dfrac{0.25 \text{ mg}}{0.125 \text{ mg}} \times 1 \text{ tab} =$
$\dfrac{0.25}{0.125} = 2 \text{ tablets}$

45. $250 \text{ mg} : 1 \text{ cap} :: 500 \text{ mg} : x \text{ cap}$
$250 : 1 :: 500 : x$
$250x = 500$
$x = \dfrac{500}{250}$
$x = 2 \text{ capsules}$

$2 \text{ cap} : 1 \text{ dose} :: x \text{ cap} : 4 \text{ dose}$
$2 : 1 :: x : 4$
$x = 8 \text{ capsules}$

$\dfrac{500 \text{ mg}}{250 \text{ mg}} \times 1 \text{ cap} =$
$\dfrac{500}{250} = 2 \text{ capsules}$

Proportion	Formula

46. 10 mg : 1 tab : : 5 mg : x tab

10 : 1 : : 5 : x

$10x = 5$

$x = \dfrac{5}{10}$

$x = \frac{1}{2}$ tablet

$\dfrac{5 \text{ mg}}{10 \text{ mg}} \times 1 \text{ tab} =$

$\dfrac{5}{10} = \frac{1}{2}$ tablet

47. 60 mg : 1 gr : : x mg : 1½ gr

60 : 1 : : x : 1½

$x = \dfrac{\overset{30}{\cancel{60}}}{1} \times \dfrac{3}{\underset{1}{\cancel{2}}}$

$x = 90$ mg

30 mg : 1 tab : : 90 mg : x tab

30 : 1 : : 90 : x

$30x = 90$

$x = 3$ tablets

$\dfrac{90 \text{ mg}}{30 \text{ mg}} \times 1 \text{ tab} =$

$\dfrac{90}{30} = 3$ tablets

48. 40 mEq : 15 ml : : 2 mEq : x ml

40 : 15 : : 2 : x

$40x = 30$

$x = \dfrac{30}{40}$

$x = 0.75$ ml

$\dfrac{2 \text{ mEq}}{40 \text{ mEq}} \times 15 \text{ ml} =$

$\dfrac{2}{40} \times \dfrac{15}{1}$

$\dfrac{2}{\underset{8}{\cancel{40}}} \times \dfrac{\overset{3}{\cancel{15}}}{1} = \dfrac{6}{8}$

$\dfrac{6}{8} = 0.75$ ml

49. 65 mg : 1 gr : : x mg : 10 gr

65 : 1 : : x : 10

$x = 650$ mg

325 mg : 1 tab : : 650 mg : x tab

325 : 1 : : 650 : x

$325x = 650$

$x = \dfrac{650}{325}$

$x = 2$ tablets

$\dfrac{650 \text{ mg}}{325 \text{ mg}} \times 1 \text{ tab} =$

$\dfrac{650}{325} = 2$ tablets

50. 5 ml : 1 ℥ : : 10 ml : x ℥

5 : 1 : : 10 : x

$5x = 10$

$x = \dfrac{10}{5}$

$x = 2$ ℥

Proportion

51. $250 \text{ mg}:5 \text{ ml}::1000 \text{ mg}:x \text{ ml}$
$250:5::1000:x$
$250x = 5000$
$x = \dfrac{5000}{250}$
$x = 20 \text{ ml}$

52. $60 \text{ mg}:1 \text{ gr}::x \text{ mg}:5 \text{ gr}$
$60:1::x:5$
$x = 300 \text{ mg}$
$0.3 \text{ g} = 300 \text{ mg}$

$324 \text{ mg}:1 \text{ tablet}::300 \text{ mg}:x \text{ tablet}$
$324:1::300:x$
$324x = 300$
$x = \dfrac{300}{324} = 0.93 \text{ tablet}$
$x = 1 \text{ tablet}$

53. $10 \text{ mg}:1 \text{ capsule}::20 \text{ mg}:x \text{ capsule}$
$10:1::20:x$
$10x = 20$
$x = \dfrac{20}{10}$
$x = 2 \text{ capsules}$

54. $10 \text{ mg}:1 \text{ t}::30 \text{ mg}:x \text{ t}$
$10:1::30:x$
$10x = 30$
$x = \dfrac{30}{10}$
$x = 3 \text{ teaspoons}$

55. $1000 \text{ mg}:1 \text{ g}::x \text{ mg}:0.75 \text{ g}$
$1000:1::x:0.75$
$x = 1000 \times 0.75$
$x = 750 \text{ mg}$

$250 \text{ mg}:1 \text{ tab}::750 \text{ mg}:x \text{ tab}$
$250:1::750:x$
$250x = 750$
$x = \dfrac{750}{250}$
$x = 3 \text{ tablets}$

Formula

$\dfrac{1000 \text{ mg}}{250 \text{ mg}} \times 5 \text{ ml} =$

$\dfrac{1000}{\cancel{250}} \times \dfrac{\cancel{5}^{1}}{1}$
$_{50}$
$\dfrac{1000}{50} = 20 \text{ ml}$

$\dfrac{300 \text{ mg}}{324 \text{ mg}} \times 1 \text{ tab} =$

$\dfrac{300}{324} = 0.93 \text{ tablet; give 1 tablet}$

$\dfrac{20 \text{ mg}}{10 \text{ mg}} \times 1 \text{ capsule} =$

$\dfrac{20}{10} = 2 \text{ capsules}$

$\dfrac{30 \text{ mg}}{10 \text{ mg}} \times 1 \text{ tsp} =$

$\dfrac{30}{10} = 3 \text{ teaspoons}$

$\dfrac{750 \text{ mg}}{250 \text{ mg}} \times 1 \text{ tab} =$

$\dfrac{750}{250} = 3 \text{ tablets}$

Proportion

Formula

56. 12.5 mg : 1 tab : : 25 mg : x tab
12.5 : 1 : : 25 : x
$12.5x = 25$
$x = \dfrac{25}{12.5}$
$x = 2$ tablets

$\dfrac{25 \text{ mg}}{12.5 \text{ mg}} \times 1 \text{ tab} =$

$\dfrac{25}{12.5} = 2$ tablets

57. 25 mg : 5 ml : : 15 mg : x ml
25 : 5 : : 15 : x
$25x = 75$
$x = \dfrac{75}{25}$
$x = 3$ ml

$\dfrac{15 \text{ mg}}{25 \text{ mg}} \times 5 \text{ ml} =$

$\underset{5}{\dfrac{15}{\cancel{25}}} \times \dfrac{\overset{1}{\cancel{5}}}{1} = \dfrac{15}{5}$

$\dfrac{15}{5} = 3$ ml

58. 1000 mg : 1 g : : x mg : 1.5 g
1000 : 1 : : x : 1.5
$x = 1500$ mg

250 mg : 1 cap : : 1500 mg : x cap
250 : 1 : : 1500 : x
$250x = 1500$
$x = \dfrac{1500}{250}$
$x = 6$ capsules stat

$\dfrac{1500 \text{ mg}}{250 \text{ mg}} \times 1 \text{ cap} =$

$\dfrac{1500}{250} = 6$ capsules stat

1000 mg : 1 g : : x mg : 0.5 g
1000 : 1 : : x : 0.5
$x = 500$
0.5 g = 500 mg

250 mg : 1 cap : : 500 mg : x cap
250 : 1 : : 500 : x
$250x = 500$
$x = \dfrac{500}{250}$
$x = 2$ capsules each q.i.d. dose

$\dfrac{500 \text{ mg}}{250 \text{ mg}} \times 1 \text{ cap} =$

$\dfrac{500}{250} = 2$ capsules each q.i.d. dose

2 cap : 1 dose : : x cap : 4 doses
2 : 1 : : x : 4
$x = 8$ capsules each day

0.5 g : : 1 dose : : 7.5 g : x dose
0.5 : 1 : : 7.5 : x
$0.5x = 7.5$
$x = \dfrac{7.5}{0.5}$
$x = 15$ doses

| Proportion | Formula |

Proportion   **Formula**

59. $500 \text{ mg}:5 \text{ ml}::250 \text{ mg}:x \text{ ml}$
$500:5::250:x$
$500x = 1250$
$x = \dfrac{1250}{500}$
$x = 2.5 \text{ ml}$

$$\dfrac{250 \text{ mg}}{500 \text{ mg}} \times 5 \text{ ml} =$$
$$\dfrac{250}{\overset{}{\underset{\cancel{500}}{}}} \times \dfrac{\overset{1}{\cancel{5}}}{1} = \dfrac{250}{100}$$
$$100$$
$$\dfrac{250}{100} = 2.5 \text{ ml}$$

60. $150 \text{ mg}:5 \text{ ml}::250 \text{ mg}:x \text{ ml}$
$150:5::250:x$
$150x = 1250$
$x = \dfrac{1250}{150}$
$x = 8.33 \text{ ml}$

$$\dfrac{250 \text{ mg}}{150 \text{ mg}} \times 5 \text{ ml} =$$
$$\dfrac{250}{\underset{30}{\cancel{150}}} \times \dfrac{\overset{1}{\cancel{5}}}{1} = \dfrac{250}{30}$$
$$\dfrac{250}{30} = 8.33 \text{ ml}$$

61. $50 \text{ mg}:5 \text{ ml}::100 \text{ mg}:x \text{ ml}$
$50:5::100:x$
$50x = 500$
$x = \dfrac{500}{50}$
$x = 10 \text{ ml}$

$$\dfrac{100 \text{ mg}}{50 \text{ mg}} \times 5 \text{ ml} =$$
$$\dfrac{100}{\underset{10}{\cancel{50}}} \times \dfrac{\overset{1}{\cancel{5}}}{1} =$$
$$\dfrac{100}{10} = 10 \text{ ml}$$

62. $50 \text{ mg}:1 \text{ tab}::25 \text{ mg}:x \text{ tab}$
$50:1::25:x$
$50x = 25$
$x = \dfrac{25}{50}$
$x = \frac{1}{2} \text{ tablet}$

$$\dfrac{25 \text{ mg}}{50 \text{ mg}} \times 1 \text{ tab} =$$
$$\dfrac{25}{50} = \frac{1}{2} \text{ tablet}$$

63. $80 \text{ mg}:1 \text{ tablet}::240 \text{ mg}:x \text{ tab}$
$80:1::240:x$
$80x = 240$
$x = \dfrac{240}{80}$
$x = 3 \text{ tablets}$

$$\dfrac{240 \text{ mg}}{80 \text{ mg}} \times 1 \text{ tab} =$$
$$\dfrac{240}{80} = 3 \text{ tablets}$$

Proportion | Formula

64. 1000 mcg:1 mg::x mcg:0.05 mg
1000:1::x:0.05
x = 50 mcg

50 mcg:1 ml::90 mcg:x ml
50:1::90:x
50x = 90
$x = \dfrac{90}{50}$
x = 1.8 ml

$\dfrac{90 \text{ mcg}}{50 \text{ mcg}} \times 1 \text{ ml} =$
$\dfrac{90}{50} = 1.8 \text{ ml}$

65. 12.5 mg:5 ml::x mg:10 ml
12.5:5::x:10
5x = 125
$x = \dfrac{125}{5}$
x = 25 mg

$\dfrac{x \text{ mg}}{12.5 \text{ mg}} \times \dfrac{5}{1} = 10 \text{ ml}$
$\dfrac{x}{12.5} \times \dfrac{5}{1} = 10$
$\dfrac{12.5}{1} \times \dfrac{x}{12.5} \times \dfrac{5}{1} = \dfrac{10}{1} \times 12.5$
$5x = 125$
$x = \dfrac{125}{5}$
$x = 25 \text{ mg}$

66. 1000 mg:1 g::x mg:0.5 g
1000:1::x:0.5
x = 500 mg

500 mg:1 tab::500 mg:x tab
500:1::500:x
500x = 500
$x = \dfrac{500}{500}$
x = 1 tablet

$\dfrac{500 \text{ mg}}{500 \text{ mg}} \times 1 \text{ tab} =$
$\dfrac{500}{500} = 1 \text{ tablet}$

67. 60 mg:1 gr::x mg:1.5 gr
60:1::x:1.5
x = 60 × 1.5
x = 90 mg

30 mg:1 capsule::90 mg:x capsule
30:1::90:x
30x = 90
$x = \dfrac{90}{30}$
x = 3 capsules

$\dfrac{90 \text{ mg}}{30 \text{ mg}} \times 1 \text{ capsule} =$
$\dfrac{90}{30} = 3 \text{ capsules}$

Proportion	Formula

68. $4\ ʒ:1\ \text{tbsp}::x\ ʒ:2\ \text{tbsp}$
$4:1::x:2$
$x = 8\ ʒ$
$8\ ʒ:1\ ʒ::8\ ʒ:x\ ʒ$
$8:1::8:x$
$8x = 8$
$x = \dfrac{8}{8}$
$x = 1\ ʒ$

69. $20\ \text{mEq}:15\ \text{ml}::10\ \text{mEq}:x\ \text{ml}$
$20:15::10:x$
$20x = 150$
$x = \dfrac{150}{20}$
$x = 7.5\ \text{ml}$

$\dfrac{10\ \text{mEq}}{20\ \text{mEq}} \times \dfrac{15\ \text{ml}}{1} =$

$\dfrac{10}{\overset{2}{\cancel{20}}} \times \dfrac{\overset{3}{\cancel{15}}}{1} = \dfrac{30}{4}$

$\dfrac{30}{4} = 7.5\ \text{ml}$

70. $600\ \text{mg}:1\ \text{tablet}::300\ \text{mg}:x\ \text{tab}$
$600:1::300:x$
$600x = 300$
$x = \dfrac{300}{600}$
$x = ½\ \text{tablet}$

$\dfrac{300\ \text{mg}}{600\ \text{mg}} \times 1\ \text{tab} =$

$\dfrac{300}{600} = ½\ \text{tablet}$

71. $0.25\ \text{mg}:1\ \text{tab}::0.5\ \text{mg}:x\ \text{tab}$
$0.25:1::0.5:x$
$0.25x = 0.5$
$x = \dfrac{0.5}{0.25}$
$x = 2\ \text{tablets}$

$\dfrac{0.5\ \text{mg}}{0.25\ \text{mg}} \times 1\ \text{tab} =$

$\dfrac{0.5}{0.25} = 2\ \text{tablets}$

72. $325\ \text{mg}:10.15\ \text{ml}::650\ \text{mg}:x\ \text{ml}$
$325:10.15::650:x$
$325x = 6597.5$
$x = \dfrac{6597.5}{325}$
$x = 20.3\ \text{ml}$

$\dfrac{650\ \text{mg}}{325\ \text{mg}} \times 10.15\ \text{ml} =$

$\dfrac{650}{325} \times \dfrac{10.15}{1} = \dfrac{6597.5}{325}$

$\dfrac{6597.5}{325} = 20.3\ \text{ml}$

73. $0.25\ \text{mg}:1\ \text{tab}::0.5\ \text{mg}:x\ \text{tab}$
$0.25:1::0.5:x$
$0.25x = 0.5$
$x = \dfrac{0.5}{0.25}$
$x = 2\ \text{tablets}$

$\dfrac{0.5\ \text{mg}}{0.25\ \text{mg}} \times 1\ \text{tab} =$

$\dfrac{0.5}{0.25} = 2\ \text{tablets}$

Proportion   **Formula**

74. $30 \text{ ml}:1\ ℥::x\ \text{ml}:½\ ℥$

$30:1::x:½$

$x = \dfrac{30}{1} \times \dfrac{1}{2}$

$x = 15 \text{ ml}$

75. $50 \text{ mg}:5 \text{ ml}::30 \text{ mg}:x \text{ ml}$

$50:5::30:x$

$50x = 150$

$x = \dfrac{150}{50}$

$x = 3 \text{ ml}$

$\dfrac{30 \text{ mg}}{50 \text{ mg}} \times 5 \text{ ml} =$

$$\dfrac{30}{\underset{10}{\cancel{50}}} \times \dfrac{\overset{1}{\cancel{5}}}{1} = \dfrac{30}{10}$$

$\dfrac{30}{10} = 3 \text{ ml}$

76. $60 \text{ mg}:1 \text{ gr}::x \text{ mg}:\dfrac{1}{200} \text{ gr}$

$60:1::x:\dfrac{1}{200}$

$x = \dfrac{60}{1} \times \dfrac{1}{200}$

$x = \dfrac{60}{200}$

$x = 0.3 \text{ mg}$

$0.15 \text{ mg}:1 \text{ tab}::0.3 \text{ mg}:x \text{ tab}$

$0.15:1::0.3:x$

$0.15x = 0.3$

$x = \dfrac{0.3}{0.15}$

$x = 2 \text{ tablets of } 0.15 \text{ mg}$

$\dfrac{0.3 \text{ mg}}{0.15 \text{ mg}} \times 1 =$

$\dfrac{0.3}{0.15} = 2 \text{ tablets of } 0.15 \text{ mg}$

77. $5 \text{ mg}:1 \text{ tab}::7.5 \text{ mg}:x \text{ tab}$

$5:1::7.5:x$

$5x = 7.5$

$x = \dfrac{7.5}{5}$

$x = 1.5 \text{ tablet}$

$\dfrac{7.5 \text{ mg}}{5 \text{ mg}} \times 1 \text{ tab} =$

$\dfrac{7.5}{5} = 1.5 \text{ tablet}$

78. $125 \text{ mg}:5 \text{ ml}::250 \text{ mg}:x \text{ ml}$

$125:5::250:x$

$125x = 1250$

$x = \dfrac{1250}{125}$

$x = 10 \text{ ml}$

$\dfrac{250 \text{ mg}}{125 \text{ mg}} \times 5 \text{ ml} =$

$$\dfrac{250}{\underset{25}{\cancel{125}}} \times \dfrac{\overset{1}{\cancel{5}}}{1} = \dfrac{250}{25}$$

$\dfrac{250}{25} = 10 \text{ ml}$

Proportion

Formula

79. $50 \text{ mg}:1 \text{ cap}::250 \text{ mg}:x \text{ cap}$
$50:1::250:x$
$50x = 250$
$x = \dfrac{250}{50}$
$x = 5 \text{ capsules}$

$$\dfrac{250 \text{ mg}}{50 \text{ mg}} \times 1 \text{ cap} =$$
$$\dfrac{250}{50} = 5 \text{ capsules}$$

80. $15 \text{ mEq}:11.25 \text{ ml}::x \text{ mEq}:15 \text{ ml}$
$15:11.25::x:15$
$11.25x = 225$
$x = \dfrac{225}{11.25}$
$x = 20 \text{ mEq}$

$$\dfrac{x \text{ mEq}}{15 \text{ mEq}} \times 11.25 =$$
$$\dfrac{x}{15} \times \dfrac{11.25}{1} = 15$$
$$\dfrac{15}{1} \times \dfrac{x}{15} \times 11.25 = \dfrac{15}{1} \times \dfrac{15}{1}$$
$$11.25x = 225$$
$$x = \dfrac{225}{11.25}$$
$$x = 20 \text{ mEq}$$

81. $20 \text{ mg}:5 \text{ ml}::55 \text{ mg}:x \text{ ml}$
$20:5::55:x$
$20x = 275$
$x = \dfrac{275}{20}$
$x = 13.75 \text{ ml}$

$$\dfrac{55 \text{ mg}}{20 \text{ mg}} \times 5 \text{ ml} =$$
$$\dfrac{55}{\overset{}{\underset{4}{20}}} \times \dfrac{\overset{1}{5}}{1} = \dfrac{55}{4}$$
$$\dfrac{55}{4} = 13.75 \text{ ml}$$

82. $125 \text{ mg}:1 \text{ tab}::250 \text{ mg}:x \text{ tab}$
$125:1::250:x$
$125x = 250$
$x = \dfrac{250}{125}$
$x = 2 \text{ tablets}$

$$\dfrac{250 \text{ mg}}{125 \text{ mg}} \times 1 \text{ tab} =$$
$$\dfrac{250}{125} = 2 \text{ tablets}$$

83. $0.05 \text{ mg}:1 \text{ tab}::0.05 \text{ mg}:x \text{ tab}$
$0.05:1::0.05:x$
$0.05x = 0.05$
$x = \dfrac{0.05}{0.05}$
$x = 1 \text{ tablet}$

$$\dfrac{0.05 \text{ mg}}{0.05 \text{ mg}} \times 1 \text{ tab} =$$
$$\dfrac{0.05}{0.05} = 1 \text{ tablet}$$

84. $1000 \text{ mg}:1 \text{ g}::x \text{ mg}:0.2\text{g}$
$1000:1::x:0.2$
$x = 200 \text{ mg}$
Give 1 tablet of 200 mg

$200 \text{ mg}:1 \text{ dose}::x \text{ mg}:3 \text{ doses}$
$x = 600 \text{ mg}$ will be given per day

$$\dfrac{200 \text{ mg}}{200 \text{ mg}} \times 1 \text{ tab} =$$
1 tablet

Proportion	Formula

85. 5 mg:1 tab::15 mg:x tab

    5:1::15:x

    5x = 15

    $x = \dfrac{15}{5}$

    x = 3 tablets

$\dfrac{15 \text{ mg}}{5 \text{ mg}} \times 1 \text{ tab} =$

$\dfrac{15}{5} = 3$ tablets

86. 300 mg:1 dose::x mg:4 doses

    300:1::x:4

    x = 1200 mg given per day

87. 15 mg:1 cap::30 mg:x cap

    15:1::30:x

    15x = 30

    $x = \dfrac{30}{15}$

    x = 2 capsules

$\dfrac{30 \text{ mg}}{15 \text{ mg}} \times 1 \text{ cap} =$

$\dfrac{30}{15} = 2$ capsules

88. 25 mg:1 tab::50 mg:x tab

    25:1::50:x

    25x = 50

    $x = \dfrac{50}{25}$

    x = 2 tablets

$\dfrac{50 \text{ mg}}{25 \text{ mg}} \times 1 \text{ tab} =$

$\dfrac{50}{25} = 2$ tablets

89. 30 mg:1 ml::40 mg:x ml

    30:1::40:x

    30x = 40

    $x = \dfrac{40}{30}$

    x = 1.33 ml

$\dfrac{40 \text{ mg}}{30 \text{ mg}} \times 1 \text{ ml} =$

$\dfrac{40}{30} = 1.33$ ml

90. 10 mg:1 ml:x mg:0.6 ml

    10:1::x:0.6

    x = 6 mg

$\dfrac{x \text{ mg}}{10 \text{ mg}} \times 1 = 0.6$ ml

$\dfrac{x}{10} \times 1 = 0.6$

$\dfrac{10}{1} \times \dfrac{x}{10} \times 1 = 0.6 \times 10$

$x = 6$ mg

91. 75 mg:1 cap::150 mg:x cap

    75:1::150:x

    75x = 150

    $x = \dfrac{150}{75}$

    x = 2 capsules

$\dfrac{150 \text{ mg}}{75 \text{ mg}} \times 1 \text{ cap} =$

$\dfrac{150}{75} = 2$ capsules

Proportion	Formula

92. $0.1 \text{ mg} : 1 \text{ tab} :: 0.05 \text{ mg} : x \text{ tab}$
$0.1 : 1 :: 0.05 : x$
$0.1x = 0.05$
$x = \dfrac{0.05}{0.1}$
$x = 0.5 \text{ or } \frac{1}{2} \text{ tablet}$

$\dfrac{0.05 \text{ mg}}{0.1 \text{ mg}} \times 1 \text{ tab} =$
$\dfrac{0.05}{0.1} = 0.5 \text{ or } \frac{1}{2} \text{ tablet}$

93. $2.5 \text{ mg} : 1 \text{ tab} :: 10 \text{ mg} : x \text{ tab}$
$2.5 : 1 :: 10 : x$
$2.5x = 10$
$x = \dfrac{10}{2.5}$
$x = 4 \text{ tablets}$

$\dfrac{10 \text{ mg}}{2.5 \text{ mg}} \times 1 \text{ tab} =$
$\dfrac{10}{2.5} = 4 \text{ tablets}$

94. $1000 \text{ mg} : 1 \text{ g} :: x \text{ mg} : 0.25 \text{ g}$
$1000 : 1 :: x : 0.25$
$x = 1000 \times 0.25$
$x = 250 \text{ mg}$

$250 \text{ mg} : 1 \text{ tab} :: 250 \text{ mg} : x \text{ tab}$
$250 : 1 :: 250 : x$
$250x = 250$
$x = 1 \text{ tablet}$

$\dfrac{250 \text{ mg}}{250 \text{ mg}} \times 1 \text{ tab} =$
$\dfrac{250}{250} = 1 \text{ tablet}$

95. $60 \text{ mg} : 1 \text{ gr} :: x \text{ mg} : \frac{1}{6} \text{ gr}$
$60 : 1 :: x : \frac{1}{6}$
$x = \dfrac{\overset{10}{\cancel{60}}}{1} \times \dfrac{1}{\underset{1}{\cancel{6}}}$
$x = 10 \text{ mg}$

$10 \text{ mg} : 1 \text{ tab} :: 25 \text{ mg} : x \text{ tab}$
$10 : 1 :: 25 : x$
$10x = 25$
$x = \dfrac{25}{10}$
$x = 2.5 \text{ tablets}$

$\dfrac{25 \text{ mg}}{10 \text{ mg}} \times 1 \text{ tab} =$
$\dfrac{25}{10} = 2.5 \text{ tablets}$

96. $500 \text{ mg} : 5 \text{ ml} :: 600 \text{ mg} : x \text{ ml}$
$500 : 5 :: 600 : x$
$500x = 3000$
$x = \dfrac{3000}{500}$
$x = 6 \text{ ml}$

$\dfrac{600 \text{ mg}}{500 \text{ mg}} \times 5 \text{ ml} =$
$\dfrac{600}{\underset{100}{\cancel{500}}} \times \dfrac{\overset{1}{\cancel{5}}}{1} = \dfrac{600}{100}$
$\dfrac{600}{100} = 6 \text{ ml}$

Proportion	Formula

97. 5 mg:1 tab::15 mg:x tab
  5:1::15:x
  $5x = 15$
  $x = \dfrac{15}{5}$
  $x = 3$ tablets

$\dfrac{15 \text{ mg}}{5 \text{ mg}} \times 1 \text{ tab} =$
  $\dfrac{15}{5} = 3$ tablets

98. 1000 mg:1 g::x mg:0.015 g
  1000:1::x:0.015
  $x = 1000 \times 0.015$
  $x = 15$ mg

  15 mg:1 cap::15 mg:x cap
  15:1::15:x
  $15x = 15$
  $x = \dfrac{15}{15}$
  $x = 1$ capsule

$\dfrac{15 \text{ mg}}{15 \text{ mg}} \times 1 \text{ capsule} =$
  $\dfrac{15}{15} = 1$ capsule

99. 20 mEq:15 ml::40 mEq:x ml
  20:15::40:x
  $20x = 600$
  $x = \dfrac{600}{20}$
  $x = 30$ ml

$\dfrac{40 \text{ mEq}}{20 \text{ mEq}} \times \dfrac{15 \text{ ml}}{1} =$
  $\dfrac{\overset{2}{\cancel{40}}}{\cancel{20}} \times \dfrac{\overset{3}{\cancel{15}}}{1} = \dfrac{120}{4}$
  $\dfrac{120}{4} = 30$ ml

100. 40 mg:1 tab::20 mg:x tab
  40:1::20:x
  $40x = 20$
  $x = \dfrac{20}{40}$
  $x = ½$ tablet

$\dfrac{20 \text{ mg}}{40 \text{ mg}} \times 1 \text{ tab} =$
  $\dfrac{20}{40} \times 1 = ½$ tablet

Chapter 11 Oral Dosages—Posttest 1, pp. 241-246

Proportion	Formula

1. 5 gr:1 tab::15 gr:x tab
  5:1::15:x
  $5x = 15$
  $x = \dfrac{15}{5}$
  $x = 3$ tablets

$\dfrac{15 \text{ gr}}{5 \text{ gr}} \times 1 \text{ tab} =$
  $\dfrac{15}{5} = 3$ tablets

Proportion   **Formula**

2. $1000 \text{ mg}:1 \text{ g}::x \text{ mg}:0.5 \text{ g}$
$1000:1::x:0.5$
$x = 500 \text{ mg}$

$500 \text{ mg}:1 \text{ cap}::500 \text{ mg}:x \text{ cap}$ $\dfrac{500 \text{ mg}}{500 \text{ mg}} \times 1 \text{ cap} =$
$500:1::500:x$
$500x = 500$ $\dfrac{500}{500} = 1 \text{ capsule}$
$\quad x = \dfrac{500}{500}$
$\quad x = 1 \text{ capsule}$

3. $500 \text{ mg}:1 \text{ cap}::1000 \text{ mg}:x \text{ cap}$ $\dfrac{1000 \text{ mg}}{500 \text{ mg}} \times 1 \text{ cap} =$
$500:1::1000:x$
$500x = 1000$ $\dfrac{1000}{500} = 2 \text{ capsules}$
$\quad x = \dfrac{1000}{500}$
$\quad x = 2 \text{ capsules}$

4. $1 \ \text{ʒ} = 1 \text{ Tbsp}$

5. $0.5 \text{ g} = 500 \text{ mg}$ $\dfrac{500 \text{ mg}}{500 \text{ mg}} \times 1 \text{ tab} =$
$500 \text{ mg}:1 \text{ tab}::500:x \text{ tab}$
$500:1::500:x$ $\dfrac{500}{500} = 1 \text{ tablet}$
$500x = 500$
$\quad x = \dfrac{500}{500}$
$\quad x = 1 \text{ tablet}$

6. $10 \text{ mg}:5 \text{ ml}::25 \text{ mg}:x \text{ ml}$ $\dfrac{25 \text{ mg}}{10 \text{ mg}} \times \dfrac{5}{1} \text{ ml} =$
$10:5::25:x$
$10x = 125$ $\quad\quad\quad 1$
$\quad x = \dfrac{125}{10}$ $\dfrac{25}{\cancel{10}} \times \dfrac{\cancel{5}}{1} = \dfrac{25}{2}$
$\quad x = 12.5 \text{ ml}$ $\quad 2$

$\quad\quad\quad\quad\quad\quad\quad\quad\quad \dfrac{25}{2} = 12.5 \text{ ml}$

7. $15 \text{ mg}:1 \text{ tab}::30 \text{ mg}:x \text{ tab}$ $\dfrac{30 \text{ mg}}{15 \text{ mg}} \times 1 \text{ tab} =$
$15:1::30:x$
$15x = 30$ $\dfrac{30}{15} = 2 \text{ tablets}$
$\quad x = \dfrac{30}{15}$
$\quad x = 2 \text{ tablets}$

Proportion

Formula

8. $60 \text{ mg}:1 \text{ gr}::x \text{ mg}:\frac{1}{2} \text{ gr}$

$60:1::x:\frac{1}{2}$

$x = \dfrac{60}{2}$

$x = 30 \text{ mg}$

$30 \text{ mg}:1 \text{ tab}::30 \text{ mg}:x \text{ tab}$

$30:1::30:x$

$30x = 30$

$x = \dfrac{30}{30}$

$x = 1 \text{ tablet}$

$\dfrac{30 \text{ mg}}{30 \text{ mg}} \times 1 \text{ tab} =$

$\dfrac{30}{30} = 1 \text{ tablet}$

9. $25 \text{ mg}:1 \text{ tsp}::50 \text{ mg}:x \text{ tsp}$

$25:1::50:x$

$25x = 50$

$x = \dfrac{50}{25}$

$x = 2 \text{ teaspoons}$

$\dfrac{50 \text{ mg}}{25 \text{ mg}} \times 1 =$

$\dfrac{50}{25} = 2 \text{ teaspoons}$

10. $1000 \text{ mg}:1 \text{ g}::x \text{ mg}:0.25 \text{ g}$

$1000:1::x:0.25$

$x = 250$

$0.25 \text{ g} = 250 \text{ mg}$

$250 \text{ mg}:1 \text{ tab}::250 \text{ mg}:x \text{ tab}$

$250:1::250:x$

$250x = 250$

$x = \dfrac{250}{250}$

$x = 1 \text{ tablet}$

$\dfrac{250 \text{ mg}}{250 \text{ mg}} \times 1 \text{ tab} =$

$\dfrac{250}{250} = 1 \text{ tablet}$

$0.25 \text{ g}:1 \text{ dose}::x \text{ g}:2 \text{ dose}$

$0.25:1::x:2$

$x = 0.5 \text{ g}$

11. $\dfrac{1}{300} \text{ gr}:1 \text{ tab}::\dfrac{1}{600} \text{ gr}:x \text{ tab}$

$\dfrac{1}{300}:1::\dfrac{1}{600}:x$

$\dfrac{1}{300}x = \dfrac{1}{600}$

$x = \dfrac{300}{600}$

$x = \frac{1}{2} \text{ tablet}$

$\dfrac{\frac{1}{600} \text{ gr}}{\frac{1}{300} \text{ gr}} \times 1 \text{ tab} =$

$\dfrac{1}{600} \div \dfrac{1}{300} =$

$\dfrac{1}{600} \times \dfrac{300}{1} = \dfrac{300}{600}$

$\dfrac{300}{600} = \frac{1}{2} \text{ tablet}$

Proportion Formula

12. 30 mEq:22.5 ml::20 mEq:x ml
30:22.5::20:x
30x = 450
$x = \dfrac{450}{30}$
x = 15 ml

$$\dfrac{20\text{ mEq}}{30\text{ mEq}} \times 22.5 =$$
$$\dfrac{20}{30} \times \dfrac{22.5}{1} = \dfrac{450}{30}$$
$$\dfrac{450}{30} = 15\text{ ml}$$

13. 0.5 g:1 tab::2 g:x tab
0.5:1::2:x
0.5x = 2
x = 2 ÷ 0.5
x = 4 tablets

$$\dfrac{2\text{ g}}{0.5\text{ g}} \times 1\text{ tab} =$$
$$\dfrac{2}{0.5} = 4\text{ tablets}$$

14. 50 mg:1 cap::100 mg:x cap
50:1::100:x
50x = 100
$x = \dfrac{100}{50}$
x = 2 capsules

$$\dfrac{100\text{ mg}}{50\text{ mg}} \times 1\text{ cap} =$$
$$\dfrac{100}{50} = 2\text{ capsules}$$

15. 10 mg:1 ml::9 mg:x ml
10:1::9:x
10x = 9
$x = \dfrac{9}{10}$ or 0.9 ml

$$\dfrac{9\text{ mg}}{10\text{ mg}} \times 1\text{ ml} =$$
$$\dfrac{9}{10} = 0.9\text{ ml}$$

16. 125 mg:5 ml::100 mg:x ml
125:5::100:x
125x = 500
$x = \dfrac{500}{125}$
x = 4 ml

$$\dfrac{100\text{ mg}}{125\text{ mg}} \times 5\text{ ml} =$$
$$\dfrac{100}{\cancel{125}} \times \dfrac{\overset{1}{\cancel{5}}}{1} = \dfrac{100}{\underset{25}{25}}$$
$$\dfrac{100}{25} = 4\text{ ml}$$

17. 1 tsp = 1 ʒ
125 mg:1 ʒ::x mg:2 ʒ
125:1::x:2
x = 250 mg

$$\dfrac{x\text{ mg}}{125\text{ mg}} \times 1\,ʒ = 2\,ʒ$$
$$\dfrac{x}{125} = 2$$
$$\dfrac{\overset{1}{\cancel{125}}}{1} \times \dfrac{x}{\underset{1}{\cancel{125}}} = \dfrac{2}{1} \times \dfrac{125}{1}$$
$$x = 250\text{ mg}$$

Proportion

18. 40 mg:1 tab::80 mg:x tab
40:1::80:x
40x = 80
$x = \dfrac{80}{40}$
x = 2 tablets

19. 10 mg:1 tab::20 mg:x tab
10:1::20:x
10x = 20
$x = \dfrac{20}{10}$
x = 2 tablets

20. 60 mg:1 gr::x mg:1½ gr
60:1::x:³⁄₂

$x = \dfrac{\overset{30}{\cancel{60}}}{1} \times \dfrac{3}{\underset{1}{\cancel{2}}}$

x = 90 mg = 1½ gr
60 mg:1 tab::90 mg:x tab
60:1::90:x
60x = 90
$x = \dfrac{90}{60}$
x = 1½ tablets per dose

1½ tab:1 dose::x tab:3 doses

³⁄₂:1::x:3

$x = \dfrac{3}{2} \times \dfrac{3}{1}$
$x = \dfrac{9}{2}$
x = 4½ tablets per day

Formula

$\dfrac{80 \text{ mg}}{40 \text{ mg}} \times 1 \text{ tab} =$
$\dfrac{80}{40}$ = 2 tablets

$\dfrac{20 \text{ mg}}{10 \text{ mg}} \times 1 \text{ tab} =$
$\dfrac{20}{10}$ = 2 tablets

$\dfrac{90 \text{ mg}}{60 \text{ mg}} \times 1 \text{ tab} =$
$\dfrac{90}{60}$ = 1½ tablets per dose

Chapter 11 Oral Dosages—Posttest 2, pp. 247-252

Proportion

1. 10 mg:1 cap::20 mg:x
10:1::20:x
10x = 20
$x = \dfrac{20}{10}$
x = 2 capsules

Formula

$\dfrac{20 \text{ mg}}{10 \text{ mg}} \times 1 \text{ cap} =$
$\dfrac{20}{10}$ = 2 capsules

Proportion	Formula

2. $8 \, \mathfrak{3} : 1 \, \mathfrak{z} : : x \, \mathfrak{z} : 4 \, \mathfrak{z}$
$8 : 1 : : x : 4$
$x = 32 \, \mathfrak{z}$

$2 \, \mathfrak{z} : 1 \text{ dose} : : 32 \, \mathfrak{z} : x \text{ doses}$
$2 : 1 : : 32 : x$
$2x = 32$
$x = \dfrac{32}{2}$
$x = 16$ doses per each bottle

3. $160 \text{ mg} : 5 \text{ ml} : : 30 \text{ mg} : x \text{ ml}$
$160 : 5 : : 30 : x$
$160x = 150$
$x = \dfrac{150}{160}$
$x = 0.9375$ ml

$15 \, \mathrm{m} : 1 \text{ ml} : : x \, \mathrm{m} : 0.9375 \text{ ml}$
$15 : 1 : : x : 0.9375$
$x = 15 \times 0.9375$
$x = 14 \, \mathrm{m}$

4. $50 \text{ mg} : 1 \text{ tab} : : 150 \text{ mg} : x \text{ tab}$
$50 : 1 : : 150 : x$
$50x = 150$
$x = \dfrac{150}{50}$
$x = 3$ tablets

$\dfrac{150 \text{ mg}}{50 \text{ mg}} \times 1 \text{ tab} =$

$\dfrac{150}{50} = 3$ tablets

5. $20 \text{ mEq} : 30 \text{ ml} : : 5 \text{ mEq} : x \text{ ml}$
$20 : 30 : : 5 : x$
$20x = 150$
$x = \dfrac{150}{20}$
$x = 7.5$ ml

$\dfrac{5 \text{ mEq}}{20 \text{ mEq}} \times 30 \text{ ml} =$

$\overset{3}{\underset{2}{\dfrac{5}{20}}} \times \dfrac{\overset{}{\cancel{30}}}{1} = \dfrac{15}{2}$

$\dfrac{15}{2} = 7.5 \text{ ml}$

6. $1000 \text{ mg} : 1 \text{ g} : : x \text{ mg} : 0.25 \text{ g}$
$1000 : 1 : : x : 0.25$
$x = 250$ mg

$250 \text{ mg} : 1 \text{ cap} : : 250 \text{ mg} : x \text{ cap}$
$250 : 1 : : 250 : x$
$250x = 250$
$x = \dfrac{250}{250}$
$x = 1$ capsule

$\dfrac{250 \text{ mg}}{250 \text{ mg}} \times 1 \text{ capsule} =$

$\dfrac{250}{250} = 1$ capsule

Proportion	Formula

7. 2.5 mg : 1 tab : : 7.5 mg : x tab
2.5 : 1 : : 7.5 : x
2.5x = 7.5
$x = \dfrac{7.5}{2.5}$
x = 3 tablets

$\dfrac{7.5 \text{ mg}}{2.5 \text{ mg}} \times 1 \text{ tab} =$
$\dfrac{7.5}{2.5} = 3 \text{ tablets}$

8. 0.05 mg : 1 ml : : 0.05 mg : x ml
0.05 : 1 : : 0.05 : x
0.05x = 0.05
$x = \dfrac{0.05}{0.05}$
x = 1 ml

$\dfrac{0.05 \text{ mg}}{0.05 \text{ mg}} \times 1 \text{ ml} =$
$\dfrac{0.5}{0.5} = 1 \text{ ml}$

9. 1000 mg : 1 g : : x mg : 0.1 g
1000 : 1 : : x : 0.1
$x = 1000 \times 0.1$
x = 100 mg

50 mg : 1 capsule : : 100 mg : x cap
50 : 1 : : 100 : x
50x = 100
$x = \dfrac{100}{50}$
x = 2 capsules

$\dfrac{100 \text{ mg}}{50 \text{ mg}} \times 1 \text{ capsule} =$
$\dfrac{100}{50} = 2 \text{ capsules}$

10. 60 mg : 1 gr : : x mg : 6 gr
60 : 1 : : x : 6
x = 360 mg

325 mg : 1 tab : : 360 mg : x tab
325 : 1 : : 360 : x
325x = 360
$x = \dfrac{360}{325}$
x = 1.11 tablet; give 1 tablet

$\dfrac{360 \text{ mg}}{325 \text{ mg}} \times 1 \text{ tab} =$
1.11 tablet; give 1 tablet

11. 60 mg : 1 gr : : x mg : ¾ gr
60 : 1 : : x : ¾
$x = \dfrac{\overset{15}{\cancel{60}}}{1} \times \dfrac{3}{\underset{1}{\cancel{4}}}$
x = 45 mg = ¾ gr

50 mg : 1 tab : : 45 mg : x tab
50 : 1 : : 45 : x
50x = 45
$x = \dfrac{45}{50}$
$x = \dfrac{9}{10}$ tablet; give 1 tablet

$\dfrac{45 \text{ mg}}{50 \text{ mg}} \times 1 \text{ tab} =$
$\dfrac{45}{50} = \dfrac{9}{10}$ tablet; give 1 tablet

Proportion

Formula

12. 125 mg:5 ml::250 mg:x ml
125:5::250:x
125x = 1250
$$x = \frac{1250}{125}$$
x = 10 ml

$$\frac{250 \text{ mg}}{125 \text{ mg}} \times 5 \text{ ml} =$$
$$\frac{250}{\underset{25}{\cancel{125}}} \times \frac{\cancel{5}^{1}}{1} = \frac{250}{25}$$
$$\frac{250}{25} = 10 \text{ ml}$$

13. 5 mg:1 tab::20 mg:x tab
5:1::20:x
5x = 20
$$x = \frac{20}{5}$$
x = 4 tablets of 5 mg/tab

$$\frac{20 \text{ mg}}{5 \text{ mg}} \times 1 \text{ tab} =$$
$$\frac{20}{5} = 4 \text{ tablets of 5 mg/tab}$$

14. 0.125 mg:1 tab::0.25 mg:x tab
0.125:1::0.25:x
0.125x = 0.25
$$x = \frac{0.25}{0.125}$$
x = 2 tablets

$$\frac{0.25 \text{ mg}}{0.125 \text{ mg}} \times 1 \text{ tab} =$$
$$\frac{0.25 \text{ mg}}{0.125} = 2 \text{ tablets}$$

15. 20 mg:5 ml::x mg:25 ml
20:5::x:25
5x = 500
$$x = \frac{500}{5}$$
x = 100 mg

$$\frac{x \text{ mg}}{20 \text{ mg}} \times 5\text{ml} = 25\text{ml}$$
$$\frac{x}{\underset{4}{\cancel{20}}} \times \frac{\cancel{5}^{1}}{1} = 25$$
$$\frac{x}{4} = 25$$
$$\frac{\cancel{4}^{1}}{1} \times \frac{x}{\cancel{4}_{1}} = \frac{25}{1} \times \frac{4}{1}$$
$$x = 100 \text{ mg}$$

16. 1000 mg:1 g::x mg:0.6 g
1000:1::x:0.6
x = 600 mg

325 mg:1 tab::600 mg:x tab
325:1::600:x
325x = 600
$$x = \frac{600}{325}$$
x = 1.85 tablets; give 2 tablets

$$\frac{600 \text{ mg}}{325 \text{ mg}} \times 1 \text{ tab} =$$
$$\frac{600}{325} = 1.85 \text{ tablets; give 2 tablets}$$

Proportion	Formula

17. 60 mg:1 gr::x mg:7.5 gr
60:1::x:7.5
$x = 7.5 \times 60$
$x = 450$ mg

450 mg:1 ʒ::500 mg:x ʒ $\dfrac{500 \text{ mg}}{450 \text{ mg}} \times 1\ ʒ =$
450:1::500:x
450x = 500 $\dfrac{500}{450} = 1.11\ ʒ$; give 1 ʒ
$\quad x = \dfrac{500}{450}$
$\quad x = 1.11\ ʒ$; give 1 ʒ

18. 0.5 g:1 tab::1.5 g:x tab $\dfrac{1.5 \text{ g}}{0.5 \text{ g}} \times 1 \text{ tab} =$
0.5:1::1.5:x
0.5x = 1.5 $\dfrac{1.5}{0.5} = 3$ tablets
$\quad x = \dfrac{1.5}{0.5}$
$\quad x = 3$ tablets

19. 15 mg:1 tab::30 mg:x tab $\dfrac{30 \text{ mg}}{15 \text{ mg}} \times 1 \text{ tab} =$
15:1::30:x
15x = 30 $\dfrac{30}{15} = 2$ tablets
$\quad x = \dfrac{30}{15}$
$\quad x = 2$ tablets

20. 250 mg:1 tablet::750 mg:x tab $\dfrac{750 \text{ mg}}{250 \text{ mg}} \times 1 \text{ tab} =$
250:1::750:x
250x = 750 $\dfrac{750}{250} = 3$ tablets
$\quad x = \dfrac{750}{250}$
$\quad x = 3$ tablets

Chapter 12 Parenteral Dosages—Work Sheet, pp. 267-292

Proportion	Formula

1. 10 mg:1 ml::30 mg:x ml $\dfrac{30}{10} \times \dfrac{1}{1} = \dfrac{30}{10} = 3$ ml
10x = 30
$\quad x = \dfrac{30}{10} = 3$ ml

2. 500 mcg:2 ml::110 mcg:x ml $\dfrac{110}{500} \times \dfrac{2}{1} = \dfrac{220}{500} = 0.44$ ml
500x = 220
$\quad x = \dfrac{220}{500}$
$\quad x = 0.44$ ml

Proportion	Formula

3. 60 mg : 1 gr : : x mg : $\frac{1}{200}$ gr

$x = \dfrac{60}{200}$

$x = 0.3$ mg

0.4 mg : 1 ml : : 0.3 mg : x ml

0.4x = 0.3

$x = \dfrac{0.3}{0.4}$

$x = 0.75$ ml

$\dfrac{0.3}{0.4} \times \dfrac{1}{1} = 0.75$ ml

4. 5 mg : 1 ml : : 10 mg : x ml

5x = 10

$x = \dfrac{10}{5} = 2$ ml

$\dfrac{10}{5} \times 1 = 2$ ml

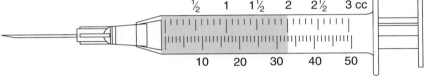

5. 75 mg : 1 ml : : 45 mg : x ml

75x = 45

$x = \dfrac{45}{75}$

$x = 0.6$ ml

$\dfrac{45}{75} \times 1 = 0.6$ ml

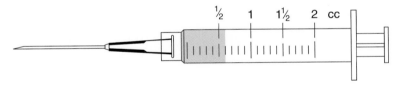

6. 1 g : 2.5 ml : : 3 g : x ml

$x = 2.5 \times 3$

$x = 7.5$ ml

$\dfrac{3}{1} \times 2.5 = 7.5$ ml

7. 10 mg : 1 ml : : 5 mg : x ml

10x = 5

$x = \dfrac{5}{10} = 0.5$ ml

$\dfrac{5}{10} \times 1 = 0.5$ ml

8. 500 mg : 6 ml : : 1000 mg : x ml

500x = 6000

$x = \dfrac{6000}{500}$

$x = 12$ ml

$\dfrac{1000}{500} \times \dfrac{6}{1} = \dfrac{6000}{500} = 12$ ml

Proportion	Formula

9. 40 mg:4 ml::30 mg:x ml

$40x = 120$

$x = \dfrac{120}{40}$

$x = 3$ ml

$$\dfrac{30}{\underset{10}{40}} \times \dfrac{\overset{1}{4}}{1} = \dfrac{30}{10} = 3 \text{ ml}$$

10. 30 ♏ = 2 ml

⅛ gr:2 ml::¹⁄₂₄ gr:x ml

$⅛x = \dfrac{2}{24}$

$x = \dfrac{2}{24} \times \dfrac{\overset{1}{8}}{\underset{3}{1}}$

$x = ⅔$

$x = 0.66$ ml

$$\dfrac{¹⁄₂₄}{⅛} \times \dfrac{2}{1} =$$

$$\dfrac{1}{24} \div \dfrac{1}{8}$$

$$\dfrac{1}{24} \times \dfrac{8}{1} = \dfrac{8}{24} = \dfrac{1}{3}$$

$$\dfrac{1}{3} \times \dfrac{2}{1} = \dfrac{2}{3} \text{ ml} =$$

$$0.66 \text{ ml}$$

11. 44.6 mEq:50 ml::25.8:x ml

$44.6x = 1290$

$x = \dfrac{1290}{44.6}$

$x = 28.9$ ml or 29 ml

$$\dfrac{25.8}{44.6} \times \dfrac{50}{1} =$$

$$0.58 \times 50 = 29 \text{ ml}$$

12. 25 mg:1 ml::100 mg:x ml

$25x = 100$

$x = \dfrac{100}{25}$

$x = 4$ ml

$$\dfrac{100}{25} \times 1 = 4 \text{ ml}$$

13. ¹⁄₁₅ gr = 4 mg

2 mg:1 ml::4 mg:x ml

$2x = 4$

$x = \dfrac{4}{2}$

$x = 2$ ml

$$\dfrac{4}{2} \times 1 = 2 \text{ ml}$$

Proportion | Formula

14. 15 gr = 900 mg
2 g = 2000 mg
2000 mg : 5 ml :: 900 mg : x ml
2000x = 4500
$x = \dfrac{4500}{2000}$
$x = 2.25$ ml

$$\dfrac{900}{\underset{400}{\cancel{2000}}} \times \dfrac{\overset{1}{\cancel{5}}}{1} = \dfrac{900}{400} = 2.25 \text{ ml}$$

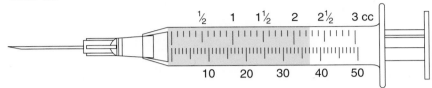

15. 250 mg : 2 ml :: 50 mg : x ml
250x = 100
$x = \dfrac{100}{250}$
$x = 0.4$ ml

$$\dfrac{50}{\underset{125}{\cancel{250}}} \times \dfrac{\overset{1}{\cancel{2}}}{1} = \dfrac{50}{125} = 0.4 \text{ ml}$$

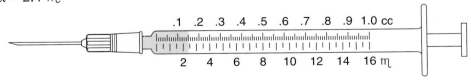

16. 120 mg : 1 ml :: 300 mg : x ml
120x = 300
$x = \dfrac{300}{120}$
$x = 2.5$ ml

$$\dfrac{300}{120} \times 1 = 2.5 \text{ ml}$$

17. 300 mg : 2 ml :: 300 mg : x ml
300x = 600
$x = \dfrac{600}{300}$
$x = 2$ ml

$$\dfrac{300}{300} \times \dfrac{2}{1} = 2 \text{ ml}$$

18. 100 mg : 30 ℳ :: 8 mg : x ℳ
100x = 240
$x = \dfrac{240}{100}$
$x = 2.4$ ℳ

$$\dfrac{8}{100} \times \dfrac{30}{1} = \dfrac{240}{100} = 2.4 \text{ ℳ}$$

Proportion	Formula

19. 2 mg : 1 ml : : 0.5 mg : x ml
    $2x = 0.5$
    $x = \dfrac{0.5}{2}$
    $x = 0.25$ ml

$\dfrac{0.5}{2} \times 1 = 0.25$ ml

20. 4 mg : 1 ml : : 1 mg : x ml
    $4x = 1$
    $x = 0.25$ ml

$\dfrac{1}{4} \times 1 = 0.25$ ml

21. 20 mg : 1 ml : : 10 mg : x ml
    $20x = 10$
    $x = \dfrac{10}{20}$
    $x = 0.5$ ml

$\dfrac{10}{20} \times 1 = 0.5$ ml

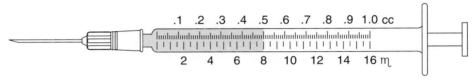

22. 40 mEq : 20 ml : : 30 mEq : x ml
    $40x = 600$
    $x = \dfrac{600}{40}$
    $x = 15$ ml

$\overset{1}{\underset{2}{\dfrac{30}{40}}} \times \dfrac{\overset{1}{20}}{1} = \dfrac{30}{2} = 15$ ml

23. 5 mg : 1 ml : : 10 mg : x ml
    $5x = 10$
    $x = \dfrac{10}{5} = 2$ ml

$\dfrac{10}{5} \times 1 = 2$ ml

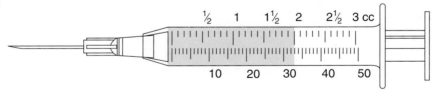

24. ½ gr : 1 ml : : ¼ gr : x ml
    $\frac{1}{2}x = \frac{1}{4}$
    $x = \dfrac{1}{4} \times \dfrac{2}{1}$
    $x = \dfrac{2}{4} = 0.5$ ml

$\dfrac{\frac{1}{4}}{\frac{1}{2}} \times 1$

$\dfrac{1}{4} \div \dfrac{1}{2}$

$\dfrac{1}{4} \times \dfrac{2}{1} = \dfrac{2}{4} = 0.5$ ml

Proportion	Formula

25. $10 \text{ mg}:1 \text{ ml}::10 \text{ mg}:x \text{ ml}$
$10x = 10$
$x = 1 \text{ ml}$

$\dfrac{10}{10} \times 1 = 1 \text{ ml}$

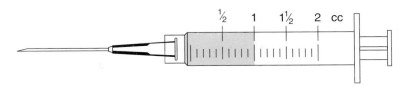

26. $2 \text{ g}:6 \text{ ml}::6 \text{ g}:x \text{ ml}$
$2x = 36$
$x = 18 \text{ ml}$

$\dfrac{6}{2} \times \dfrac{6}{1} = \dfrac{36}{2} = 18 \text{ ml}$

27. $15 \text{ mg}:1 \text{ ml}::12 \text{ mg}:x \text{ ml}$
$15x = 12$
$x = \dfrac{12}{15}$
$x = 0.8 \text{ ml}$

$\dfrac{12}{15} \times 1 = 0.8 \text{ ml}$

28. $50 \text{ mg}:1 \text{ ml}::100 \text{ mg}:x \text{ ml}$
$50x = 100$
$x = \dfrac{100}{50}$
$x = 2 \text{ ml}$

$\dfrac{100}{50} \times 1 = 2 \text{ ml}$

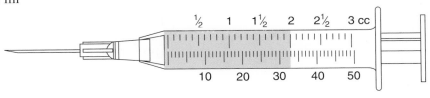

29. $500 \text{ mcg}:2 \text{ ml}::100 \text{ mcg}:x \text{ ml}$
$500x = 200$
$x = \dfrac{200}{500}$
$x = 0.4 \text{ ml}$

$\dfrac{100}{500} \times 2 = 0.4 \text{ ml}$

30. $225 \text{ mg}:1 \text{ ml}::500 \text{ mg}:x \text{ ml}$
$225x = 500$
$x = \dfrac{500}{225}$
$x = 2.22 \text{ ml}$

$\dfrac{500}{225} \times 1 = 2.22 \text{ ml}$

31. $120 \text{ mg}:1 \text{ ml}::300 \text{ mg}:x \text{ ml}$
$120x = 300$
$x = \dfrac{300}{120}$
$x = 2.5 \text{ ml}$

$\dfrac{300}{120} \times 1 = 2.5 \text{ ml}$

Proportion	Formula

32. 250 mg:2 ml::100 mg:x ml
$250x = 200$
$x = \dfrac{200}{250}$
$x = 0.8$ ml

$$\dfrac{100}{\cancel{250}}^{\;1} \times \dfrac{\cancel{2}}{1} = 0.8 \text{ ml}$$
$$_{125}$$

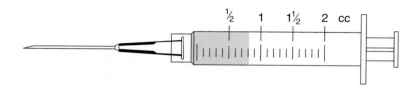

33. 2.5 mEq:1 ml::7.5 mEq:x ml
$2.5x = 7.5$
$x = \dfrac{7.5}{2.5}$
$x = 3$ ml

$$\dfrac{7.5}{2.5} \times \dfrac{1}{1} = 3 \text{ ml}$$

34. 50 mg:1 ml::x mg:3 ml
$x = 150$ mg

$$\dfrac{x}{50} \times 1 = 3$$
$$x = 150 \text{ mg}$$

35. $\frac{1}{150}$ gr:1 ml::$\frac{1}{100}$ gr:x ml

$\dfrac{1}{150}x = \dfrac{1}{100}$
$x = \dfrac{150}{100}$
$x = 1.5$ ml

$$\dfrac{\dfrac{1}{100}}{\dfrac{1}{150}} \times \dfrac{1}{1} =$$
$$\dfrac{1}{100} \div \dfrac{1}{150}$$
$$\dfrac{1}{100} \times \dfrac{150}{1} = \dfrac{150}{100} = 1.5 \text{ ml}$$

36. 50 mg:1 ml::50 mg:x ml
$50x = 50$
$x = \dfrac{50}{50} = 1$ ml

$$\dfrac{50}{50} \times 1 = 1 \text{ ml}$$

37. 100 mg:2 ml::75 mg:x ml
$100x = 150$
$x = \dfrac{150}{100}$
$x = 1.5$ ml

$$\dfrac{75}{100} \times 2 = \dfrac{150}{100} = 1.5 \text{ ml}$$

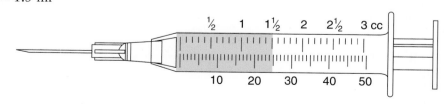

Proportion	Formula

38. 25 mg : 1 ml : : 75 mg : x ml
25x = 75
$x = \dfrac{75}{25}$
x = 3 ml

$$\dfrac{75}{25} \times \dfrac{1}{1} = 3 \text{ ml}$$

39. 100 mg : 2 ml : : 75 mg : x ml
100x = 150
$x = \dfrac{150}{100}$
x = 1.5 ml

$$\dfrac{75}{100} \times \dfrac{2}{1} = \dfrac{150}{100} = 1.5 \text{ ml}$$

40. 5 mg : 1 ml : : 15 mg : x ml
5x = 15
$x = \dfrac{15}{5}$
x = 3 ml

$$\dfrac{15}{5} \times 1 = 3 \text{ ml}$$

41. 100 mg : 2 ml : : 25 mg : x ml
100x = 50
$x = \dfrac{50}{100}$
x = 0.5 ml

$$\dfrac{25}{100} \times \dfrac{2}{1} = \dfrac{50}{100} = 0.5 \text{ ml}$$

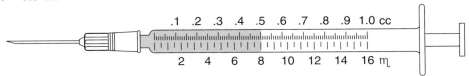

42. 500 mg : 2 ml : : 400 mg : x ml
500x = 800
$x = \dfrac{800}{500}$
x = 1.6 ml

$$\dfrac{400}{500} \times \dfrac{2}{1} = \dfrac{800}{500} = 1.6 \text{ ml}$$

43. 500 mg : 1 ml : : 250 mg : x ml
500x = 250
$x = \dfrac{250}{500}$
x = 0.5 ml

$$\dfrac{250}{500} \times \dfrac{1}{1} = 0.5 \text{ ml}$$

Proportion

Formula

44. 13.6 mEq : 10 ml : : 5 mEq : x ml

13.6x = 50

$x = \dfrac{50}{13.6}$

x = 3.68 ml

$\dfrac{5}{13.6} \times \dfrac{10}{1} = \dfrac{50}{13.6} = 3.68$ ml

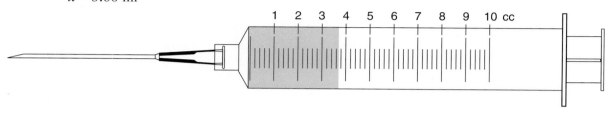

45. 65 mg : 1 ml : : 70 mg : x ml

65x = 70

$x = \dfrac{70}{65}$

x = 1.07 or 1.1 ml

$\dfrac{70}{65} \times \dfrac{1}{1} = 1.07$ or 1.1 ml

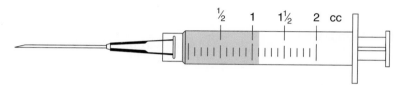

46. 10 mg : 1 ml : : 200 mg : x ml

10x = 200

$x = \dfrac{200}{10}$

x = 20 ml

$\dfrac{200}{10} \times \dfrac{1}{1} = 20$ ml

47. $\frac{1}{30}$ gr = 2 mg

4 mg : 1 ml : : 2 mg : x ml

4x = 2

$x = \dfrac{2}{4} = 0.5$ ml

$\dfrac{2}{4} \times \dfrac{1}{1} = \dfrac{2}{4} = 0.5$ ml

48. 0.5 mg : 2 ml : : 0.2 mg : x ml

0.5x = 0.4

$x = \dfrac{0.4}{0.5}$

x = 0.8 ml

$\dfrac{0.2}{0.5} \times \dfrac{2}{1} = \dfrac{0.4}{0.5} = 0.8$ ml

Proportion   Formula

49. $\frac{1}{4}$ gr : 15 $\mathfrak{m}$: : $\frac{1}{6}$ gr : x $\mathfrak{m}$

$\frac{1}{4}x = \frac{15}{6}$

$$x = \frac{15}{\overset{}{6}} \times \frac{\overset{2}{\cancel{4}}}{1}$$
$$\underset{3}{}$$

$x = \frac{30}{3} = 10$ $\mathfrak{m}$

$$\frac{\frac{1}{6}}{\frac{1}{4}} \times \frac{15}{1} =$$

$$\frac{1}{6} \div \frac{1}{4} =$$

$$\frac{1}{6} \times \frac{4}{1} = \frac{4}{\overset{}{6}} \times \frac{\overset{5}{\cancel{15}}}{1} = \frac{20}{2} = 10 \ \mathfrak{m}$$
$$\underset{2}{}$$

50. 5 mg : 15 $\mathfrak{m}$: : 3 mg : x $\mathfrak{m}$
$5x = 45$
$x = \frac{45}{5}$
$x = 9$ $\mathfrak{m}$

$$\frac{3}{\cancel{5}} \times \frac{\overset{3}{\cancel{15}}}{1} = \frac{9}{1} = 9 \ \mathfrak{m}$$
$$\underset{1}{}$$

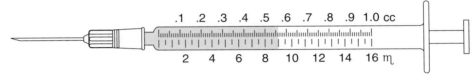

51. 50 mg : 1 ml : : x mg : 0.6 ml
$x = 30$ mg

$$\frac{x}{50} \times \frac{1}{1} = 0.6$$
$$\frac{x}{50} = 0.6$$
$$x = 0.6 \times 50$$
$$x = 30 \text{ mg}$$

52. 0.4 mg : 1 ml : : 0.9 mg : x ml
$0.4x = 0.9$
$x = \frac{0.9}{0.4}$
$x = 2.25$ ml

$$\frac{0.9}{0.4} \times \frac{1}{1} = 2.25 \text{ ml}$$

53. $\frac{1}{2}$ gr : 1 ml : : $\frac{1}{2}$ gr : x ml
$\frac{1}{2}x = \frac{1}{2}$
$x = 1$ ml

$$\frac{\frac{1}{2}}{\frac{1}{2}} \times 1 =$$

$$\frac{1}{2} \div \frac{1}{2} =$$
$$\frac{1}{2} \times \frac{2}{1} = 1 \text{ ml}$$

Proportion	Formula

54. ¼ gr = 15 mg
65 mg : 15 ℳ : : 15 mg : x ℳ
65x = 225
$x = \dfrac{225}{65}$
x = 3.46 ℳ

$\dfrac{15}{65} \times \dfrac{15}{1} = \dfrac{225}{65} = 3.46\ \text{ℳ}$

55. 0.89 mEq : 1 ml : : 6 mEq : x ml
0.89x = 6
$x = \dfrac{6}{0.89}$
x = 6.74 ml

$\dfrac{6}{0.89} \times 1 = 6.74\ \text{ml}$

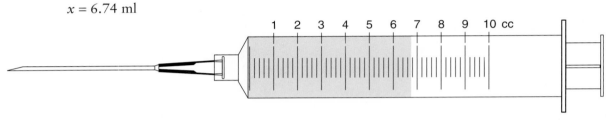

56. 40 mg : 1 ml : : 20 mg : x ml
40x = 20
$x = \dfrac{20}{40}$
x = 0.5 ml

$\dfrac{20}{40} \times 1 = 0.5\ \text{ml}$

57. 25 mg : 1 ml : : x mg : 0.2 ml
x = 25 × 0.2
x = 5 mg

$\dfrac{x}{25} \times 1 = 0.2$
$\dfrac{x}{25} = 0.2$
x = 0.2 × 25
x = 5 mg

58. 100 mg : 1 ml : : 500 mg : x ml
100x = 500
$x = \dfrac{500}{100}$
x = 5 ml

$\dfrac{500}{100} \times \dfrac{1}{1} = 5\ \text{ml}$

59. 100 mg : 1 ml : : 50 mg : x ml
100x = 50
$x = \dfrac{50}{100}$
x = 0.5 ml

$\dfrac{50}{100} \times \dfrac{1}{1} = 0.5\ \text{ml}$

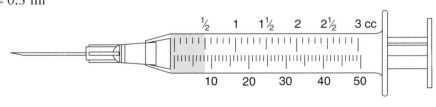

Proportion	Formula

60. $2 \text{ mg} : 1 \text{ ml} :: 0.5 \text{ mg} : x \text{ ml}$

$2x = 0.5$

$x = \dfrac{0.5}{2}$

$x = 0.25 \text{ ml}$

$$\dfrac{0.5}{2} \times 1 = 0.25 \text{ ml}$$

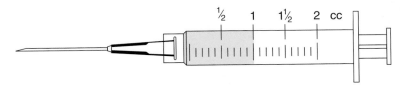

61. $0.25 \text{ g} : 10 \text{ ml} :: 0.2 \text{ g} : x \text{ ml}$

$0.25x = 2$

$x = \dfrac{2}{0.25}$

$x = 8 \text{ ml}$

$$\dfrac{0.2}{0.25} \times \dfrac{10}{1} = \dfrac{2}{0.25} = 8 \text{ ml}$$

62. $30 \text{ mg} : 1 \text{ ml} :: 15 \text{ mg} : x \text{ ml}$

$30x = 15$

$x = \dfrac{15}{30}$

$x = 0.5 \text{ ml}$

$$\dfrac{15}{30} \times \dfrac{1}{1} = 0.5 \text{ ml}$$

63. $50 \text{ mg} : 1 \text{ ml} :: 100 \text{ mg} : x \text{ ml}$

$50x = 100$

$x = \dfrac{100}{50}$

$x = 2 \text{ ml}$

$$\dfrac{100}{50} \times \dfrac{1}{1} = 2 \text{ ml}$$

64. $0.5 \text{ mg} : 2 \text{ ml} :: 0.25 : x \text{ ml}$

$0.5x = 0.5$

$x = \dfrac{0.5}{0.5}$

$x = 1 \text{ ml}$

$$\dfrac{0.25}{0.50} \times \dfrac{2}{1} = \dfrac{0.5}{0.5} = 1 \text{ ml}$$

65. $25 \text{ mg} : 0.5 \text{ ml} :: 35 \text{ mg} : x \text{ ml}$

$25x = 17.5$

$x = \dfrac{17.5}{25}$

$x = 0.7 \text{ ml}$

$$\dfrac{35}{25} \times \dfrac{0.5}{1} = \dfrac{17.5}{25} = 0.7 \text{ ml}$$

<table>
<tr><th align="center">Proportion</th><th align="center">Formula</th></tr>
</table>

66. $4.8 \text{ mEq}:10 \text{ ml}::5 \text{ mEq}:x \text{ ml}$
$4.8x = 50$
$x = \dfrac{50}{4.8}$
$x = 10.42 \text{ ml}$

$$\dfrac{5}{4.8} \times \dfrac{10}{1} = \dfrac{50}{4.8} = 10.42 \text{ ml}$$

67. $150 \text{ mg}:1 \text{ ml}::50 \text{ mg}:x \text{ ml}$
$150x = 50$
$x = \dfrac{50}{150}$
$x = 0.33 \text{ ml}$

$$\dfrac{50}{150} \times \dfrac{1}{1} = \dfrac{50}{150} = 0.33 \text{ ml}$$

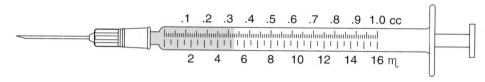

68. $1 \text{ mg}:1 \text{ ml}::0.2 \text{ mg}:x \text{ ml}$
$1x = 0.2$
$x = 0.2 \text{ ml}$

$$\dfrac{0.2}{1} \times \dfrac{1}{1} = 0.2 \text{ ml}$$

69. $40 \text{ mg}:1 \text{ ml}::55 \text{ mg}:x \text{ ml}$
$40x = 55$
$x = \dfrac{55}{40}$
$x = 1.38 \text{ ml}$

$$\dfrac{55}{40} \times \dfrac{1}{1} = 1.38 \text{ ml}$$

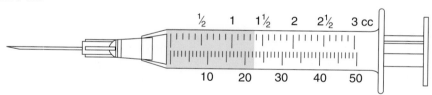

70. $65 \text{ mg}:1 \text{ ml}::22 \text{ mg}:x \text{ ml}$
$65x = 22$
$x = \dfrac{22}{65}$
$x = 0.34 \text{ ml}$

$$\dfrac{22}{65} \times \dfrac{1}{1} = 0.34 \text{ ml}$$

71. $15 \text{ mg}:1 \text{ ml}::10 \text{ mg}:x \text{ ml}$
$15x = 10$
$x = \dfrac{10}{15}$
$x = 0.66 \text{ ml}$

$$\dfrac{10}{15} \times \dfrac{1}{1} = 0.66 \text{ ml}$$

Proportion   **Formula**

72. $1000 \text{ mcg}:1 \text{ ml}::1000 \text{ mcg}:x \text{ ml}$

$$1000x = 1000$$

$$x = \frac{1000}{1000}$$

$$x = 1 \text{ ml}$$

$$\frac{1000}{1000} \times \frac{1}{1} = 1 \text{ ml}$$

73. $\frac{1}{8} \text{ gr}:15 \text{ m}::\frac{1}{30} \text{ gr}:x \text{ m}$

$$\frac{1}{8}x = \frac{15}{30}$$

$$x = \frac{15}{30} \times \frac{8}{1}$$

$$x = \frac{120}{30}$$

$$x = 4 \text{ m}$$

74. $25 \text{ mg}:1 \text{ ml}::6.5 \text{ mg}:x \text{ ml}$

$$25x = 6.5$$

$$x = \frac{6.5}{25}$$

$$x = 0.26 \text{ ml}$$

$$\frac{6.5}{25} \times \frac{1}{1} = 0.26 \text{ ml}$$

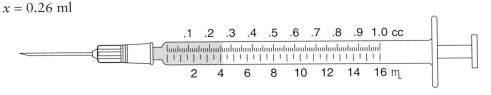

75. $0.2 \text{ mg}:1 \text{ ml}::0.28 \text{ mg}:x \text{ ml}$

$$0.2x = 0.28$$

$$x = \frac{0.28}{0.2}$$

$$x = 1.4 \text{ ml}$$

$$\frac{0.28}{0.2} \times \frac{1}{1} = 1.4 \text{ ml}$$

76. $25 \text{ mg}:1 \text{ ml}::10 \text{ mg}:x \text{ ml}$

$$25x = 10$$

$$x = \frac{10}{25}$$

$$x = 0.4 \text{ ml}$$

$$\frac{10}{25} \times \frac{1}{1} = 0.4 \text{ ml}$$

77. $100 \text{ mEq}:40 \text{ ml}::15 \text{ mEq}:x \text{ ml}$

$$100x = 600$$

$$x = \frac{600}{100}$$

$$x = 6 \text{ ml}$$

$$\frac{15}{100} \times \frac{40}{1} = \frac{600}{100} = 6 \text{ ml}$$

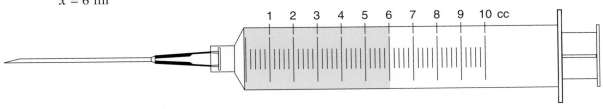

Proportion	Formula

78. $125 \text{ mg} : 1 \text{ ml} :: 250 \text{ mg} : x \text{ ml}$

$125x = 250$

$x = \dfrac{250}{125}$

$x = 2 \text{ ml}$

$\dfrac{250}{125} \times \dfrac{1}{1} = 2 \text{ ml}$

79. $600 \text{ mg} : 4 \text{ ml} :: 300 \text{ mg} : x \text{ ml}$

$600x = 1200$

$x = \dfrac{1200}{600}$

$x = 2 \text{ ml}$

$\dfrac{300}{600} \times \dfrac{4}{1} = \dfrac{1200}{600} = 2 \text{ ml}$

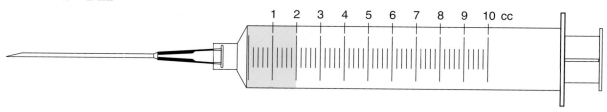

80. $100 \text{ mg} : 75 \, \text{m} :: 75 \text{ mg} : x \, \text{m}$

$100x = 5625$

$x = \dfrac{5625}{100}$

$x = 56.25 \, \text{m}$

$\dfrac{75}{100} \times \dfrac{75}{1} = \dfrac{5625}{100} = 56.25 \, \text{m}$

81. $120 \text{ mg} : 1 \text{ ml} :: 20 \text{ mg} : x \text{ ml}$

$120x = 20$

$x = \dfrac{20}{120}$

$x = 0.17 \text{ ml}$

$\dfrac{20}{120} \times \dfrac{1}{1} = 0.17 \text{ ml}$

82. $125 \text{ mg} : 2 \text{ ml} :: 100 \text{ mg} : x \text{ ml}$

$125x = 200$

$x = \dfrac{200}{125}$

$x = 1.6 \text{ ml}$

$\dfrac{100}{125} \times \dfrac{2}{1} = \dfrac{200}{125} = 1.6 \text{ ml}$

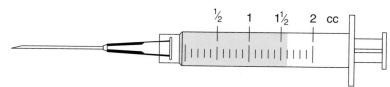

Proportion

Formula

83. $50 \text{ mg} : 1 \text{ ml} : : 25 \text{ mg} : x \text{ ml}$
$50x = 25$
$x = \dfrac{25}{50}$
$x = 0.5 \text{ ml}$

$\dfrac{25}{50} \times \dfrac{1}{1} = 0.5 \text{ ml}$

84. $0.4 \text{ mg} : 1 \text{ ml} : : 0.4 \text{ mg} : x \text{ ml}$
$0.4x = 0.4$
$x = \dfrac{0.4}{0.4}$
$x = 1 \text{ ml}$

$\dfrac{0.4}{0.4} \times \dfrac{1}{1} = 1 \text{ ml}$

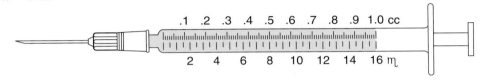

85. $25 \text{ mg} : 1 \text{ ml} : : x \text{ mg} : 0.2 \text{ ml}$
$x = 5 \text{ mg}$

$\dfrac{x}{25} \times \dfrac{1}{1} = 0.2$
$\dfrac{x}{25} = 0.2$
$x = 0.2 \times 25$
$x = 5 \text{ mg}$

86. $10 \text{ mg} : 1 \text{ ml} : : 1 \text{ mg} : x \text{ ml}$
$10x = 1$
$x = \dfrac{1}{10} \text{ or } 0.1 \text{ ml}$

$\dfrac{1}{10} \times \dfrac{1}{1} = \dfrac{1}{10} = 0.1 \text{ ml}$

87. $100 \text{ mg} : 2 \text{ ml} : : 50 \text{ mg} : x \text{ ml}$
$100x = 100$
$x = \dfrac{100}{100}$
$x = 1 \text{ ml}$

$\dfrac{50}{100} \times \dfrac{2}{1} = \dfrac{100}{100} = 1 \text{ ml}$

88. $2 \text{ mEq} : 1 \text{ ml} : : 8 \text{ mEq} : x \text{ ml}$
$2x = 8$
$x = \dfrac{8}{2}$
$x = 4 \text{ ml}$

$\dfrac{8}{\overset{}{\underset{2}{40}}} \times \dfrac{\overset{1}{20}}{1} = \dfrac{8}{2} = 4 \text{ ml}$

Proportion

Formula

89. gr $\frac{1}{150}$: 15 m̃ : : gr $\frac{1}{120}$: x m̃

$$\frac{1}{150}x = \frac{15}{120}$$

$$x = \frac{15}{\cancel{120}} \times \frac{\cancel{150}^{\ 5}}{1}$$
^{4}

$$x = \frac{75}{4}$$

$$x = 18.75 \text{ m̃}$$

$$\frac{\dfrac{1}{120}}{\dfrac{1}{150}} \times \frac{15}{1}$$

$$\frac{1}{120} \div \frac{1}{150}$$

$$\frac{1}{\cancel{120}} \times \frac{\cancel{150}^{\ 5}}{1} = \frac{5}{4}$$
^{4}

$$\frac{5}{4} \times \frac{15}{1} = \frac{75}{4} = 18.75 \text{ m̃}$$

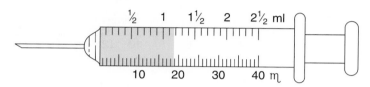

90. 25 mg : 1 ml : : 15 mg : x ml

$$25x = 15$$

$$x = \frac{15}{25}$$

$$x = 0.6 \text{ ml}$$

$$\frac{15}{25} \times \frac{1}{1} = 0.6 \text{ ml}$$

91. 250 mg : 5 ml : : 500 mg : x ml

$$250x = 2500$$

$$x = \frac{2500}{250}$$

$$x = 10 \text{ ml}$$

$$\frac{500}{250} \times \frac{5}{1} = \frac{2500}{250} = 10 \text{ ml}$$

92. 80 mg : 2 ml : : 90 mg : x ml

$$80x = 180$$

$$x = 2.25 \text{ ml}$$

$$\frac{90}{\cancel{80}} \times \frac{\cancel{2}^{\ 1}}{1} = \frac{90}{40} = 2.25 \text{ ml}$$
^{40}

93. 5 mg : 1 ml : : 2 mg : x ml

$$5x = 2$$

$$x = \frac{2}{5}$$

$$x = 0.4 \text{ ml}$$

$$\frac{2}{5} \times \frac{1}{1} = 0.4 \text{ ml}$$

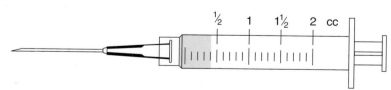

Proportion   Formula

94. $100 \text{ mg} : 1 \text{ ml} :: 500 \text{ mg} : x \text{ ml}$ $\dfrac{500}{100} \times \dfrac{1}{1} = 5 \text{ ml}$

$100x = 500$

$x = \dfrac{500}{100}$

$x = 5 \text{ ml}$

95. $400 \text{ mg} : 1 \text{ ml} :: 640 \text{ mg} : x \text{ ml}$ $\dfrac{640}{400} \times \dfrac{1}{1} = 1.6 \text{ ml}$

$400x = 640$

$x = \dfrac{640}{400}$

$x = 1.6 \text{ ml}$

96. $250 \text{ mg} : 1 \text{ ml} :: 500 \text{ mg} : x \text{ ml}$ $\dfrac{500}{250} \times \dfrac{1}{1} = 2 \text{ ml}$

$250x = 500$

$x = \dfrac{500}{250}$

$x = 2 \text{ ml}$

97. $1 \text{ mg} : 5 \text{ ml} :: 0.2 \text{ mg} : x \text{ ml}$ $\dfrac{0.2}{1} \times \dfrac{5}{1} = \dfrac{1.0}{1} = 1 \text{ ml}$

$x = 1.0 \text{ ml}$

98. $25 \text{ mg} : 0.5 \text{ ml} :: 100 \text{ mg} : x \text{ ml}$ $\dfrac{100}{25} \times \dfrac{0.5}{1} = \dfrac{50}{25} = 2 \text{ ml}$

$25x = 50$

$x = \dfrac{50}{25}$

$x = 2 \text{ ml}$

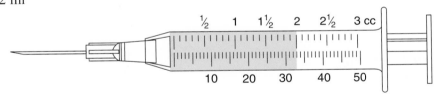

99. $50 \text{ mg} : 1 \text{ ml} :: 10 \text{ mg} : x \text{ ml}$ $\dfrac{10}{50} \times \dfrac{1}{1} = 0.2 \text{ ml}$

$50x = 10$

$x = \dfrac{10}{50}$

$x = 0.2 \text{ ml}$

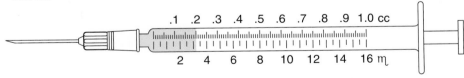

100. $10 \text{ mg} : 1 \text{ ml} :: 4 \text{ mg} : x \text{ ml}$ $\dfrac{4}{10} \times \dfrac{1}{1} = 0.4 \text{ ml}$

$10x = 4$

$x = \dfrac{4}{10}$

$x = 0.4 \text{ ml}$

Chapter 12 Parenteral Dosages—Posttest 1, pp. 293-298

| Proportion | Formula |

1. 50 mg : 1 ml : : 25 mg : x ml

$50x = 25$

$x = \dfrac{25}{50}$

$x = 0.5$ ml

$\dfrac{25}{50} \times \dfrac{1}{1} = 0.5$ ml

2. 25 mg : 15 ℳ : : 5.5 mg : x ℳ

$25x = 82.5$

$x = \dfrac{82.5}{25}$

$x = 3.3$ ℳ

$\dfrac{5.5}{25} \times \dfrac{15}{1} = \dfrac{82.5}{25} = 3.3$ ℳ

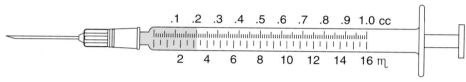

3. 15 mg : 1 ml : : 30 mg : x ml

$15x = 30$

$x = \dfrac{30}{15}$

$x = 2$ ml

$\dfrac{30}{15} \times \dfrac{1}{1} = 2$ ml

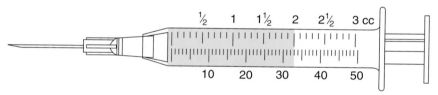

4. 1000 mg : 10 ml : : 500 mg : x ml

$1000x = 5000$

$x = \dfrac{5000}{1000}$

$x = 5$ ml

$\dfrac{500}{1000} \times \dfrac{10}{1} = \dfrac{5000}{1000} = 5$ ml

5. 100 mg : 2 ml : : 50 mg : x ml

$100x = 100$

$x = \dfrac{100}{100}$

$x = 1$ ml

$\dfrac{50}{100} \times \dfrac{2}{1} = \dfrac{100}{100} = 1$ ml

6. 2 mg : 1 ml : : 0.5 mg : x ml

$2x = 0.5$

$x = \dfrac{0.5}{2}$

$x = 0.25$ ml

$\dfrac{0.5}{2} \times \dfrac{1}{1} = 0.25$ ml

Proportion	Formula

7. 120 mg : 1 ml : : 240 mg : x ml

120x = 240

$x = \dfrac{240}{120}$

x = 2 ml

$\dfrac{240}{120} \times \dfrac{1}{1} = 2$ ml

8. 0.4 mg : 1 ml : : 0.2 mg : x ml

0.4x = 0.2

$x = \dfrac{0.2}{0.4}$

x = 0.5 ml

$\dfrac{0.2}{0.4} \times \dfrac{1}{1} = 0.5$ ml

9. 25 mg : 1 ml : : 100 mg : x ml

25x = 100

$x = \dfrac{100}{25}$

x = 4 ml

$\dfrac{100}{25} \times \dfrac{1}{1} = 4$ ml

10. 5 mg : 1 ml : : 2 mg : x ml

5x = 2

$x = \dfrac{2}{5}$

x = 0.4 ml

$\dfrac{2}{5} \times \dfrac{1}{1} = 0.4$ ml

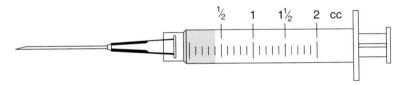

11. 0.5 mg : 1 ml : : 0.7 : x ml

0.5x = 0.7

$x = \dfrac{0.7}{0.5}$

x = 1.4 ml

$\dfrac{0.7}{0.5} \times \dfrac{1}{1} = 1.4$ ml

12. 50 mg : 1 ml : : 25 mg : x ml

50x = 25

$x = \dfrac{25}{50}$

x = 0.5 ml

$\dfrac{25}{50} \times \dfrac{1}{1} = 0.5$ ml

| Proportion | Formula |

13. 25 mg:0.5 ml::42 mg:x ml

25x = 21

$x = \dfrac{21}{25}$

$x = 0.84$ ml

$$\dfrac{42}{25} \times \dfrac{0.5}{1} = \dfrac{21}{25} = 0.84 \text{ ml}$$

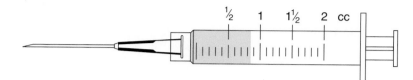

14. 2500 mg:10 ml::500 mg:x ml

2500x = 5000

$x = \dfrac{5000}{2500}$

$x = 2$ ml

$$\dfrac{500}{2500} \times \dfrac{10}{1} = \dfrac{5000}{2500} = 2 \text{ ml}$$

15. 100 mg:5 ml::x mg:0.5 ml

5x = 50

$x = \dfrac{50}{5}$

$x = 10$ mg

$$\dfrac{x}{100} \times \dfrac{5}{1} = 0.5$$

$$\dfrac{5x}{100} = 0.5$$

$$5x = 50$$

$$x = \dfrac{50}{5}$$

$$x = 10 \text{ mg}$$

16. 10 mg:1 ml::6 mg:x ml

10x = 6

$x = \dfrac{6}{10}$

$x = 0.6$ ml

$$\dfrac{6}{10} \times \dfrac{1}{1} = 0.6 \text{ ml}$$

17. 500 mg:10 ml::300 mg:x ml

500x = 3000

$x = \dfrac{3000}{500}$

$x = 6$ ml

$$\dfrac{300}{500} \times \dfrac{10}{1} = \dfrac{3000}{500} = 6 \text{ ml}$$

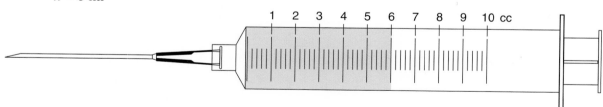

Proportion Formula

18. 40 mg:4 ml::10 mg:x ml
$40x = 40$
$x = 1$ ml

$$\frac{10}{\overset{1}{\cancel{40}}} \times \frac{\overset{1}{\cancel{4}}}{1} = \frac{10}{10} = 1 \text{ ml}$$

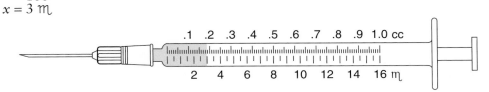

19. 100 mcg:15 ℳ::20 mcg:x ℳ
$100x = 300$
$x = \dfrac{300}{100}$
$x = 3$ ℳ

$$\frac{20}{100} \times \frac{15}{1} = \frac{300}{100} = 3 \text{ ℳ}$$

20. 20 mEq:1 ml::5 mEq:x ml
$20x = 5$
$x = \dfrac{5}{20}$
$x = 0.25$ ml

$$\frac{5}{20} \times \frac{1}{1} = 0.25 \text{ ml}$$

Chapter 12 Parenteral Dosages—Posttest 2, pp. 299-304

Proportion Formula

1. 4 mg:1 ml::2 mg:x ml
$4x = 2$
$x = \dfrac{2}{4}$
$x = 0.5$ ml

$$\frac{2}{4} \times \frac{1}{1} = 0.5 \text{ ml}$$

2. 4 mg:1 ml::2 mg:x ml
$4x = 2$
$x = \dfrac{2}{4}$
$x = 0.5$ ml

$$\frac{2}{4} \times \frac{1}{1} = 0.5 \text{ ml}$$

Proportion	Formula

3. 500 mg:10 ml::400 mg:x ml $\qquad$ $\dfrac{400}{500} \times \dfrac{10}{1} = \dfrac{4000}{500} = 8$ ml

$500x = 4000$

$x = \dfrac{4000}{500}$

$x = 8$ ml

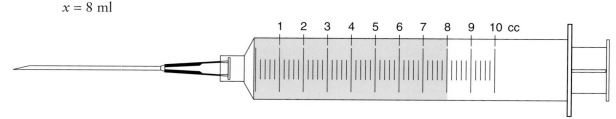

4. 50 mg:1 ml::75 mg:x ml $\qquad$ $\dfrac{75}{50} \times \dfrac{1}{1} = 1.5$ ml

$50x = 75$

$x = \dfrac{75}{50}$

$x = 1.5$ ml

5. 30 mg:1 ml::60 mg:x ml $\qquad$ $\dfrac{60}{30} \times \dfrac{1}{1} = 2$ ml

$30x = 60$

$x = \dfrac{60}{30}$

$x = 2$ ml

6. 25 mg:0.5 ml::15 mg:x ml $\qquad$ $\dfrac{5}{25} \times \dfrac{0.5}{1} = \dfrac{2.5}{25} = 0.1$ ml

$25x = 7.5$

$x = \dfrac{7.5}{25}$

$x = 0.3$ ml

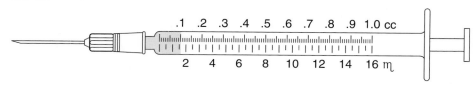

7. 0.4 mg:1 ml::0.3 mg:x ml $\qquad$ $\dfrac{0.3}{0.4} \times \dfrac{1}{1} = 0.75$ ml

$0.4x = 0.3$

$x = \dfrac{0.3}{0.4}$

$x = 0.75$ ml

8. 10 mg:1 ml::25 mg:x ml $\qquad$ $\dfrac{25}{10} \times \dfrac{1}{1} = 2.5$ ml

$10x = 25$

$x = \dfrac{25}{10}$

$x = 2.5$ ml

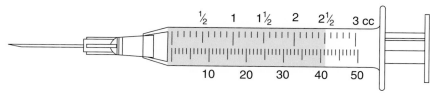

<table>
<tr><td align="center">**Proportion**</td><td align="center">**Formula**</td></tr>
</table>

9. 40 mg:1 ml::55 mg:x ml

   $40x = 55$

     $x = \dfrac{50}{40}$

     $x = 1.375$ ml

$\dfrac{55}{40} \times \dfrac{1}{1} = 1.375$ ml

10. 25 mg:1 ml::30 mg:x ml

   $25x = 30$

     $x = \dfrac{30}{25}$

     $x = 1.2$ ml

$\dfrac{30}{25} \times \dfrac{1}{1} = 1.2$ ml

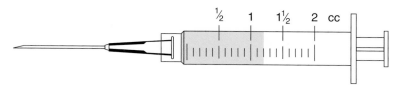

11. 100 mg:1 ml::200 mg:x ml

   $100x = 200$

     $x = \dfrac{200}{100}$

     $x = 2$ ml

$\dfrac{200}{100} \times \dfrac{1}{1} = 2$ ml

12. ¹⁄₂₀₀ gr:15 ♏::¹⁄₁₅₀ gr:x ♏

   $\dfrac{1}{200}x = \dfrac{15}{150}$

     $x = \dfrac{15}{\overset{3}{\cancel{150}}} \times \dfrac{\overset{4}{\cancel{200}}}{1}$

     $x = \dfrac{60}{3}$

     $x = 20$ ♏

$\dfrac{\dfrac{1}{150}}{\dfrac{1}{200}} \times \dfrac{15}{1} =$

$\dfrac{1}{150} \times \dfrac{200}{1} = \dfrac{200}{150}$

$\dfrac{200}{\underset{10}{\cancel{150}}} \times \dfrac{\overset{1}{\cancel{15}}}{1} = \dfrac{200}{10} = 20$ ♏

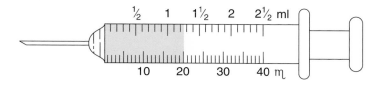

13. 1 g:2.5 ml::2 g:x ml

     $x = 5$ ml

$\dfrac{2}{1} \times \dfrac{2.5}{1} = 5$ ml

14. 40 mg:15 ♏::26 mg:x ♏

   $40x = 390$

     $x = 9.75$ ♏

$\dfrac{26}{40} \times \dfrac{15}{1} = \dfrac{390}{40} = 9.75$ ♏

Proportion	Formula

15. $50 \text{ mg}:15 \text{ m}::x \text{ mg}:6 \text{ m}$
$15x = 300$
$x = \dfrac{300}{15}$
$x = 20 \text{ mg}$

$$\dfrac{x}{\overset{}{\underset{10}{\cancel{50}}}} \times \dfrac{\overset{3}{\cancel{15}}}{1} = 6$$

$$\dfrac{3x}{10} = 6$$
$$3x = 6 \times 10$$
$$3x = 60$$
$$x = 20 \text{ mg}$$

16. $500 \text{ mcg}:30 \text{ m}::8 \text{ mcg}:x \text{ m}$
$500x = 240$
$x = \dfrac{240}{500}$
$x = 0.48 \text{ m or } 0.5 \text{ m}$

$$\dfrac{8}{500} \times \dfrac{30}{1} = \dfrac{240}{500} = 0.48 \text{ m or } 0.5 \text{ m}$$

17. $8 \text{ mg}:15 \text{ m}::4 \text{ mg}:x \text{ m}$
$8x = 60$
$x = \dfrac{60}{8}$
$x = 7.5 \text{ or } 8 \text{ m}$

$$\dfrac{4}{8} \times \dfrac{15}{1} = \dfrac{60}{8} = 7.5 \text{ or } 8 \text{ m}$$

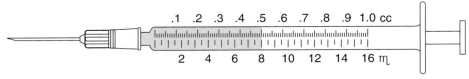

18. $50 \text{ mg}:2 \text{ ml}::100 \text{ mg}:x \text{ ml}$
$50x = 200$
$x = \dfrac{200}{50}$
$x = 4 \text{ ml}$

$$\dfrac{100}{50} \times \dfrac{2}{1} = \dfrac{200}{50} = 4 \text{ ml}$$

19. $120 \text{ mg}:1 \text{ ml}::200 \text{ mg}:x \text{ ml}$
$120x = 200$
$x = \dfrac{200}{120}$
$x = 1.66 \text{ ml}$

$$\dfrac{200}{120} \times \dfrac{1}{1} = 1.66 \text{ ml}$$

20. $13.6 \text{ mEq}:10 \text{ ml}::10 \text{ mEq}:x \text{ ml}$
$13.64x = 100$
$x = \dfrac{100}{13.6}$
$x = 7.35 \text{ ml}$

$$\dfrac{10}{13.6} \times \dfrac{10}{1} = \dfrac{100}{13.6} = 7.35 \text{ ml}$$

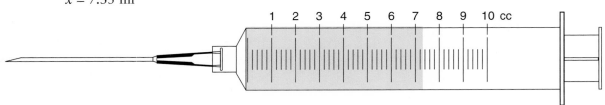

Chapter 13 Dosages Measured in Units—Work Sheet, pp. 311-316

Proportion | Formula

1. $400{,}000\ \text{U} : 5\ \text{ml} : : 200{,}000\ \text{U} : x\ \text{ml}$
$400{,}000x = 1{,}000{,}000$
$x = \dfrac{1{,}000{,}000}{400{,}000}$
$x = 2.5\ \text{ml}$

$\dfrac{200{,}000}{\cancel{400{,}000}} \times \dfrac{\overset{1}{\cancel{5}}}{1} =$
$80{,}000$
$\dfrac{200{,}000}{80{,}000} = 2.5\ \text{ml}$

2. $5000\ \text{U} : 1\ \text{ml} : : 7500\ \text{U} : x\ \text{ml}$
$5000x = 7500$
$x = \dfrac{7500}{5000}$
$x = 1.5\ \text{ml}$

$\dfrac{7500}{5000} \times \dfrac{1}{1} = 1.5\ \text{ml}$

3.

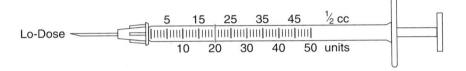

Lo-Dose

4. diluent 9.6 ml, 100,000 U/ml
$100{,}000\ \text{U} : 1\ \text{ml} : : 500{,}000\ \text{U} : x\ \text{ml}$
$100{,}000x = 500{,}000$
$x = \dfrac{500{,}000}{100{,}000}$
$x = 5\ \text{ml}$

$\dfrac{500{,}000}{100{,}000} \times \dfrac{1}{1} = 5\ \text{ml}$

diluent 4.6 ml, 200,000 U/ml
$200{,}000\ \text{U} : 1\ \text{ml} : : 500{,}000\ \text{U} : x\ \text{ml}$
$200{,}000x = 500{,}000$
$x = \dfrac{500{,}000}{200{,}000}$
$x = 2.5\ \text{ml}$

$\dfrac{500{,}000}{200{,}000} \times \dfrac{1}{1} = 2.5\ \text{ml}$

diluent 1.6 ml, 500,000 U/ml
$500{,}000\ \text{U} : 1\ \text{ml} : : 500{,}000\ \text{U} : x\ \text{ml}$
$500{,}000x = 500{,}000$
$x = \dfrac{500{,}000}{500{,}000}$
$x = 1\ \text{ml}$

$\dfrac{500{,}000}{500{,}000} \times \dfrac{1}{1} = 1\ \text{ml}$

5. $5000\ \text{U} : 1\ \text{ml} : : 2500\ \text{U} : x\ \text{ml}$
$5000x = 2500$
$x = \dfrac{2500}{5000}$
$x = 0.5\ \text{ml}$

$\dfrac{2500}{5000} \times \dfrac{1}{1} = 0.5\ \text{ml}$

Proportion	Formula

6.

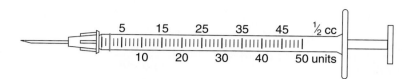

7. 10,000 U:1 ml::5000 U:*x* ml
10,000*x* = 5000
$$x = \frac{5000}{10,000}$$
x = 0.5 ml

$$\frac{5000}{10,000} \times \frac{1}{1} = 0.5 \text{ ml}$$

8. 200,000 U:5 ml::400,000 U:*x* ml
200,000*x* = 2,000,000
$$x = \frac{2,000,000}{200,000}$$
x = 10 ml

$$\frac{400,000}{200,000} \times \frac{5}{1} = \frac{2,000,000}{200,000} = 10 \text{ ml}$$

9.

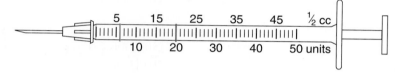

10. 400,000 U:5 ml::300,000 U:*x* ml
400,000*x* = 1,500,000
$$x = \frac{1,500,000}{400,000}$$
x = 3.75 ml

$$\frac{300,000}{400,000} \times \frac{5}{1} =$$
$$\frac{1,500,000}{400,000} = 3.75 \text{ ml}$$

11. 10,000 U:1 ml::6000 U:*x* ml
10,000*x* = 6000
$$x = \frac{6000}{10,000}$$
x = 0.6 ml

$$\frac{6000}{10,000} \times \frac{1}{1} = 0.6 \text{ ml}$$

12.

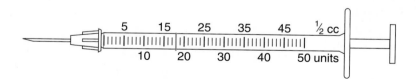

13.

Lo-Dose

Proportion	Formula

14. Diluent 9.6 ml, 100,000 U/ml
100,000 U : 1 ml : : 600,000 U : x ml

$$\frac{600,000}{100,000} \times \frac{1}{1} = 6 \text{ ml}$$

$$100,000x = 600,000$$
$$x = \frac{600,000}{100,000}$$
$$x = 6 \text{ ml}$$

diluent 4.6 ml, 200,000 U/ml
200,000 U : 1 ml : : 600,000 U : x ml
$$200,000x = 600,000$$
$$x = \frac{600,000}{200,000}$$
$$x = 3 \text{ ml}$$

$$\frac{600,000}{200,000} \times \frac{1}{1} = 3 \text{ ml}$$

diluent 1.6 ml, 500,000 U/ml
500,000 U : 1 ml : : 600,000 : x ml
$$500,000x = 600,000$$
$$x = \frac{600,000}{500,000}$$
$$x = 1.2 \text{ ml}$$

$$\frac{600,000}{500,000} \times \frac{1}{1} = 1.2 \text{ ml}$$

15. 5000 U : 1 ml : : 10,000 U : x ml
$$5000x = 10,000$$
$$x = \frac{10,000}{5000}$$
$$x = 2 \text{ ml}$$

$$\frac{10,000}{5000} \times \frac{1}{1} = 2 \text{ ml}$$

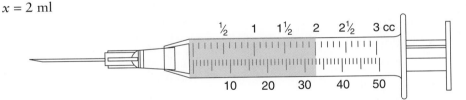

16. 10,000 U : 1 ml : : 5000 U : x ml
$$10,000x = 5000$$
$$x = \frac{5000}{10,000}$$
$$x = 0.5 \text{ ml}$$

$$\frac{5000}{10,000} \times \frac{1}{1} = 0.5 \text{ ml}$$

Proportion   Formula

17. $200,000 \, U:5 \, ml::300,000 \, U:x \, ml$

$200,000x = 1,500,000$

$x = \dfrac{1,500,000}{200,000}$

$x = 7.5 \, ml$

$\dfrac{300,000}{200,000} \times \dfrac{5}{1} =$

$\dfrac{1,500,000}{200,000} = 7.5 \, ml$

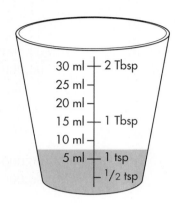

18.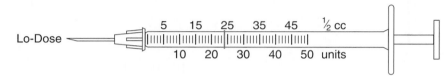

19. $10,000 \, U:1 \, ml::x \, U:0.5 \, ml$

$x = 5000 \, U$

$\dfrac{x}{10,000} \times \dfrac{1}{1} = 0.5 \, ml$

$\dfrac{x}{10,000} = 0.5$

$x = 0.5 \times 10,000$

$x = 5000 \, U$

20. $250,000 \, U:1 \, ml::200,000 \, U:x \, ml$

$250,000x = 200,000$

$x = \dfrac{200,000}{250,000}$

$x = 0.8 \, ml$

$\dfrac{200,000}{250,000} \times \dfrac{1}{1} = 0.8 \, ml$

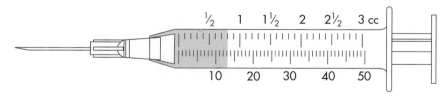

Chapter 13 Dosages Measured in Units—Posttest 1, pp. 317-320

Proportion   Formula

1. $400,000 \, U:5 \, ml::500,000 \, U:x \, ml$

$400,000x = 2,500,000$

$x = \dfrac{2,500,000}{400,000}$

$x = 6.25 \, ml$

$\dfrac{500,000}{400,000} \times \dfrac{5}{1} =$

$\dfrac{2,500,000}{400,000} = 6.25 \, ml$

2.   Insulin

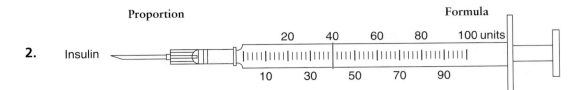

Proportion   Formula

3. $5000 \text{ U} : 1 \text{ ml} :: 7500 \text{ U} : x \text{ ml}$
$5000x = 7500$
$x = \dfrac{7500}{5000}$
$x = 1.5 \text{ ml}$

$$\frac{7500}{5000} \times \frac{1}{1} = 1.5 \text{ ml}$$

4.

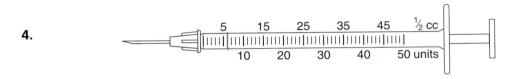

5. 11.5 ml best amount of diluent to add
1,000,000 U/ml
$1,000,000 \text{ U} : 1 \text{ ml} :: 3,000,000 \text{ U} : x \text{ ml}$
$1,000,000x = 3,000,000$
$x = \dfrac{3,000,000}{1,000,000}$
$x = 3 \text{ ml}$

$$\frac{3,000,000}{1,000,000} \times \frac{1}{1} = 3 \text{ ml}$$

6.   Insulin

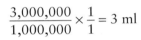

7. $10,000 \text{ U} : 1 \text{ ml} :: 20,000 \text{ U} : x \text{ ml}$
$10,000x = 20,000$
$x = \dfrac{20,000}{10,000}$
$x = 2 \text{ ml}$

$$\frac{20,000}{10,000} \times \frac{1}{1} = 2 \text{ ml}$$

8.

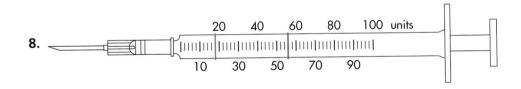

Proportion	Formula

9. $200,000 \text{ U} : 5 \text{ ml} :: 300,000 \text{ U} : x \text{ ml}$

$200,000x = 1,500,000$

$x = \dfrac{1,500,000}{200,000}$

$x = 7.5 \text{ ml}$

$\dfrac{300,000}{200,000} \times \dfrac{5}{1} =$

$\dfrac{1,500,000}{200,000} = 7.5 \text{ ml}$

10. Diluent added 9 ml

Concentration is 400 mg/ml

$400,000 \text{ mg} : 1 \text{ ml} :: 500,000 \text{ mg} : x \text{ ml}$

$400,000x = 500,000$

$x = \dfrac{500,000}{400,000}$

$x = 1.25 \text{ ml}$

$\dfrac{500,000}{400,000} \times \dfrac{1}{1} = 1.25 \text{ ml}$

11. $400,000 \text{ U} : 5 \text{ ml} :: 200,000 \text{ U} : x \text{ ml}$

$400,000x = 1,000,000$

$x = \dfrac{1,000,000}{400,000}$

$x = 2.5 \text{ ml}$

$\dfrac{200,000}{400,000} \times \dfrac{5}{1} =$

$\dfrac{1,000,000}{400,000} = 2.5 \text{ ml}$

12. $5000 \text{ U} : 1 \text{ ml} :: 7500 \text{ U} : x \text{ ml}$

$5000x = 7500$

$x = \dfrac{7500}{5000}$

$x = 1.5 \text{ ml}$

$\dfrac{7500}{5000} \times \dfrac{1}{1} = 1.5 \text{ ml}$

13. $1,000,000 \text{ U} : 1 \text{ ml} :: 500,000 \text{ U} : x \text{ ml}$

$1,000,000x = 500,000$

$x = \dfrac{500,000}{1,000,000}$

$x = 0.5 \text{ ml}$

$\dfrac{500,000}{1,000,000} \times \dfrac{1}{1} = 0.5 \text{ ml}$

14. Diluent added 6.6 ml

Concentration of 250 mg/ml

$250 \text{ mg} : 1 \text{ ml} :: 600 \text{ mg} : x \text{ ml}$

$250x = 600$

$x = \dfrac{600}{250}$

$x = 2.4 \text{ ml}$

$\dfrac{600}{250} \times \dfrac{1}{1} = 2.4 \text{ ml}$

15. $10,000 \text{ U} : 1 \text{ ml} :: 5000 \text{ U} : x \text{ ml}$

$10,000x = 5000$

$x = \dfrac{5000}{10,000}$

$x = 0.5 \text{ ml}$

$\dfrac{5000}{10,000} \times \dfrac{1}{1} = 0.5 \text{ ml}$

Chapter 13 Dosages Measured in Units—Posttest 2, pp. 321-325

Proportion   Formula

1.

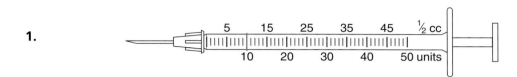

2. $10,000 \text{ U}:15 \text{ m}::1000 \text{ U}:x \text{ m}$
$10,000x = 15,000$
$x = \dfrac{15,000}{10,000}$
$x = 1.5 \text{ m}$

$\dfrac{1000}{10,000} \times \dfrac{15}{1} =$
$\dfrac{15,000}{10,000} = 1.5 \text{ m}$

3. $200,000 \text{ U}:1 \text{ ʒ}::500,000:x \text{ ʒ}$
$200,000x = 500,000$
$x = \dfrac{500,000}{200,000}$
$x = 2.5 \text{ ʒ}$

$\dfrac{500,000}{200,000} \times \dfrac{1}{1} = 2.5 \text{ ʒ}$

4.

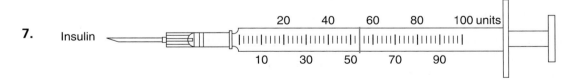

5. $1000 \text{ U}:1 \text{ ml}::1500 \text{ U}:x \text{ ml}$
$1000x = 1500$
$x = \dfrac{1500}{1000}$
$x = 1.5 \text{ ml}$

$\dfrac{1500}{1000} \times \dfrac{1}{1} = 1.5 \text{ ml}$

6. $1,000,000 \text{ U}:1 \text{ ml}::1,200,000 \text{ U}:x \text{ ml}$
$1,000,000x = 1,200,000$
$x = \dfrac{1,200,000}{1,000,000}$
$x = 1.2 \text{ ml}$

$\dfrac{1,200,000}{1,000,000} \times \dfrac{1}{1} = 1.2 \text{ ml}$

7. Insulin

8. Lo-Dose

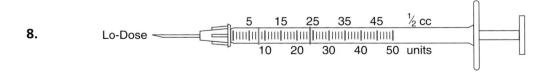

Proportion	Formula

9. $400{,}000\,U:5\,ml::300{,}000\,U:x\,ml$
$400{,}000x = 1{,}500{,}000$
$x = \dfrac{1{,}500{,}000}{400{,}000}$
$x = 3.75\,ml$

$\dfrac{300{,}000}{400{,}000} \times \dfrac{5}{1} =$
$\dfrac{1{,}500{,}000}{400{,}000} = 3.75\,ml$

10. $5000\,U:1\,ml::6000\,U:x\,ml$
$5000x = 6000$
$x = \dfrac{6000}{5000}$
$x = 1.2\,ml$

$\dfrac{6000}{5000} \times \dfrac{1}{1} = 1.2\,ml$

11. $9.6\,ml$ diluent, $100{,}000\,U/ml$
$100{,}000\,U:1\,ml::600{,}000\,U:x\,ml$
$100{,}000x = 600{,}000$
$x = \dfrac{600{,}000}{100{,}000}$
$x = 6\,ml$

$\dfrac{600{,}000}{100{,}000} \times \dfrac{1}{1} = 6\,ml$

$4.6\,ml$ diluent, $200{,}000\,U/ml$
$200{,}000\,U:1\,ml::600{,}000\,U:x\,ml$
$200{,}000x = 600{,}000$
$x = \dfrac{600{,}000}{200{,}000}$
$x = 3\,ml$

$\dfrac{600{,}000}{200{,}000} \times \dfrac{1}{1} = 3\,ml$

$1.6\,ml$ diluent, $500{,}000\,U/ml$
$500{,}000\,U:1\,ml::600{,}000\,U:x\,ml$
$500{,}000x = 600{,}000$
$x = \dfrac{600{,}000}{500{,}000}$
$x = 1.2\,ml$

$\dfrac{600{,}000}{500{,}000} \times \dfrac{1}{1} = 1.2\,ml$

12. $5000\,U:1\,ml::10{,}000\,U:x\,ml$
$5000x = 10{,}000$
$x = \dfrac{10{,}000}{5{,}000}$
$x = 2\,ml$

$\dfrac{10{,}000}{5000} \times \dfrac{1}{1} = 2\,ml$

13.

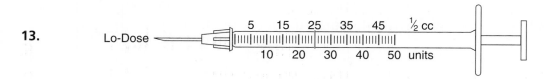

Proportion	Formula

14. 5000 U : 1 ml : : 7500 U : x ml

$5000x = 7500$

$x = \dfrac{7500}{5000}$

$x = 1.5$ ml

$\dfrac{7500}{5000} \times \dfrac{1}{1} = 1.5$ ml

15. 10,000 U : 1 ml : : 20,000 U : x ml

$10,000x = 20,000$

$x = \dfrac{20,000}{10,000}$

$x = 2$ ml

$\dfrac{20,000}{10,000} \times \dfrac{1}{1} = 2$ ml

Chapter 14 IV Flow Rates—Work Sheet, pp. 343-348

1. 1000 ml : 8 h. : : x ml : 1 h.

$8x = 1000$

$x = \dfrac{1000}{8}$

$x = 125$ ml/h.

125 ml : 60 min : : x ml : 1 min

$60x = 125$

$x = \dfrac{125}{60}$

$x = 2.08$ ml/min

12 gtt : 1 ml : : x gtt : 2.08 ml

$x = 24.96$ or 25 gtt/min

2. 800 ml : 8 h. : : x ml : 1 h.

$8x = 800$

$x = \dfrac{800}{8}$

$x = 100$ ml/h.

100 ml : 60 min : : x ml : 1 min

$60x = 100$

$x = \dfrac{100}{60}$

$x = 1.67$ ml/min

10 gtt : 1 ml : : x gtt : 1.67 ml

$x = 16.7$ or 17 gtt/min

3. 250 ml : 2 h. : x ml : 1 h.

$2x = 250$

$x = \dfrac{250}{2}$

$x = 125$ ml/h.

125 ml : 60 min : : x ml : 1 min

$60x = 125$

$x = \dfrac{125}{60}$

$x = 2.08$ ml/min

15 gtt : 1 ml : : x gtt : 2.08 ml

$x = 31.2$ or 31 gtt/min

4. 1500 ml : 10 h. : : x ml : 1 h.

$10x = 1500$

$x = \dfrac{1500}{10}$

$x = 150$ ml/h.

150 ml : 60 min : : x ml : 1 min

$60x = 150$

$x = \dfrac{150}{60}$

$x = 2.5$ ml/min

15 gtt : 1 ml : : x gtt : 2.5 ml

$x = 37.5$ or 38 gtt/min

5. 3000 ml : 48 h. : : x ml : 1 h.
   48x = 3000
   $$x = \frac{3000}{48}$$
   x = 62.5 ml/h.

   62.5 ml : 60 min : : x ml : 1 min
   60x = 62.5
   $$x = \frac{62.5}{60}$$
   x = 1.04 ml/min

   10 gtt : 1 ml : : x gtt : 1.04 ml
   x = 10.4 or 10 gtt/min

6. 100 ml/h. from problem 6

   100 ml : 60 min : : x ml : 1 min
   60x = 100
   $$x = \frac{100}{60}$$
   x = 1.67 ml/min

   12 gtt : 1 ml : : x gtt : 1.67
   x = 20.04 or 20 gtt/min

7. 500 ml : 4 h. : : x ml : 1 h.
   4x = 500
   $$x = \frac{500}{4}$$
   x = 125 ml/h.

   125 ml : 60 min : : x ml : 1 min
   60x = 125
   $$x = \frac{125}{60}$$
   x = 2.08 ml/min

   15 gtt : 1 ml : : x gtt : 2.08 ml
   x = 31.2 or 31 gtt/min

8. 1500 ml : 16 h. : : x ml : 1 h.
   16x = 1500
   $$x = \frac{1500}{16}$$
   x = 93.75 ml/h.

   93.75 ml : 60 min : : x ml : 1 min
   60x = 93.75
   $$x = \frac{93.75}{60}$$
   x = 1.56 ml/min

   10 gtt : 1 ml : : x gtt : 1.56 ml
   x = 15.6 or 16 gtt/min

9. 10 ml/h. from problem 9

   10 ml : 60 min : : x ml : 1 min
   60x = 10
   $$x = \frac{10}{60}$$
   x = 0.17 ml/min

   60 gtt : 1 ml : : x gtt : 0.17 ml
   x = 10.2 or 10 gtt/min

10. 500 ml : 6 h. : : x ml : 1 h.
   6x = 500
   $$x = \frac{500}{6}$$
   x = 83.33 ml/h.

   83.33 ml : 60 min : : x ml : 1 min
   60x = 83.33
   $$x = \frac{83.33}{60}$$
   x = 1.39 ml/min

   12 gtt : 1 ml : : x gtt : 1.39 ml
   x = 16.68 or 17 gtt/min

11. 800 ml : 6 h. : : x ml : 1 h.
   6x = 800
   $$x = \frac{800}{6}$$
   x = 133.33 ml/h.

   133.33 ml : 60 min : : x ml : 1 min
   60x = 133.33
   $$x = \frac{133.33}{60}$$
   x = 2.22 ml/min

   15 gtt : 1 ml : : x gtt : 2.22 ml
   x = 33.3 or 33 gtt/min

12. 2 ml/h. from problem 12

   2 ml : 60 min : : x ml : 1 min
   60x = 2
   $$x = \frac{2}{60}$$
   x = 0.03 ml/min

   60 gtt : 1 ml : : x gtt : 0.03 ml
   x = 1.8 or 2 gtt/min

13. $250 \text{ ml}:100 \text{ U}::1 \text{ ml}:x \text{ U}$
$250x = 100$
$$x = \frac{100}{250}$$
$x = 0.4 \text{ U/ml}$

$0.4 \text{ U}:1 \text{ ml}::12 \text{ U}:x \text{ ml}$
$0.4x = 12$
$$x = \frac{12}{0.4}$$
$x = 30 \text{ ml/h.}$

$30 \text{ ml}:60 \text{ min}::x \text{ ml}:1 \text{ min}$
$60x = 30$
$$x = \frac{30}{60}$$
$x = 0.5 \text{ ml/min}$

$60 \text{ gtt}:1 \text{ ml}::x \text{ gtt}:0.5 \text{ ml}$
$x = 30 \text{ gtt/min}$

14. $500 \text{ ml}:100 \text{ U}::1 \text{ ml}:x \text{ U}$
$500x = 100$
$$x = \frac{100}{500}$$
$x = 0.2 \text{ U/ml}$

$0.2 \text{ U}:1 \text{ ml}::8 \text{ U}:x \text{ ml}$
$0.2x = 8$
$$x = \frac{8}{0.2}$$
$x = 40 \text{ ml/h.}$

$40 \text{ ml}:60 \text{ min}::x \text{ ml}:1 \text{ min}$
$60x = 40$
$$x = \frac{40}{60}$$
$x = 0.67 \text{ ml/min}$

$60 \text{ gtt}:1 \text{ ml}::x \text{ gtt}:0.67 \text{ ml}$
$x = 40.2 \text{ or } 40 \text{ gtt/min}$

15. $500 \text{ ml}:10{,}000 \text{ U}::x \text{ ml}:1 \text{ U}$
$10{,}000 \, x = 500$
$$x = \frac{500}{10{,}000}$$
$x = 0.05 \text{ ml/U}$

$0.5 \text{ ml}:1 \text{ U}::x \text{ ml}:100 \text{ U}$
$x = 50 \text{ ml/h.}$
$50 \text{ ml}:60 \text{ min}::x \text{ ml}:1 \text{ min}$
$60x = 50$
$$x = \frac{50}{60}$$
$x = 0.83 \text{ ml/min}$

$60 \text{ gtt}:1 \text{ ml}::x \text{ gtt}:0.83 \text{ ml}$
$x = 49.8 \text{ or } 50 \text{ gtt/min}$

16. $1000 \text{ ml}:30{,}000 \text{ U}::x \text{ ml}:1 \text{ U}$
$30{,}000x = 1000$
$$x = \frac{1000}{30{,}000}$$
$x = 0.03 \text{ ml/U}$

$0.03 \text{ ml}:1 \text{ U}::x \text{ ml}:1000 \text{ U}$
$x = 30 \text{ ml/h.}$

$30 \text{ ml}:60 \text{ min}::x \text{ ml}:1 \text{ min}$
$60x = 30$
$$x = \frac{30}{60}$$
$x = 0.5 \text{ ml/min}$

$60 \text{ gtt}:1 \text{ ml}::x \text{ gtt}:0.5 \text{ ml}$
$x = 30 \text{ gtt/min}$

17. $12 \text{ mcg}:1 \text{ kg}::x \text{ mcg}:75 \text{ kg}$
$x = 900 \text{ mcg for } 75 \text{ kg patient/min}$

$1{,}000{,}000 \text{ mcg}:250 \text{ ml}::x \text{ mcg}:1 \text{ ml}$
$250x = 1{,}000{,}000$
$$x = \frac{1{,}000{,}000}{250}$$
$x = 4000 \text{ mcg/ml}$

$4000 \text{ mcg}:1 \text{ ml}::900 \text{ mcg}:x \text{ ml}$
$4000x = 900$
$$x = \frac{900}{4000}$$
$x = 0.23 \text{ ml/min}$

$60 \text{ gtt}:1 \text{ ml}::x \text{ gtt}:0.23 \text{ ml}$
$x = 60 \times 0.23$
$x = 13.8 \text{ or } 14 \text{ gtt/min}$

18. $0.4 \text{ mg}:1 \text{ kg}::x \text{ mg}:55 \text{ kg}$
$x = 0.4 \times 55$
$x = 22 \text{ mg}/55 \text{ kg/h}.$

$22 \text{ mg}:60 \text{ min}::x \text{ mg}:1 \text{ min}$
$60x = 22$
$x = \dfrac{22}{60}$
$x = 0.37 \text{ mg/min}$

$2000 \text{ mg}:1000 \text{ ml}::x \text{ mg}:1 \text{ ml}$
$1000x = 2000$
$x = \dfrac{2000}{1000}$
$x = 2 \text{ mg/ml}$

$2 \text{ mg}:1 \text{ ml}::0.37 \text{ mg}:x \text{ ml}$
$2x = 0.37$
$x = \dfrac{0.37}{2}$
$x = 0.185 \text{ or } 0.19 \text{ ml/min}$

$60 \text{ gtt}:1 \text{ ml}::x \text{ gtt}:0.19 \text{ ml}$
$x = 60 \times 0.19$
$x = 11.4 \text{ or } 11 \text{ gtt/min}$

19. $3 \text{ mcg}:1 \text{ kg}::x \text{ mcg}:66 \text{ kg}$
$x = 198 \text{ mcg}/66 \text{ kg patient/min}$

$100,000 \text{ mcg}:500 \text{ ml}::x \text{ mcg}:1 \text{ ml}$
$500x = 100,000$
$x = \dfrac{100,000}{500}$
$x = 200 \text{ mcg/ml}$

$200 \text{ mcg}:1 \text{ ml}::198 \text{ mcg}:x \text{ ml}$
$200x = 198$
$x = \dfrac{198}{200}$
$x = 0.99 \text{ ml/min}$

$60 \text{ gtt}:1 \text{ ml}::x \text{ gtt}:0.99 \text{ ml}$
$x = 59.4 \text{ gtt/min or } 59 \text{ gtt/min}$

20. $5 \text{ mcg}:1 \text{ kg}::x \text{ mcg}:80 \text{ kg}$
$x = 400 \text{ mcg}/80 \text{ kg patient}$

$250,000 \text{ mcg}:250::x \text{ mcg}:1 \text{ ml}$
$250x = 250,000$
$x = \dfrac{250,000}{250}$
$x = 1000 \text{ mcg}:1 \text{ ml}$

$1000 \text{ mcg}:1 \text{ ml}::400 \text{ mcg}:x \text{ ml}$
$1000x = 400$
$x = \dfrac{400}{1000}$
$x = 0.4 \text{ ml/min}$

$60 \text{ gtt}:1 \text{ ml}::x \text{ gtt}:0.4 \text{ ml}$
$x = 24 \text{ gtt/min}$

21. $500 \text{ ml}:200 \text{ U}::x \text{ ml}:10 \text{ U}$
$200x = 5000$
$x = \dfrac{5000}{200}$
$x = 25 \text{ ml/h}.$

$25 \text{ ml}:60 \text{ min}::x \text{ ml}:1 \text{ min}$
$60x = 25$
$x = \dfrac{25}{60}$
$x = 0.42 \text{ ml/min}$

$60 \text{ gtt}:1 \text{ ml}::x \text{ gtt}:0.42$
$x = 25.2 \text{ or } 25 \text{ gtt/min}$

22. $500 \text{ ml}:6 \text{ h.}::x \text{ ml}:1 \text{ h.}$
$6x = 500$
$x = \dfrac{500}{6}$
$x = 83.33 \text{ ml/h}.$

$83.33 \text{ ml}:60 \text{ min}::x \text{ ml}:1 \text{ min}$
$60x = 83.33$
$x = \dfrac{83.33}{60}$
$x = 1.388 \text{ or } 1.39 \text{ ml/min}$

$12 \text{ gtt}:1 \text{ ml}::x \text{ gtt}:1.39 \text{ ml}$
$x = 16.68 \text{ or } 17 \text{ gtt/min}$

23. 1000 ml:40,000 U::x ml:1 U
40,000x = 1000
$$x = \frac{1000}{40,000}$$
x = 0.025 ml/U

0.25 ml:1 U::x ml:200 U
x = 50 ml/h.

50 ml:60 min::x ml:1 min
60x = 50
$$x = \frac{50}{60}$$
x = 0.83 ml/min

60 gtt:1 ml::x gtt:0.83 ml
x = 49.8 or 50 gtt/min

24. 500 ml:4 h.::x ml:1 h.
4x = 500
$$x = \frac{500}{4}$$
x = 125 ml/h.

125 ml:60 min::x ml:1 min
60x = 125
$$x = \frac{125}{60}$$
x = 2.08 ml/min

12 gtt:1 ml::x gtt:2.08 ml
x = 24.96 or 25 gtt/min

25. 1000 ml:12 h.::x ml:1 h.
12x = 1000
x = 83.33 ml/h.

83.33:60 min::x ml:1 min
60x = 83.33
$$x = \frac{83.33}{60}$$
x = 1.39 ml/min

15 gtt:1 ml::x gtt:1.39 ml
x = 20.85 or 21 gtt/min

Chapter 14 IV Flow Rates—Posttest 1, pp. 349-352

1. 1000 ml:12 h.::x ml:1 h.
12x = 1000
$$x = \frac{1000}{12}$$
x = 83.33 ml/h.

83.33 ml:60 min::x ml:1 min
60x = 83.33
$$x = \frac{83.33}{60}$$
x = 1.39 ml/min

15 gtt:1 ml::x gtt:1.39 ml
x = 20.85 or 21 gtt/min

2. 500 ml:4 h.::x ml:1 h.
4x = 500
$$x = \frac{500}{4}$$
x= 125 ml/h.

125 ml:60 min::x ml:1 min
60x = 125
$$x = \frac{125}{60}$$
x = 2.08 ml/min

12 gtt:1 ml::x gtt:2.08 ml
x = 24.96 or 25 gtt/min

3. 150 ml/h. from problem 3

150 ml:60 min::x ml:1 min
$60x = 150$
$$x = \frac{150}{60}$$
$x = 2.5$ ml/min

15 gtt:1 ml::x gtt:2.5 ml
$x = 37.5$ or 38 gtt/min

4. 750 ml:10 h.::x ml:1 h.
$10x = 750$
$$x = \frac{750}{10}$$
$x = 75$ ml/h.

75 ml:60 min::x ml:1 min
$60x = 75$
$$x = \frac{75}{60}$$
$x = 1.25$ ml/min

10 gtt:1 ml::x gtt:1.25 ml
$x = 12.5$ or 13 gtt/min

5. 50 ml:30 min::x ml:1 min
$30x = 50$
$$x = \frac{50}{30}$$
$x = 1.67$ ml/min

12 gtt:1 ml::x gtt:1.67 ml
$x = 20$ gtt/min

6. 1000 ml:500 U::1 ml:x U
$1000x = 500$
$$x = \frac{500}{1000}$$
$x = 0.5$ U/ml

0.5 U:1 ml::9 U:x ml
$0.5x = 9$
$$x = \frac{9}{0.5}$$
$x = 18$ ml/h.

18 ml:60 min::x ml:1 min
$60x = 18$
$$x = \frac{18}{60}$$
$x = 0.3$ ml/min

60 gtt:1 ml::x gtt:0.3 ml
$x = 18$ gtt/min

7. 1000 ml:30,000 U::1 ml:x U
$1000x = 30,000$
$$x = \frac{30,000}{1000}$$
$x = 30$ U/ml

30 U:1 ml::500 U:x ml
$30x = 500$
$$x = \frac{500}{30}$$
$x = 16.67$ ml/h.

16.67 ml:60 min::x ml:1 min
$60x = 16.67$
$$x = \frac{16.67}{60}$$
$x = 0.28$ ml/min

60 gtt:1 ml::x gtt:0.28 ml
$x = 16.8$ or 17 gtt/min

8. 3 mcg:1 kg::x mcg:82 kg
$x = 246$ mcg/min/82 kg patient

250 ml:50,000 mcg::1 ml:x mcg
$250x = 50,000$
$$x = \frac{50,000}{250}$$
$x = 200$ mcg/ml

200 mcg:1 ml::246 mcg:x ml
$200x = 246$
$$x = \frac{246}{200}$$
$x = 1.23$ ml/min

60 gtt:1 ml::x gtt:1.23 ml
$x = 73.8$ or 74 gtt/min

9. 500 ml:10,000 U::1 ml:x U
$500x = 10,000$
$$x = \frac{10,000}{500}$$
$x = 20$ U/ml

20 U:1 ml::100 U:x ml
$20x = 100$
$$x = \frac{100}{20}$$
$x = 5$ ml/h.

5 ml:60 min::x ml:1 min
$60x = 5$
$$x = \frac{5}{60}$$
$x = 0.08$ ml/min

60 gtt:1 ml::x gtt:0.08 ml
$x = 4.8$ or 5 gtt/min

10. 30 ml/h. from problem 10

30 ml:60 min::x ml:1 min
60x = 30
$$x = \frac{30}{60}$$
x = 0.5 ml/min

20 gtt:1 ml::x gtt:0.5 ml
x = 10 gtt/min

11. 250 ml:250 U::1 ml:x U
250x = 250
$$x = \frac{250}{250}$$
x = 1 U/ml

1 U:1 ml::7 U:x ml
x = 7 ml/h.

7 ml:60 min::x ml:1 min
60x = 7
$$x = \frac{7}{60}$$
x = 0.12 ml/min

60 gtt:1 ml::x gtt:0.12 ml
x = 7.2 or 7 gtt/min

12. 1000 ml:30,000 U::1 ml:x U
1000x = 30,000
$$x = \frac{30,000}{1000}$$
x = 30 U/ml

30 U:1 ml::1500 U:x ml
30x = 1500
$$x = \frac{1500}{30}$$
x = 50 ml/h.

50 ml:60 min::x ml:1 min
60x = 50
$$x = \frac{50}{60}$$
x = 0.83 ml/min

60 gtt:1 ml::x gtt:0.83 ml
x = 49.8 or 50 gtt/min

13. 1000 ml:18 h.::x ml:1 h.
18x = 1000
$$x = \frac{1000}{18}$$
x = 55.56 ml/h.

55.56 ml:60 min::x ml:1 min
60x = 55.56
$$x = \frac{55.56}{60}$$
x = 0.93 ml/min

10 gtt:1 ml::x gtt:0.93 ml
x = 9.3 or 9 gtt/min

14. 250 ml:24 h.::x ml:1 h.
24x = 250
$$x = \frac{250}{24}$$
x = 10.42 ml/h.

10.42 ml:60 min::x ml:1 min
60x = 10.42
$$x = \frac{10.42}{60}$$
x = 0.17 ml/min

60 gtt:1 ml::x gtt:0.17 ml
x = 10.2 or 10 gtt/min

15. 1500 ml:16 h.::x ml:1 h.
16x = 1500
$$x = \frac{1500}{16}$$
x = 93.75 ml/h.

93.75 ml:60 min::x ml:1 min
60x = 93.75
$$x = \frac{93.75}{60}$$
x = 1.56 ml/min

10 gtt:1 ml::x gtt:1.56 ml
x = 15.6 or 16 gtt/min

Chapter 14 IV Flow Rates—Posttest 2, pp. 353-356

1. $500 \text{ ml}:6 \text{ h}.::x \text{ ml}:1 \text{ h}.$
$6x = 500$
$x = \dfrac{500}{6}$
$x = 83.33 \text{ ml/h}.$

$83.33:60 \text{ min}::x \text{ ml}:1 \text{ min}$
$60x = 83.33$
$x = \dfrac{83.33}{60}$
$x = 1.39 \text{ ml/min}$

$15 \text{ gtt}:1 \text{ ml}::x \text{ gtt}:1.39 \text{ ml}$
$x = 20.85 \text{ or } 21 \text{ gtt/min}$

2. 30 ml/h. from problem 2

$30 \text{ ml}:60 \text{ min}::x \text{ ml}:1 \text{ min}$
$60x = 30$
$x = \dfrac{30}{60}$
$x = 0.5 \text{ ml/min}$

$20 \text{ gtt}:1 \text{ ml}::x \text{ gtt}:0.5 \text{ ml}$
$x = 10 \text{ gtt/min}$

3. $3000 \text{ ml}:24 \text{ h}.::x \text{ ml}:1 \text{ h}.$
$24x = 3000$
$x = \dfrac{3000}{24}$
$x = 125 \text{ ml/h}.$

$125 \text{ ml}:60 \text{ min}::x \text{ ml}:1 \text{ min}$
$60x = 125$
$x = \dfrac{125}{60}$
$x = 2.08 \text{ ml/min}$

$12 \text{ gtt}:1 \text{ ml}::x \text{ gtt}:2.08 \text{ ml}$
$x = 24.96 \text{ or } 25 \text{ gtt/min}$

4. 3 ml/h. from problem 4

$3 \text{ ml}:60 \text{ min}::x \text{ ml}:1 \text{ min}$
$60x = 3$
$x = \dfrac{3}{60}$
$x = 0.05 \text{ ml/min}$

$60 \text{ gtt}:1 \text{ ml}::x \text{ gtt}:0.05 \text{ ml}$
$x = 3 \text{ gtt/min}$

5. $1000 \text{ ml}:18 \text{ h}.::x \text{ ml}:1 \text{ h}.$
$18x = 1000$
$x = \dfrac{1000}{18}$
$x = 55.56 \text{ ml/h}.$

$55.56 \text{ ml}:60 \text{ min}::x \text{ ml}:1 \text{ min}$
$60x = 55.56$
$x = \dfrac{55.56}{60}$
$x = 0.93 \text{ ml/min}$

$10 \text{ gtt}:1 \text{ ml}::x \text{ gtt}:0.93 \text{ ml}$
$x = 9.3 \text{ or } 9 \text{ gtt/min}$

6. 1 U/ml from problem 6

$1 \text{ U}:1 \text{ ml}::7 \text{ U}:x \text{ ml}$
$x = 7 \text{ ml/h}.$

$7 \text{ ml}:60 \text{ min}::x \text{ ml}:1 \text{ min}$
$60x = 7$
$x = \dfrac{7}{60}$
$x = 0.12 \text{ ml/min}$

$60 \text{ gtt}:1 \text{ ml}::x \text{ gtt}:0.12 \text{ ml}$
$x = 7.2 \text{ or } 7 \text{ gtt/min}$

7. $1000 \text{ ml}:30,000 \text{ U}::1 \text{ ml}:x \text{ U}$
$1000x = 30,000$
$x = \dfrac{30,000}{1000}$
$x = 30 \text{ U/ml}$

$30 \text{ U}:1 \text{ ml}::1500 \text{ U}:x \text{ ml}$
$30x = 1500$
$x = \dfrac{1500}{30}$
$x = 50 \text{ ml/h}.$

$50 \text{ ml}:60 \text{ min}::x \text{ ml}:1 \text{ min}$
$60x = 50$
$x = \dfrac{50}{60}$
$x = 0.83 \text{ ml/min}$

$60 \text{ gtt}:1 \text{ ml}::x \text{ gtt}:0.83 \text{ ml}$
$x = 49.8 \text{ or } 50 \text{ gtt/min}$

8. $0.5 \text{ mcg} : 1 \text{ kg} : : x \text{ mcg} : 75 \text{ kg}$
$x = 37.5 \text{ mcg/min/75 kg patient}$

$50,000 \text{ mcg} : 500 \text{ ml} : : x \text{ mcg} : 1 \text{ ml}$
$500x = 50,000$
$x = \dfrac{50,000}{500}$
$x = 100 \text{ mcg/ml}$

$100 \text{ mcg} : 1 \text{ ml} : : 37.5 \text{ mcg} : x \text{ ml}$
$100x = 37.5$
$x = \dfrac{37.5}{100}$
$x = 0.375 \text{ ml/min}$

$60 \text{ gtt} : 1 \text{ ml} : : x \text{ gtt} : 0.375 \text{ ml}$
$x = 22.5 \text{ or } 23 \text{ gtt/ml}$

9. $250 \text{ ml} : 12 \text{ h.} : : x \text{ ml} : 1 \text{ h.}$
$12x = 250$
$x = \dfrac{250}{12}$
$x = 20.83 \text{ ml/h.}$

$20.83 \text{ ml} : 60 \text{ min} : : x \text{ ml} : 1 \text{ min}$
$60x = 20.83$
$x = \dfrac{20.83}{60}$
$x = 0.35 \text{ ml/min}$

$60 \text{ gtt} : 1 \text{ ml} : : x \text{ gtt} : 0.35 \text{ ml}$
$x = 21 \text{ gtt/min}$

10. $500 \text{ ml} : 12 \text{ h.} : : x \text{ ml} : 1 \text{ h.}$
$12x = 500$
$x = \dfrac{500}{12}$
$x = 41.67 \text{ ml/h.}$

$41.67 \text{ ml} : 60 \text{ min} : : x \text{ ml} : 1 \text{ min}$
$60x = 41.67$
$x = \dfrac{41.67}{60}$
$x = 0.69 \text{ ml/min}$

$12 \text{ gtt} : 1 \text{ ml} : : x \text{ gtt} : 0.69 \text{ ml}$
$x = 8.28 \text{ or } 8 \text{ gtt/min}$

11. $500 \text{ ml} : 100 \text{ U} : : 1 \text{ ml} : x \text{ U}$
$500x = 100$
$x = \dfrac{100}{500}$
$x = 0.2 \text{ U/ml}$

$0.2 \text{ U} : 1 \text{ ml} : : 2 \text{ U} : x \text{ ml}$
$0.2x = 2$
$x = \dfrac{2}{0.2}$
$x = 10 \text{ ml/h.}$

$10 \text{ ml} : 60 \text{ min} : : x \text{ ml} : 1 \text{ min}$
$60x = 10$
$x = \dfrac{10}{60}$
$x = 0.17 \text{ ml/min}$

$60 \text{ gtt} : 1 \text{ ml} : : x \text{ gtt} : 0.17 \text{ ml}$
$x = 10.2 \text{ or } 10 \text{ gtt/min}$

12. 250 ml/h. from problem 12
$250 \text{ ml} : 60 \text{ min} : : x \text{ ml} : 1 \text{ min}$
$60x = 250$
$x = \dfrac{250}{60}$
$x = 4.17 \text{ ml/min}$

$10 \text{ gtt} : 1 \text{ ml} : : x \text{ gtt} : 4.17 \text{ ml}$
$x = 41.7 \text{ or } 42 \text{ gtt/min}$

13. $250 \text{ ml} : 50,000 \text{ U} : : 1 \text{ ml} : x \text{ U}$
$250x = 50,000$
$x = \dfrac{50,000}{250}$
$x = 200 \text{ U/ml}$

$200 \text{ U} : 1 \text{ ml} : : 1200 \text{ U} : x \text{ ml}$
$200x = 1200$
$x = \dfrac{1200}{200}$
$x = 6 \text{ ml/h.}$

$6 \text{ ml} : 60 \text{ min} : : x \text{ ml} : 1 \text{ min}$
$60x = 6$
$x = \dfrac{6}{60}$
$x = 0.1 \text{ ml/min}$

$60 \text{ gtt} : 1 \text{ ml} : : x \text{ gtt} : 0.1 \text{ ml}$
$x = 6 \text{ gtt/min}$

14. 120 ml/h. from problem 14

$120\ ml:60\ min::x\ ml:1\ min$
$60x = 120$
$x = \dfrac{120}{60}$
$x = 2\ ml/min$

$12\ gtt:1\ ml::x\ gtt:2\ ml$
$x = 24\ gtt/min$

15. $500\ ml:6\ h.::x\ ml:1\ h.$
$6x = 500$
$x = \dfrac{500}{6}$
$x = 83.33\ ml/h.$

$83.33:60\ min::x\ ml:1\ min$
$60x = 83.33$
$x = \dfrac{83.33}{60}$
$x = 1.39\ ml/min$

$12\ gtt:1\ ml::x\ gtt:1.39\ ml$
$x = 16.68\ or\ 17\ gtt/ml$

Chapter 15 Dimensional Analysis and the Calculation of Drug Dosages— Work Sheet, pp. 361-362

1. $x\ tablet = \dfrac{1\ tablet}{5\ mg} \times 10\ mg$
$x = \dfrac{1 \times 10}{5}$
$x = 2\ tablets$

2. $x\ ml = \dfrac{5\ ml}{25\ mg} \times 60\ mg$
$x = \dfrac{5 \times 60}{25}$
$x = 12\ ml$

3. $x\ tablet = \dfrac{1\ tablet}{50\ mg} \times \dfrac{1000\ mg}{1\ g} \times 0.025\ g$
$x = \dfrac{1 \times 1000 \times 0.025}{50}$
$x = \dfrac{25}{50}$
$x = \tfrac{1}{2}\ tablet$

4. $x\ tablet = \dfrac{1\ tablet}{\frac{1}{4}\ gr} \times \dfrac{1\ gr}{60\ mg} \times 30\ mg$
$x = \dfrac{1 \times 1 \times 30}{\frac{1}{4} \times 60}$
$x = \dfrac{30}{15}$
$x = 2\ tablets$

5. $x\ capsule = \dfrac{1\ capsule}{250\ mg} \times \dfrac{1000\ mg}{1\ g} \times 0.5\ g$
$x = \dfrac{1 \times 1000 \times 0.5}{250}$
$x = \dfrac{500}{250}$
$x = 2\ capsules$

6. $x\ ml = \dfrac{1\ ml}{4\ mg} \times 3\ mg$
$x = \dfrac{1 \times 3}{4}$
$x = \dfrac{3}{4}\ or\ 0.75\ ml$

7. $x\ ml = \dfrac{1\ ml}{0.1\ mg} \times \dfrac{1\ mg}{1000\ mcg} \times 40\ mcg$
$x = \dfrac{1 \times 1 \times 40}{0.1 \times 1000}$
$x = \dfrac{40}{100}$
$x = 0.4\ ml$

8. $x\ ml = \dfrac{1\ ml}{2\ mg} \times 1\ mg$
$x = \dfrac{1}{2}$
$x = 0.5\ ml$

9. $x \text{ ml} = \dfrac{1 \text{ ml}}{5000 \text{ V}} \times 2500 \text{ V}$

$x = \dfrac{1 \times 2500}{5000}$

$x = \dfrac{2500}{5000}$ or 0.5 ml

10. $x \text{ tablet} = \dfrac{1 \text{ tablet}}{500 \text{ mg}} \times \dfrac{1000 \text{ mg}}{1 \text{ g}} \times 2 \text{ g}$

$x = \dfrac{1 \times 1000 \times 2}{500 \times 1}$

$x = \dfrac{2000}{500}$

$x = 4 \text{ tablets}$

Chapter 17 Pediatric Dosages—Work Sheet, pp. 373-375

1. $2.2 \text{ lb} : 1 \text{ kg} :: 50 \text{ lb} : x \text{ kg}$
$2.2x = 50$
$x = \dfrac{50}{2.2}$
$x = 22.73 \text{ kg}$

$25 : 1 :: x : 22.73$
$x = 568.25$ or
$x = 568 \text{ mg}$

$50 : 1 :: x : 22.73$
$x = 1136.5$ or
$x = 1137 \text{ mg}$
The safe range is 568-1137 mg
   in a 24-hour period

$250 \text{ mg} : 1 \text{ dose} :: x \text{ mg} : 4 \text{ doses}$
$x = 1000 \text{ mg}$ in a 24-hour period
Yes, the order is safe.

$250 \text{ mg} : 1 \text{ cap} :: 250 \text{ mg} : x \text{ cap}$
$250x = 250$
$x = \dfrac{250}{250}$
$x = 1 \text{ capsule}$

2. $2.2 \text{ lb} : 1 \text{ kg} : 6.5 \text{ lb} : x \text{ kg}$
$2.2x = 6.5$
$x = \dfrac{6.5}{2.2}$
$x = 2.95 \text{ kg}$

$0.035 \text{ mg} : 1 \text{ kg} :: x \text{ mg} : 2.95 \text{ kg}$
$x = 0.103 \text{ mg}$

$0.06 \text{ mg} : 1 \text{ kg} :: x \text{ mg} : 2.95 \text{ kg}$
$x = 0.177 \text{ mg}$
The safe range is 0.103-0.177 mg/day.

$12.5 \text{ mg} : 1 \text{ dose} :: x \text{ mg} : 1 \text{ dose}$
$x = 12.5 \text{ mg per day}$
No, the order is not safe.

3. $2.2 \text{ lb} : 1 \text{ kg} :: 50 \text{ lb} : x \text{ kg}$
$2.2x = 50$
$x = \dfrac{50}{2.2}$
$x = 22.73 \text{ kg}$

$5 \text{ mg} : 1 \text{ kg} :: x \text{ mg} : 22.73 \text{ kg}$
$x = 113.65 \text{ mg/day}$
$25 \text{ mg} : 1 \text{ dose} :: x \text{ mg} : 4 \text{ doses}$
$x = 100 \text{ mg}$
Yes, the order is safe.

$10 \text{ mg} : 1 \text{ ml} :: 25 \text{ mg} : x \text{ ml}$
$10x = 25$
$x = \dfrac{25}{10}$
$x = 2.5 \text{ ml/dose}$

4. $2.2 \text{ lb} : 1 \text{ kg} :: 44 \text{ lb} : x \text{ kg}$
$2.2x = 44$
$x = \dfrac{44}{2.2}$
$x = 20 \text{ kg}$

$0.55 \text{ mg} : 1 \text{ kg} :: x \text{ mg} : 20 \text{ kg}$
$x = 11 \text{ mg q.6-8h./day}$
Total of 33-44 mg/day

$10 \text{ mg} : 1 \text{ dose} :: x \text{ mg} : 4 \text{ doses}$
$x = 40 \text{ mg/day}$
Yes, the order is safe.

$25 \text{ mg} : 1 \text{ ml} :: 10 \text{ mg} : x \text{ ml}$
$25x = 10$
$x = \dfrac{10}{25}$
$x = 0.4 \text{ ml}$

5. 2.2 lb:1 kg::78 lb:x kg
$2.2x = 78$
$$x = \frac{78}{2.2}$$
$x = 35.45$ kg

2 mg:1 kg::x mg:35.45 kg
$x = 70.9$ mg/day
60 mg <70.9 mg
Therefore, yes, the order is safe.

40 mg:1 tab::60 mg:x tab
$40x = 60$
$$x = \frac{60}{40}$$
$x = 1.5$ tablets

6. 2.2 lb:1 kg:30.31 lb:x kg
$2.2x = 30.31$
$x = 13.77$ kg

2 mg:1 kg::x mg:13.77 kg
$x = 27.54$ mg

10 mg/day is <27.54 mg
Therefore, yes, the order is safe.

5 mg:1 ml::10 mg:x ml
$5x = 10$
$$x = \frac{10}{5}$$
$x = 2$ ml

7. 2.2 lb:1 kg::28 lb:x kg
$2.2x = 28$
$$x = \frac{28}{2.2}$$
$x = 12.73$ kg

12 mg:1 kg::x mg:12.73 kg
$x = 152.76$ mg/day

16 mg:1 dose::x mg:4 doses
$x = 64$ mg/day
Yes, the order is safe.

11.25 mg:1 ml::16 mg:x ml
$11.25x = 16$
$$x = \frac{16}{11.25}$$
$x = 1.42$ ml

8. 2.2 lb:1 kg::66 lb:x kg
$2.2x = 66$
$$x = \frac{66}{2.2}$$
$x = 30$ kg

5 mg:1 kg::x mg:30 kg
$x = 150$ mg

7 mg:1 kg::x mg:30 kg
$x = 210$ mg
150-210 mg/day

75 mg:1 dose::x mg:2 doses
$x = 150$ mg
Yes, the order is safe.

50 mg:1 tab::75 mg:x tab
$50x = 75$
$$x = \frac{75}{50}$$
$x = 1.5$ tablets

Chapter 17 Pediatric Dosages—Posttest 1, pp. 377-378

1. 2.2 lb : 1 kg : : 55 lb : x kg
$2.2x = 55$
$$x = \frac{55}{2.2}$$
$x = 25$ kg

4 mg : 1 kg : : x mg : 25 kg
$x = 100$ mg

6 mg : 1 kg : : x mg : 25 kg
$x = 150$ mg
100-150 mg/day

60 mg : 1 dose : : x mg : 2 doses
$x = 120$ mg/day
Yes, the order is safe.

20 mg : 5 ml : : 60 mg : x ml
$20x = 300$
$$x = \frac{300}{20}$$
$x = 15$ ml

2. 2.2 lb : 1 kg : : 44 lb : x kg
$2.2x = 44$
$$x = \frac{44}{2.2}$$
$x = 20$ kg

30 mg : 1 kg : : x mg : 20 kg
$x = 600$ mg

60 mg : 1 kg : : x mg : 20 kg
$x = 1200$ mg
600-1200 mg/day

500 mg : 1 dose : : x mg : 4 dose
$x = 2000$ mg
No, the order is not safe.

3. 2.2 lb : 1 kg : : 6.75 lb : x kg
$2.2x = 6.75$
$$x = \frac{6.75}{2.2}$$
$x = 3.07$ kg

50,000 U : 1 kg : : x U : 3.07 kg
$x = 153,500$ U/day
150,000 U < 153,500
Therefore, yes, the order is safe.

300,000 U : 1 ml : : 150,000 U : x ml
$300,000x = 150,000$
$$x = \frac{150,000}{300,000}$$
$x = 0.5$ ml

4. 2.2 lb : 1 kg : : 44 lb : x kg
$2.2x = 44$
$$x = \frac{44}{2.2}$$
$x = 20$ kg

20 mg : 1 kg : : x mg : 20 kg
$x = 400$ mg

40 mg : 1 kg : : x mg : 20 kg
$x = 800$ mg
400-800 mg/day

250 mg : 1 dose : : x mg : 3 doses
$x = 750$ mg
Yes, the order is safe.

125 mg : 5 ml : : 250 mg : x ml
$125x = 1250$
$$x = \frac{1250}{125}$$
$x = 10$ ml

5. 2.2 lb : 1 kg : : 78 lb : x kg
$2.2x = 78$
$$x = \frac{78}{2.2}$$
$x = 35.45$ kg

0.1 mg : 1 kg : : x mg : 35.45 kg
$x = 3.55$ mg

0.2 mg : 1 kg : : x mg : 35.45 kg
$x = 7.09$ mg
3.55-7.09 mg/day
4 mg < 7.09 mg
Therefore, yes, the order is safe.

15 mg : 1 ml : : 4 mg : x ml
$15x = 4$
$$x = \frac{4}{15}$$
$x = 0.27$ ml

Chapter 17 Pediatric Dosages—Posttest 2, pp. 379-380

1. $2.2 \text{ lb}:1 \text{ kg}::58 \text{ lb}:x \text{ kg}$
$2.2x = 58$
$$x = \frac{58}{2.2}$$
$x = 26.36 \text{ kg}$

$15 \text{ mg}:1 \text{ kg}::x \text{ mg}:26.36 \text{ kg}$
$x = 395 \text{ mg}$

$40 \text{ mg}:1 \text{ kg}:x \text{ mg}:26.36 \text{ kg}$
$x = 1054 \text{ mg}$
$395\text{-}1054 \text{ mg/day}$

$225 \text{ mg}:1 \text{ dose}:x \text{ mg}:4 \text{ doses}$
$x = 1000 \text{ mg}$
Yes, the order is safe.

$150 \text{ mg}:1 \text{ ml}::225 \text{ mg}:x \text{ ml}$
$150x = 225$
$$x = \frac{225}{150}$$
$x = 1.5 \text{ ml}$

2. $2.2 \text{ lb}:1 \text{ kg}::70 \text{ lb}:x \text{ kg}$
$2.2x = 70$
$$x = \frac{70}{2.2}$$
$x = 31.81 \text{ kg}$

$5 \text{ mg}:1 \text{ kg}::x \text{ mg}:31.81 \text{ kg}$
$x = 159 \text{ mg}$

$7 \text{ mg}:1 \text{ kg}::x \text{ mg}:31.81 \text{ kg}$
$x = 222.67 \text{ mg}$
$159\text{-}222.67 \text{ mg/day}$

$50 \text{ mg}:1 \text{ dose}::x \text{ mg}:2 \text{ doses}$
$x = 100 \text{ mg}$
No, 100 mg <159 is recommended.

3. $2.2 \text{ lb}:1 \text{ kg}::58 \text{ lb}:x \text{ kg}$
$2.2x = 58$
$$x = \frac{58}{2.2}$$
$x = 26.36 \text{ kg}$

$20 \text{ mg}:1 \text{ kg}::x \text{ mg}:26.36 \text{ kg}$
$x = 527 \text{ mg}$

$40 \text{ mg}:1 \text{ kg}::x \text{ mg}:26.36 \text{ kg}$
$x = 1054$
$527\text{-}1054 \text{ mg/day}$

$250 \text{ mg}:1 \text{ dose}:x \text{ mg}:3 \text{ doses}$
$x = 750 \text{ mg/day}$
Yes, the order is safe.

$125 \text{ mg}:5 \text{ ml}::250 \text{ mg}:x \text{ ml}$
$125x = 1250$
$$x = \frac{1250}{125}$$
$x = 10 \text{ ml}$

4. $2.2 \text{ lb}:1 \text{ kg}::99 \text{ lb}:x \text{ kg}$
$2.2x = 99$
$$x = \frac{99}{2.2}$$
$x = 45 \text{ kg}$

$25 \text{ mg}:1 \text{ kg}::x \text{ mg}:45 \text{ kg}$
$x = 1125 \text{ mg}$

$50 \text{ mg}:1 \text{ kg}::x \text{ mg}:45 \text{ kg}$
$x = 2250 \text{ mg}$
$1125\text{-}2250 \text{ mg/day}$

$500 \text{ mg}:1 \text{ dose}::x \text{ mg}:4 \text{ doses}$
$x = 2000$
Yes, the order is safe.

$250 \text{ mg}:1 \text{ cap}::500 \text{ mg}:x \text{ cap}$
$250x = 500$
$$x = \frac{500}{250}$$
$x = 2 \text{ capsules}$

5. $2.2 \text{ lb}:1 \text{ kg}::66 \text{ lb}:x \text{ kg}$
$2.2x = 66$
$$x = \frac{66}{2.2}$$
$x = 30 \text{ kg}$

$50 \text{ mg}:1 \text{ kg}::x \text{ mg}:30 \text{ kg}$
$x = 1500 \text{ mg}$

$100 \text{ mg}:1 \text{ kg}::x \text{ mg}:30 \text{ kg}$
$x = 3000 \text{ mg}$
$1500\text{-}3000 \text{ mg/day}$

$500 \text{ mg}:1 \text{ dose}::x \text{ mg}:4 \text{ doses}$
$x = 2000 \text{ mg}$
Yes, the order is safe.

$125 \text{ mg}:1 \text{ ml}::500 \text{ mg}:x \text{ ml}$
$125x = 500$
$$x = \frac{500}{125}$$
$x = 4 \text{ ml}$

Comprehensive Posttest, pp. 393-407

Case 1

1. 2 tablets
2. Digoxin 0.25 mg
E.C. ASA gr v
Cimetidine 300 mg
Slow-K 10 mEq
3. 400 ml of $D_5\frac{1}{2}$ N.S. per shift
4.

2/3	Percocet								
	$\overset{..}{11}$ dose	p.o. route	q.4 h. interval	prn pain					
2/3	Tylenol								
	grX dose	p.o. route	q.4 h. interval	prn pain or Temp >38°					
2/3	MOM								
	30 cc dose	p.o. route	q.day interval	prn constipation					
2/3	Mylanta								
	30 cc dose	p.o. route	q.4 h. interval	prn indigestion					
2/3	Restoril								
	15 mg dose	p.o. route	q.h.s. interval	prn insomnia					

5.

2/3	Digoxin								
	0.25 mg dose	p.o. route	q.day interval	09					
2/3	E.C. ASA								
	gr V dose	p.o. route	q.day interval	09					
2/3	Cimetidine								
	300 mg dose	p.o. route	t.i.d. interval	09	13	17			
2/3	Lasix								
	20 mg dose	I.V. route	q.8 h. interval	08		16		24	
2/3	Slow-K								
	10 mEq dose	p.o. route	b.i.d. interval	09		17			

6. Restoril 15 mg p.o.
7. 100 gtt/min
8. Milk of Magnesia 30 cc
9. Lasix 20 mg

Case 2

1. Synthroid 0.15 mg
Tagamet 300 mg
2. 1 ml
3. 600 ml/shift
1800 ml/day
4. ½ tablet
5. Demerol
Tylenol
6. 0.5 ml
7. 2 tablets

8.

1	Synthroid										
	0.15 mg dose	p.o. route	q.day interval								
2	Tagamet										
	300 mg dose	p.o. route	q.day interval								

Case 3

1. Med. FESO$_4$
    amt. 0.3 g
2. 300 cc
3. 0.5 ml

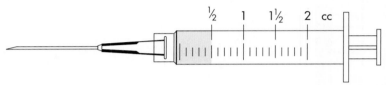

4. ½ tablet
5.

10	Ibuprofen										
	600 mg dose	p.o. route	q.6 h. interval	prn pain							
11	Seconal										
	100 mg dose	p.o. route	q.h.s. interval	prn							
12	Tucks										
	one dose	Peri route	 interval	prn @ bedside							
13	Senokot										
	one dose	p.o. route	qd prn interval								
14	Tylenol										
	650 mg dose	p.o. route	q.4 h. interval	prn pain							

6. 2½ tablets

Case 4

1.

1	Allopurinol										
	50 mg dose	p.o. route	t.i.d. interval								
2	Theophylline										
	16 mg dose	p.o. route	q.6 h. interval								
3	Prednisone										
	2 mg/kg dose	p.o. route	q.day interval								
4	Vincristine										
	5.0 mg/m² dose	I.V. route	x ÷ now interval								
5	MVI										
	÷ dose	p.o. route	q.day interval								

2.

7	Compazine							
	0.07 mg/kg dose	IM route	q.day interval	PRN Nausea				
8	Tylenol							
	120 mg dose	p.o. route	t.i.d. interval	PRN pain				

3. 1.42 ml

4. 0.5 ml

5. 12.73 kg
2.5 ml

6. 50 gtt/min

7. 0.90 ml

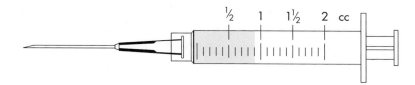

8. 200 cc

9. 0.66 ml

Case 5

1.

1	Heparin									
	5000 U dose	SC route	b.i.d. interval	09		21				
2	Cefuroxime									
	1 g dose	IVPB route	q.4 h. interval	08	16	24				

2.

3	Torecan						
	10 mg dose	IM route	q.4 h. interval	prn nausea			
4	Mylanta						
	30 cc dose	p.o. route	interval	prn indigestion			
5	Dulcolax Supp.						
	1 dose	pr route	q.shift interval	prn			
6	Restoril						
	15 mg dose	p.o. route	q.h.s. interval	prn insomnia			
7	Tylenol #3						
	2 dose	p.o. route	q.4 h. interval	prn pain			
8	Tylenol #3						
	1 dose	p.o. route	q.4 h. interval	prn pain			
9	PCA-Demerol						
	10 mg dose	IV route	q.10 min interval	250 mg/4 h. lockout			

3. 0.5 ml

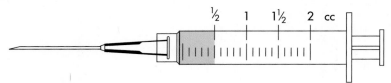

4. 1 ml/10 min
5. 1.0 ml
6. 400 cc/shift
1200 cc/day
7. 200 ml/h.
3.33 ml/min
200 gtt/min

Index

Abbreviations and Symbols*

$\bar{a}$	before		NaCl	sodium chloride
$\overrightarrow{aa}$	of each		$NaHCO_3$	sodium bicarbonate
a.c.	before meals		NGT, ng	nasogastric tube
A.M.	morning, before noon		NKDA	no known drug allergies
aq.	water		NPO	nothing by mouth
A.S.A.	acetylsalicylic acid (aspirin)		N.S.	normal saline
BSA	body surface area		OD	right eye
b.i.d.	twice a day		OS	left eye
C	Celsius, centigrade		OU	both eyes
$\bar{c}$	with		oz	ounce
Ca	calcium		$\bar{p}$	after
$CaCl_2$	calcium chloride		p.c.	after meals
cap(s)	capsule		PCA	patient-controlled analgesia
cc	cubic centimeter		per	by
Cl	chlorine		P.M.	after noon
d.c., d/c	discontinue		p.o.	orally
dil.	dilute		p.r.	by rectum
D.W.	dextrose water; distilled water		p.r.n.	as needed
elix.	elixir		pt	pint
F	Fahrenheit		q.	every
$FeSO_4$	ferrous sulfate		q.d.	once a day
fl., fld	fluid		q.h.	every hour
gal	gallon		q.i.d.	four times a day
g	gram		q.o.d.	every other day
gr	grain		q.o.h.	every other hour
gtt	drops		q.s.	quantity sufficient
h., hr	hour		qt	quart
H_2O	water		R	a medical prescription
H_2O_2	hydrogen peroxide		$\bar{s}$	without
h.s.	at bedtime		sc	subcutaneous
I	iodine		sl	sublingual
I.M.	intramuscular		sol.	solution
inf.	infusion		S.O.S.	once if necessary
inj.	injection		SQ	subcutaneous
I.V.	intravenous		SR	slow release
I.V.P.B.	intravenous piggy back		ss, $\overline{ss}$	one half
I.V.S.S.	intravenous soluset		STAT, stat	immediately
K	potassium		subq.	subcutaneous
KCl	potassium chloride		supp	suppository
kg	kilogram		susp.	suspension
L	liter		syr.	syrup
LA	long acting		tab	tablet
lb	pound		Tbsp.	tablespoon
liq.	liquid		t.i.d.	three times a day
$\mathfrak{m}$, m	minim		tr., tinct.	tincture
mcg, μg	microgram		tsp.	teaspoon
mEq	milliequivalent		U	unit
mg	milligram		ʒ	dram
Mg	magnesium		ʒ	ounce
min	minute		>	greater than
ml	milliliter		<	less than
Na	sodium		/	per

*Where two acceptable options are provided for abbreviations, the first abbreviation listed is most often used throughout the book.